Diagnosis and Management of Endocrine Disorders in Interventional Radiology

AF400233

Hyeon Yu • Charles T. Burke
Clayton W. Commander

Editors

Diagnosis and Management of Endocrine Disorders in Interventional Radiology

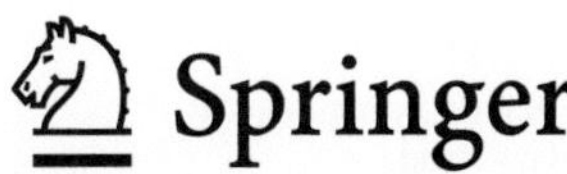 Springer

Editors
Hyeon Yu
Division of Vascular and Interventional
Radiology
Department of Radiology
University of North Carolina at Chapel Hill
School of Medicine
Chapel Hill, NC
USA

Charles T. Burke
Division of Vascular and Interventional
Radiology
Department of Radiology
University of North Carolina at Chapel Hill
School of Medicine
Chapel Hill, NC
USA

Clayton W. Commander
Division of Vascular and Interventional
Radiology
Department of Radiology
University of North Carolina at Chapel Hill
School of Medicine
Chapel Hill, NC
USA

ISBN 978-3-030-87191-8 ISBN 978-3-030-87189-5 (eBook)
https://doi.org/10.1007/978-3-030-87189-5

© The Editor(s) (if applicable) and The Author(s), under exclusive license to Springer Nature
Switzerland AG 2022, corrected publication 2022
This work is subject to copyright. All rights are solely and exclusively licensed by the Publisher, whether
the whole or part of the material is concerned, specifically the rights of translation, reprinting, reuse of
illustrations, recitation, broadcasting, reproduction on microfilms or in any other physical way, and
transmission or information storage and retrieval, electronic adaptation, computer software, or by similar
or dissimilar methodology now known or hereafter developed.
The use of general descriptive names, registered names, trademarks, service marks, etc. in this publication
does not imply, even in the absence of a specific statement, that such names are exempt from the relevant
protective laws and regulations and therefore free for general use.
The publisher, the authors and the editors are safe to assume that the advice and information in this book
are believed to be true and accurate at the date of publication. Neither the publisher nor the authors or the
editors give a warranty, expressed or implied, with respect to the material contained herein or for any
errors or omissions that may have been made. The publisher remains neutral with regard to jurisdictional
claims in published maps and institutional affiliations.

This Springer imprint is published by the registered company Springer Nature Switzerland AG
The registered company address is: Gewerbestrasse 11, 6330 Cham, Switzerland

Preface

Diseases of the endocrine system involve an imbalance in the natural homeostasis of the hormones produced by the glands in the body. There are a variety of endocrine conditions characterized by either hormonal hyposecretion or hypersecretion. Often, these conditions can lead to debilitating or, in some instances, life-threatening situations that can be challenging to diagnose and treat. While one doesn't often consider interventional radiology a critical part of the endocrine clinic setting, there are several conditions for which interventional radiologists can play a valuable role. These disorders include primary aldosteronism, primary hyperparathyroidism, Cushing's disease, hormone-secreting pancreatic adenomas, and androgen-secreting ovarian tumors. A collaboration of multiple specialties, including endocrinologists, surgeons, and radiologists, is often needed to diagnose and manage these conditions.

Radiologists play a prominent role in the evaluation of patients with suspected endocrine disorders. CT and MRI are commonly used first-line imaging modalities; however, cross-sectional imaging lacks physiologic information resulting in poor specificity of these tests for many endocrine conditions. Thus, percutaneous selective venous sampling is a useful diagnostic tool for the medical and surgical management of patients with select endocrine disorders. Selective venous sampling is a minimally invasive interventional procedure performed by interventional radiologists to localize sites of abnormal hormone secretion. These tests can confirm a suspected clinical diagnosis and, in some instances, direct curative surgical therapy.

As venous sampling procedures are increasingly performed worldwide, the collaboration between interventional radiology, endocrinology, surgical endocrinology, surgical oncology, neurosurgery, and gynecology teams is essential. Currently, there are limited guidelines from The Endocrine Society and relatively few published papers for each venous sampling procedure. Furthermore, except for the book "Percutaneous Venous Blood Sampling in Endocrine Diseases" published in 1992 by Springer, there is no modern comprehensive guide for all traditional and newly emerging selective venous sampling procedures.

To correct this information gap, we have put together a book focusing on selective venous sampling, including the interventional techniques for diagnosis and chapters on the pathophysiology, epidemiology, clinical diagnosis, and medical, surgical, and interventional treatments of endocrine disorders. We have recruited experts from endocrinology, endocrine surgery, radiology, and interventional radiology to provide a comprehensive and state-of-the-art textbook surrounding the diseases in which venous sampling is typically used. We have also included chapters on the latest percutaneous therapies that may be the future for treating some common endocrine disorders, such as hyperthyroidism and hyperparathyroidism. And given the rise in pediatric interventional radiology in recent years, we felt it was important to dedicate a chapter to venous sampling in this patient population.

This book is organized into five parts: Clinical, Laboratory, and Radiological Diagnosis, Selective Venous Sampling, Medical and Surgical Management, and Intervention Treatments, with chapters in each part addressing primary aldosteronism, hyperparathyroidism, hyperandrogenism, hypercortisolism, and pancreatic islet cell tumors. This type of organization allows the reader to read the book straight through to get a comprehensive overview from the initial evaluation through the different management options for these disease processes. Alternatively, the reader can select specific chapters to answer a particular question or focus on a single disease process.

As interventional radiologists, we have experienced firsthand the value and complexity that venous sampling procedures can provide. These procedures can be gratifying and significantly improve patient care. Understanding the relevant disease processes from the perspective of the other members of the multi-disciplinary teams and learning the selective venous sampling techniques from the experts will help guide the interventional radiologist to be a more valuable team member. We have thoroughly enjoyed the process of bringing this book together, and we hope that all readers who are involved in the management of these patients will find this book a valuable reference for many years.

Chapel Hill, NC, USA   Hyeon Yu
Chapel Hill, NC, USA   Charles T. Burke
Chapel Hill, NC, USA   Clayton W. Commander

The original version of this book was revised: The incorrect author affiliation has been corrected. The correction to this book can be found at https://doi.org/10.1007/978-3-030-87189-5_22

Contents

Contributors

Osman Ahmed Department of Interventional Radiology, University of Chicago Medical Center, Chicago, IL, USA

Jung Hwan Baek Department of Radiology and Research Institute of Radiology, University of Ulsan College of Medicine, Asan Medical Center, Seoul, South Korea

Charles T. Burke Division of Vascular and Interventional Radiology, Department of Radiology, University of North Carolina at Chapel Hill School of Medicine, Chapel Hill, NC, USA

Lauren M. B. Burke Department of Radiology, Division of Abdominal Imaging, University of North Carolina School of Medicine, Chapel Hill, NC, USA

Kent A. Cabatingan Interventional Radiology, Children's Minnesota, Minneapolis, MN, USA

Jennifer H. Choe Division of Hematology and Medical Oncology, Department of Medicine, Duke University Medical Center, Durham, NC, USA

Clayton W. Commander Division of Vascular and Interventional Radiology, Department of Radiology, University of North Carolina at Chapel Hill School of Medicine, Chapel Hill, NC, USA

Jessica L. Dahle Endocrine Surgery, Department of Surgery, Ochsner Health, LA, USA

Christos Georgiades Department of Radiology & Radiological Sciences, Johns Hopkins University, Baltimore, MD, USA

Jashalynn German Department of Medicine, Division of Endocrinology, Metabolism and Nutrition, Duke University, Durham, NC, USA

Paul A. Guido Department of Endocrinology, University of North Carolina, Chapel Hill, NC, USA

James P. Ho Department of Neurology, University of North Carolina at Chapel Hill, Chapel Hill, NC, USA

Kelvin Hong Department of Radiology & Radiological Sciences, Johns Hopkins University, Baltimore, MD, USA

Tim Huber Dotter Department of Interventional Radiology, Oregon Health and Science University, Portland, OR, USA

Jeffrey Johnson Division of Surgical Oncology and Endocrine Surgery, University of North Carolina at Chapel Hill, Chapel Hill, NC, USA

Hadiza S. Kazaure Division of Endocrine Surgery, Department of Surgery, Duke University Medical Center, Durham, NC, USA

Joseph Kearney Department of Surgery, University of North Carolina at Chapel Hill, Chapel Hill, NC, USA

Hong Jin Kim Division of Surgical Oncology and Endocrine Surgery, University of North Carolina at Chapel Hill, Chapel Hill, NC, USA

Lawrence Kim Division of Surgical Oncology and Endocrine Surgery, Department of Surgery, University of North Carolina, Chapel Hill, NC, USA

Adam J. Kimple Department of Otolaryngology-Head and Neck Surgery, University of North Carolina Medical Center, Chapel Hill, NC, USA

Akiyuki Kotoku Department of Radiology, St. Marianna University School of Medicine, Yokohama City Seibu Hospital, Yokohama, Kanagawa, Japan

Panagiotis Liasides USC Medical Center, Los Angeles, CA, USA

Division of Trauma and Surgical Critical Care, University of Southern California Keck School of Medicine, Los Angeles, CA, USA

Megan Elizabeth Lombardi Department of Surgery, University of North Carolina, Chapel Hill, NC, USA

Jennifer D. Merrill Division of Endocrinology, Diabetes, and Metabolism, Department of Internal Medicine, The Ohio State University College of Medicine, Columbus, OH, USA

Juan Camilo Mira Division of Surgical Oncology and Endocrine Surgery, Department of Surgery, University of North Carolina, Chapel Hill, NC, USA

Justin C. Morse Department of Otolaryngology-Head and Neck Surgery, University of North Carolina Medical Center, Chapel Hill, NC, USA

Jorge D. Oldan Division of Molecular Imaging and Therapeutics, Department of Radiology, University of North Carolina School of Medicine, Chapel Hill, NC, USA

Auh Whan Park Department of Radiology, University of Virginia Health System, Charlottesville, VA, USA

Chengzhong Peng Department of Ultrasound, Zhejiang Provincial People's Hospital, and Hangzhou Medical College, Hangzhou, Zhejiang, China

Jennifer M. Perkins Division of Endocrinology, University of California San Francisco Medical Center, San Francisco, CA, USA

Ali Qamar Division of Endocrinology, Diabetes and Metabolism, Duke University School of Medicine, Durham, NC, USA

Daniel J. Rocke Division of Head and Neck Surgery & Communication Sciences, Department of Surgery, Duke University Medical Center, Durham, NC, USA

Jennifer V. Rowell Department of Medicine, Division of Endocrinology, Metabolism and Nutrition, Duke University, Durham, NC, USA

Alan Alper Sag Division of Vascular and Interventional Radiology, Department of Radiology, Duke University Medical Center, Durham, NC, USA

Randall P. Scheri Division of Endocrine Surgery, Department of Surgery, Duke University Medical Center, Durham, NC, USA

Sona Sharma Division of Endocrinology and Metabolism, Department of Medicine, Duke University Medical Center, Durham, NC, USA

Tony P. Smith Division of Vascular and Interventional Radiology, Department of Radiology, Duke University Medical Center, Durham, NC, USA

Sten Y. Solander Department of Radiology, University of North Carolina at Chapel Hill, Chapel Hill, NC, USA

Diana Soliman Division of Endocrinology, Diabetes and Metabolism, Duke University School of Medicine, Durham, NC, USA

Michael T. Stang Division of Endocrine Surgery, Department of Surgery, Duke University Medical Center, Durham, NC, USA

Brian D. Thorp Department of Otolaryngology-Head and Neck Surgery, University of North Carolina Medical Center, Chapel Hill, NC, USA

Anne Weaver Division of Endocrinology and Metabolism, Department of Medicine, Duke University Medical Center, Durham, NC, USA

Takayuki Yamada Department of Radiology, St. Marianna University School of Medicine, Yokohama City Seibu Hospital, Yokohama, Kanagawa, Japan

Qian Yang Laboratory for Investigatory Imaging, School of Health and Rehabilitation Sciences, The Ohio State University, Columbus, USA

Jen Jen Yeh Department of Surgery, University of North Carolina, Chapel Hill, NC, USA

Hyeon Yu Division of Vascular and Interventional Radiology, Department of Radiology, University of North Carolina at Chapel Hill School of Medicine, Chapel Hill, NC, USA

Kurt Zacharias Department of Radiology, University of Chicago Medical Center, Chicago, IL, USA

Carlos A. Zamora Division of Neuroradiology, Department of Radiology, University of North Carolina at Chapel Hill, Chapel Hill, NC, USA

Part I
Clinical, Laboratory, and Radiological Diagnosis of Endocrine Disorders

Chapter 1
Clinical, Laboratory, and Radiological Diagnosis of Primary Aldosteronism

Ali Qamar and Lauren M. B. Burke

Introduction

Primary aldosteronism (PA) is the most common [1] cause of secondary hypertension. Despite its relatively high prevalence, it is commonly underdiagnosed. Patients with untreated PA have an increased risk of stroke, atrial fibrillation, heart failure, coronary artery disease [1], and chronic kidney disease [2] when compared to patients with essential hypertension. Aldosterone-producing adenoma and bilateral idiopathic hyperplasia are the most common subtypes of PA. Familial hyperaldosteronism is rare and will not be discussed in detail.

History

Dr. J.W. Conn was a Professor of Medicine at the University of Michigan. His research focused on the mechanisms of human acclimatization to humid heat [3]. He concluded that the body's acclimatization involved rapidly diminishing renal salt and water loss. He suggested that these responses were the result of the increased adrenocortical function of salt-retaining steroids as intramuscular administration of

A. Qamar (✉)
Division of Endocrinology, Diabetes and Metabolism, Duke University School of Medicine, Durham, NC, USA
e-mail: ali.qamar@duke.edu

L. M. B. Burke
Department of Radiology, Division of Abdominal Imaging, University of North Carolina School of Medicine, Chapel Hill, NC, USA
e-mail: lauren_burke@med.unc.edu

© The Author(s), under exclusive license to Springer Nature Switzerland AG 2022

H. Yu et al. (eds.), *Diagnosis and Management of Endocrine Disorders in Interventional Radiology*, https://doi.org/10.1007/978-3-030-87189-5_1

deoxycorticosterone acetate (DOCA) produced similar changes in the electrolyte composition of urine, sweat, and saliva.

In April 1954, he saw a 34-year-old woman with a 7-year history of muscle spasms, temporary paralysis, tetany, and weakness and a 4-year history of hypertension. She was found to have a blood pressure of 176/104 mm Hg, severe hypokalemia (1.6 to 2.5 mEq/L), mild hypernatremia (146 to 151 mEq/L), and alkalosis (serum pH 7.62). Because there were no signs or symptoms of glucocorticoid or androgen excess, Dr. Conn suspected that her clinical presentation was related to adrenal salt-retaining corticoid [4] and studied DOCA level in the patient's urine which averaged 1333 µg/day equivalent compared with normotensive control subjects who averaged 61.4 µg/day.

In December 1954, his study patient was scheduled for bilateral adrenalectomy, but surgeons found a 13-g right adrenal tumor which was removed while leaving the contralateral gland intact. "The patient's postoperative studies showed an almost total reversal of the preoperative metabolic and clinical abnormalities. Conn had achieved irrefutable proof of the validity of his investigative conclusions and established for the first time the relationship between an adrenal aldosterone-producing tumor and hypertension with hypokalemia. A new era had arrived in the study of hypertension and adrenal mineralocorticoids" [5].

In his Presidential Address Primary aldosteronism (PA) history to the 1955 Society of Clinical Research, Dr. Conn stated: "It is believed that these studies delineate a new clinical syndrome which is designated *temporarily* as Primary Aldosteronism" [4].

Prevalence

Historically, the diagnosis of PA was not considered unless a patient had spontaneous hypokalemia, and then the diagnostic evaluation would require discontinuation of antihypertensive medications for at least 2 weeks. This resulted in predicted prevalence rates of less than 0.5% of hypertensive patients. Based on the available literature review, most patients with PA are not hypokalemic, and screening can be completed while the patient is taking antihypertensive drugs. Current prevalence estimates for PA suspect the diagnosis in 5–10% of all patients with hypertension [6–8]. Recently published data from four US academic centers showed a high prevalence of biochemically overt PA that parallels the severity of hypertension [9].

Hypokalemia and Primary Aldosteronism

Only 9–37% of patients with PA have hypokalemia [10, 11], and the absence of hypokalemia in no way should deter clinicians from screening for primary hyperaldosteronism. The prevalence of target-organ damage to the heart and kidney is increased in patients with PA compared to those with essential hypertension [1].

Case Detection: Who Should Be Tested?

The Endocrine Society guidelines for PA recommend case detection in the following patients [11]:

1. Blood pressure over 150/100 on three measurements on different days
2. Uncontrolled blood pressure >140/90 on three conventional drugs, including a diuretic
3. Controlled blood pressure <140/90 on four or more conventional drugs, including a diuretic
4. Hypertension and hypokalemia (spontaneous or diuretic-induced)
5. Hypertension and adrenal incidentaloma
6. Hypertension and sleep apnea [12]
7. Hypertension and a family history of early-onset hypertension or cerebrovascular accident at a young age (<40 years)
8. All hypertensive first-degree relatives of patients with PA

Of note, patients with obstructive sleep apnea for unclear reasons have a very high prevalence of primary hyperaldosteronism [12].

How to Test

Plasma aldosterone concentration (PAC) and plasma renin activity or plasma renin concentration (PRC) are measured in *a patient with seating position in the morning.*
Renin can be measured based on its enzymatic activity (PRA) or its mass (PRC).
PRA is determined by measurement of angiotensin I generation and expressed as the amount of angiotensin I generated per unit of time (e.g., ng/mL/h).

Interfering Medications

Concern about medication interference has deterred clinicians from screening for PA. Many medications can interfere with PAC, PRA, and PRC, but screening tests can be completed when patients are taking interfering medications, including mineralocorticoid receptor antagonist (MRA), angiotensin-converting enzyme inhibitors (ACEi), and angiotensin receptor blockers (ARB) as long as PRA is non-suppressed (>1) [2, 11].

MRA, ACEi, ARB, and direct renin inhibitors can potentially elevate PRC or PRA. Therefore, if PRA or PRC is suppressed, interfering medications should be held for 4–6 weeks before repeating case detection studies.

Medications like beta-blockers, calcium channel blockers, alpha-blockers, and vasodilators like hydralazine have minimal interference. Therefore, they can be used while patients are being evaluated for primary aldosteronism.

Hypokalemia should be repleted before testing. PRC can be affected by estrogen status and false-positive results on case detection testing for PA can occur when PRC is measured in women receiving estrogen-containing preparations. PRA is not affected by estrogen preparations and is the recommended screening test [13].

Lab Interpretation

Case detection testing for PA is considered positive when PRA is suppressed to <1 ng/mL/h (or PRC below the lower limit of normal) and PAC is $\geq$10 ng/dL [11]. PAC/PRA ratio is generally >20, and in one study, a PAC/PRA ratio more than 30 and a PA value of more than 20 ng/dL provided a sensitivity of 90%, specificity of 91%, the positive predictive value of 69%, and negative predictive value of 98% [14].

If both PAC and PRA are elevated (after stopping interfering medications), diagnosis of renovascular hypertension should be explored. If both PAC and PRA are suppressed on case detection studies, diagnosis of Cushing syndrome, Liddle syndrome, and Licorice use should be considered.

Confirmatory Testing

Most patients with positive case detection will need confirmatory testing. Only patients who have PAC > 20 and PRA below detection levels and spontaneous hypokalemia [11] can proceed with subtype classification without confirmatory testing. Confirmatory tests include oral sodium loading test, saline infusion test, fludrocortisone suppression test, and captopril challenge test [11]. Fludrocortisone suppression test and captopril challenge test are very rarely used and falling out of favor in most parts of the world.

Oral Sodium Load This is the preferred test at most centers. After controlling hypertension and hypokalemia, patients are started on a high-sodium diet (this can be accomplished by adding three 1-gram salt tablets twice a day) for 3 days. On day 3, 24-hour urine creatinine, sodium, and aldosterone, and serum electrolytes are measured. Urine sodium>200 mEq /24 h (to document adequate sodium load) and urine aldosterone >12 mcg/24 h confirm the diagnosis of PA.

Saline Infusion Test This test is used in some centers. Patients stay recumbent for at least 1 h before and during the infusion of 0.9 saline IV over 4 h, starting in the morning, usually between the hours of 8:00 and 9:30 am. PAC will fall below 5 ng/dL (140 pmol/L) in normal patients. Values above 10 ng/dL (280 pmol/L) are consistent with PA. Values between 5 and 10 ng/dl are indeterminate. This test should not be used in patients with uncontrolled hypertension, renal insufficiency, and cardiac arrhythmia. Further, patients should be monitored for hypokalemia if this test is used [11].

Radiological Diagnosis

All patients with confirmed PA should undergo testing for subtype classification [11], including computed tomography (CT) or magnetic resonance imaging (MRI) and adrenal venous sampling (AVS), if they are surgical candidates and considering surgery as a potential treatment option.

Multiphasic CT or MRI are typically first-line imaging examinations to help detect the presence of an adrenal adenoma or adrenal hyperplasia. Unfortunately, both imaging techniques have limitations. First, adenomas can be small and below the resolution of the examination [15]. Furthermore, the presence of an adenoma does not distinguish between functioning and non-functioning adenomas. Also, many adrenal glands demonstrate diffuse nodularity with increasing age and hypertension, and it can be challenging to distinguish nodular hyperplasia from a discrete adrenal adenoma [16]. For these reasons, there is a wide range in the reported sensitivity of CT and MRI, with sensitivities ranging between 40% and 100% for CT and 70% and 100% for MRI in the detection of aldosterone-producing adenomas [17].

Adrenal adenomas do have a characteristic appearance on both CT and MRI secondary to the presence of intracellular fat [18]. On unenhanced CT images, adenomas demonstrate low Hounsfield units of 10 or lower. Contrast-enhanced CT imaging obtained in portal venous phase and at 15 min can further describe the washout characteristics of the adrenal nodule with greater than 40% relative washout and 60% absolute washout indicative of an adrenal adenoma. On chemical shift MRI, there is loss of signal on out-of-phase imaging indicative of an intracellular fat component (Fig. 1.1). Unfortunately, research has not yet determined a method to further distinguish between non-functioning and functioning adrenal adenomas.

Adrenal hyperplasia, by definition, is diffuse thickening of the adrenal gland with a length greater than 5 cm and thickness greater than 10 mm [19]. The adrenal thickening can be smooth or nodular in contour (Fig. 1.2). This has been recently challenged by Lingam et al., who describe a 100% specificity and sensitivity for

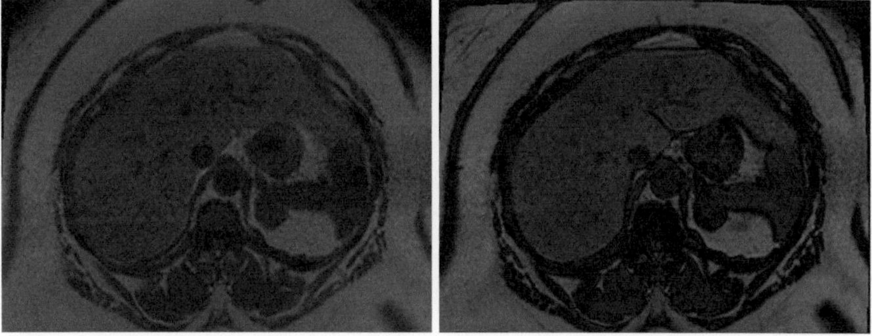

Fig. 1.1 Axial in and out-of-phase MR imaging through the upper abdomen demonstrating a 2.6 cm left adrenal nodule with loss of signal on out-of-phase imaging, compatible with intracellular lipid and an adrenal adenoma

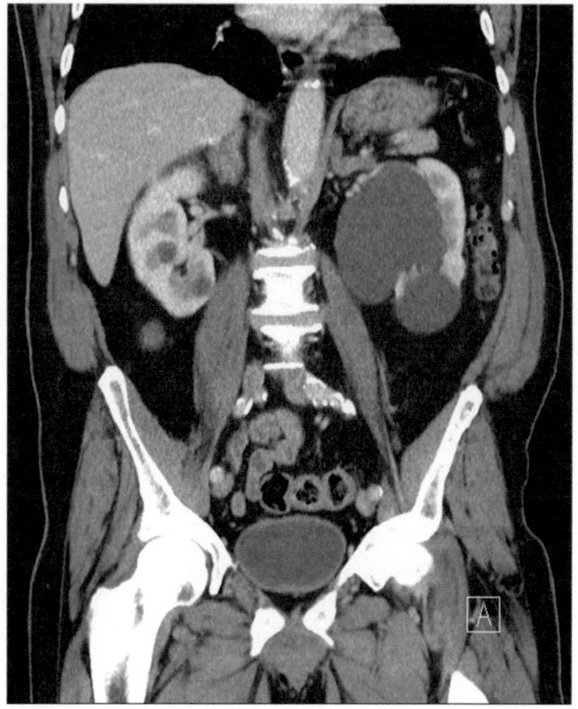

Fig. 1.2 Single coronal CT image through the mid-abdomen in portal venous phase demonstrating nodular thickening of both adrenal glands, measuring greater than 1 cm in thickness. No discrete nodule was visualized. Findings are compatible with adrenal hyperplasia

limb width greater than or equal to 5 mm and 3 mm, respectively [20]. Adrenal hyperplasia is typically a diagnosis of exclusion if no discrete adrenal nodule is detected.

Adrenal venous sampling involves obtaining blood samples from the IVC and both adrenal veins to measure aldosterone and cortisol levels and is considered the gold standard for detecting the underlying cause of PA. Specifics of this technique, including the detection rate, sensitivity, specificity, and complications, are discussed at length in Chap. 6.

References

1. Monticone S, D'Ascenzo F, Moretti C, Williams TA, Veglio F, Gaita F, Mulatero P. Cardiovascular events and target organ damage in primary aldosteronism compared with essential hypertension: a systematic review and meta-analysis. Lancet Diabetes Endocrinol. 2018;6(1):41–50.
2. Young WF Jr. Diagnosis and treatment of primary aldosteronism: practical clinical perspectives. J Intern Med. 2019;285(2):126–48. https://doi.org/10.1111/joim.12831. Epub 2018 Sep 25
3. Melmed S, Koenig R, Rosen C, Auchus R, Goldfine A, Williams R. Williams textbook of endocrinology. 13th ed. Philadelphia: Elsevier; 2016.

4. Conn JW. Presidential address: part I; painting background, part II; primary aldosternism: a new clinical syndrome. J Lab Clin Med. 1955;45:3–17.
5. Gittler RD, Fajans SS. Primary aldosteronism (Conn's syndrome). J Clin Endocrinol Metab. 1995;80(12):3438–41.
6. Mulatero P, Stowasser M, Loh KC, Fardella CE, Gordon RD, Mosso L, Gomez-Sanchez CE, Veglio F, Young WF Jr. Increased diagnosis of primary aldosteronism, including surgically correctable forms, in centers from five continents. J Clin Endocrinol Metab. 2004;89(3):1045–50. https://doi.org/10.1210/jc.2003-031337.
7. Douma S, Petidis K, Doumas M, Papaefthimiou P, Triantafyllou A, Kartali N, Papadopoulos N, Vogiatzis K, Zamboulis C. Prevalence of primary hyperaldosteronism in resistant hypertension: a retrospective observational study. Lancet. 2008;371(9628):1921–6.
8. Monticone S, Burrello J, Tizzani D, Bertello C, Viola A, Buffolo F, Gabetti L, Mengozzi G, Williams TA, Rabbia F, Veglio F, Mulatero P. Prevalence and clinical manifestations of primary aldosteronism encountered in primary care practice. J Am Coll Cardiol. 2017;69(14):1811–20.
9. Brown JM, Siddiqui M, Calhoun DA, Carey RM, Hopkins PN, Williams GH, Vaidya A. The unrecognized prevalence of primary aldosteronism: a cross-sectional study. Ann Intern Med. 2020;173(1):10–20.
10. Rossi GP, Bernini G, Caliumi C, Desideri G, Fabris B, Ferri C, Ganzaroli C, Giacchetti G, Letizia C, Maccario M, Mallamaci F, Mannelli M, Mattarello MJ, Moretti A, Palumbo G, Parenti G, Porteri E, Semplicini A, Rizzoni D, Rossi E, Boscaro M, Pessina AC, Mantero F, PAPY Study Investigators. A prospective study of the prevalence of primary aldosteronism in 1,125 hypertensive patients. J Am Coll Cardiol. 2006;48(11):2293–300.
11. Romero DG, Yanes Cardozo LL. Clinical practice guideline for management of primary aldosteronism: what is new in the 2016 update? Int J Endocrinol Metab Disord. 2016;2(3) https://doi.org/10.16966/2380-548X.129.
12. Di Murro A, Petramala L, Cotesta D, Zinnamosca L, Crescenzi E, Marinelli C, Saponara M, Letizia C. Renin-angiotensin-aldosterone system in patients with sleep apnoea: prevalence of primary aldosteronism. J Renin-Angiotensin-Aldosterone Syst. 2010;11(3):165–72. https://doi.org/10.1177/1470320310366581. Epub 2010 May 20
13. Ahmed AH, Gordon RD, Taylor PJ, Ward G, Pimenta E, Stowasser M. Effect of contraceptives on aldosterone/renin ratio may vary according to the components of contraceptive, renin assay method, and possibly route of administration. J Clin Endocrinol Metab. 2011;96(6):1797–804.
14. Weinberger MH, Fineberg NS. The diagnosis of primary aldosteronism and separation of two major subtypes. Arch Intern Med. 1993;153(18):2125–9.
15. Rossi GP, Sacchetto A, Chiesura-Corona M, et al. Identification of the etiology of primary aldosteronism with adrenal vein sampling in patients with equivocal computed tomography and magnetic resonance findings; results in 104 consecutive cases. J Clin Endocrinol Metab. 2001;86:1083–90.
16. Lingam RK, Sohaib SA, Rockall AG, et al. Diagnostic performance of CT versus MR in detecting aldosterone-producing adenoma in primary hyperaldosteronism (Conn's syndrome). Eur Radiol. 2004;14:1787–92.
17. Patel SM, Lingam RK, Beaconsfield TI, et al. Role of radiology in the management of primary aldosteronism. Radiographics. 2007;27:1145–57.
18. Korobkin M, Giordano TJ, Brodeur FJ, et al. Adrenal adenomas: relationship between histologic lipid and CT and MR findings. Radiology. 1996;200:743–7.
19. Michelle MA, Jensen CT, Habra MA, Menias CO, Shaaban AM, Wagner-Bartak NA, Roman-Colon AM, Elsayes KM. Adrenal cortical hyperplasia: diagnostic workup, subtypes, imaging features and mimics. Br J Radiol. 2017;90(1079):20170330.
20. Lingam RK, Sohaib SA, Vlahos I, et al. CT of primary hyperaldosteronism (Conn's syndrome): the value of measuring the adrenal gland. AJR Am J Roentgenol. 2003;181:843–9.

Chapter 2
Clinical, Laboratory, and Radiological Diagnosis of Hyperparathyroidism

Jennifer D. Merrill, Carlos A. Zamora, and Jorge D. Oldan

Introduction

Primary hyperparathyroidism (PHPT) is the most common cause of hypercalcemia in outpatients. It is typically characterized by a high serum calcium and high or inappropriately normal parathyroid hormone (PTH). Most PHPT is caused by a single parathyroid adenoma, but multiple parathyroid adenomas, parathyroid hyperplasia, and parathyroid carcinoma are also important causes. Although most patients present without symptoms, severe or long-standing hyperparathyroidism can cause symptomatic hypercalcemia, osteoporosis, and nephrolithiasis. A biochemical diagnosis should be confirmed before imaging studies for localization, and secondary causes of PTH elevation should be excluded. After biochemical confirmation of the diagnosis, further laboratory and imaging evaluation should center on identifying adverse impacts from the inappropriately elevated PTH. Once laboratory and imaging evaluation have confirmed the diagnosis and adverse impact from it, removal of the offending parathyroid gland is the most common treatment. Presurgical localization of the gland has allowed for the development of minimally invasive surgical techniques. Parathyroid ultrasound and SPECT-CT are the most common imaging modalities used to identify the gland and offer good sensitivity and specificity.

J. D. Merrill (✉)
Division of Endocrinology, Diabetes, and Metabolism, Department of Internal Medicine, The Ohio State University College of Medicine, Columbus, OH, USA

C. A. Zamora
Division of Neuroradiology, Department of Radiology, University of North Carolina at Chapel Hill, Chapel Hill, NC, USA
e-mail: carlos_zamora@med.unc.edu

J. D. Oldan
Division of Molecular Imaging and Therapeutics, Department of Radiology, University of North Carolina School of Medicine, Chapel Hill, NC, USA
e-mail: jorge_oldan@med.unc.edu

© The Author(s), under exclusive license to Springer Nature Switzerland AG 2022

H. Yu et al. (eds.), *Diagnosis and Management of Endocrine Disorders in Interventional Radiology*, https://doi.org/10.1007/978-3-030-87189-5_2

Etiology

PHPT represents an autonomous spontaneous overproduction of PTH. PHPT is almost always due to a benign overgrowth of parathyroid tissue, either of single or multiple glands. Parathyroid adenomas are the most common cause of PHPT and occur in 85–90% of cases. About 5% of these patients have multiple parathyroid adenomas, and 5% have adenomas of ectopic glands. Four-gland hyperplasia and parathyroid carcinoma account for 10–15% and about 1% of PHPT cases, respectively [1–3]. PHPT caused by ectopic secretion of PTH from a non-parathyroid tumor may occur but is exceedingly rare [4].

Most cases of PHPT occur sporadically as single-gland parathyroid adenomas that are monoclonal [5], though PHPT may also occur as part of several inherited syndromes [4]. These syndromes include multiple endocrine neoplasia types 1, 2a, and 4; hyperparathyroidism-jaw tumor syndrome; and familial isolated hyperparathyroidism [4]. It is estimated that more than 10% of patients with PHPT have a mutation in one of the 11 implicated genes [6, 7].

Some of the genes responsible for heritable forms of PHPT also contribute to sporadic PHPT through a somatic mutation or a predisposing germline mutation. MEN1 and CCND1/cyclin D1 are the two molecular defects with the most established role in the pathogenesis of sporadic parathyroid adenomas [3, 4]. Cyclin D1 is a major cell cycle regulator. A pericentromeric inversion on chromosome 11 causes the relocation of cyclin D1 so that it is positioned adjacent to the PTH gene. This change causes a regulatory element of the PTH gene to cause overexpression of the cyclin D1 protein, which forces the cells to proliferate [3]. Between 10% and 20% of adenomas have this clonal gene defect, and cyclin D1 is overexpressed in approximately 40% of parathyroid adenomas [3]. Between 20% and 30% of parathyroid tumors not associated with MEN1 have mutations in both copies of the MEN1 gene [3]. Sporadic parathyroid carcinoma appears to arise through distinct pathways from parathyroid adenomas mostly. It is most frequently driven by mutational inactivation of the CDC73 (HRPT2) tumor suppressor gene, though there are many other mutations known to contribute to the pathogenesis [4].

Epidemiology

PHPT is one of the most common endocrine disorders and is the most common cause of hypercalcemia diagnosed in the outpatient setting [3, 8]. The annual incidence is estimated to be about 25 cases per 100,000 in the United States and Europe, with as many as 80% identified as outpatients by elevated calcium on routine measurement of serum electrolytes [3]. PHPT is more common in women than men, with a female to male ratio of 3–4:1 [9–11]. The demographics of PHPT vary significantly depending on whether it presents asymptomatically or as a symptomatic disease with nephrolithiasis or bone involvement. Most asymptomatic cases occur in the 6th decade or later in life, and PHPT rarely presents before the age of 15 [3, 12]. Symptomatic patients tend to present in their 7th decade with a female to male ratio of 4:1. Patients who present with nephrolithiasis tend to present at a younger age, and females tend to predominate. In one study, patients with evidence of PHPT on skeletal radiographs at presentation presented at a mean age of 38.7 years. In this group, slightly more men presented than women [13].

Anatomy and Pathophysiology

Parathyroid Gland Anatomy

Most people have four parathyroid glands. The parathyroid glands originate in the 3rd and 4th pharyngeal pouches during embryologic development and migrate to the lower neck, which causes variation in their location [14]. About 5% of people have more than four glands, and some people only have two. The parathyroid glands typically lay external to the fibrous capsule on the posterior surface of the thyroid [15]. The superior glands are more constant in their location and are often embedded in the posterior capsule of the upper 2/3 of the left and right thyroid lobes. They may also be found in the pharynx or the tracheoesophageal groove. The location of the inferior glands is more variable due to a longer developmental migration path from the 3rd pharyngeal pouches. Almost half are located within 1 cm of the lower pole of the thyroid. They may also be found at the carotid bifurcation, in the carotid sheath, within the thymus, or near the superior portion of it, intrathyroidal, retropharyngeal, or within the thorax [16, 17].

The parathyroid glands are typically tan to reddish-brown and kidney-shaped, measuring 2–7 mm long and 2–4 mm wide and surrounded by a thin capsule [3]. They are composed of 70% chief cells and 30% fat and have a vascular supply that is anatomically distinct from the thyroid [3]. The chief cells of the parathyroid glands make PTH. Parathyroid cells have G-protein-coupled calcium-sensing receptors (CaSR) on their surface, which respond to serum concentrations of ionized calcium [18].

Parathyroid cells typically replicate during mammalian growth but rarely replicate in adulthood except when chronically stimulated by hypocalcemia, low calcitriol, hyperphosphatemia, or uremia [12, 19].

Physiologic Roles of Calcium and Organic Phosphate

Calcium and phosphorus are the main constituents of bone. Bone contains nearly all of the calcium and phosphorus in the body, but the small amounts of calcium and phosphorus in the extracellular fluid and within cells play crucial roles in normal physiologic processes [12].

Calcium has a wide range of essential intracellular and extracellular roles. Extracellular calcium serves as a cofactor for various enzymes, including the enzymes of the coagulation cascade. Calcium ions also serve as the signaling molecules for muscle contraction, neurotransmitter release, and endocrine and exocrine function [12]. Many of these functions require a large gradient between intracellular and extracellular calcium as well as tight regulation of the extracellular calcium level. About 1% of bone calcium is rapidly exchangeable with calcium in the intra and extracellular fluid. Roughly half of the calcium in the blood is bound to albumin and serum globulins. The remaining ionized fraction is biologically active and thus tightly controlled by hormonal mechanisms. A complex feedback system involving PTH, parathyroid glands, bone, kidney, small intestine, calcitonin, and parafollicular cells of the thyroid is responsible for regulating serum calcium and organic phosphate levels (Fig. 2.1).

Organic phosphate is an essential component of nucleic acids, phospholipids, complex carbohydrates, glycolysis intermediaries, a cofactor for enzymes and adenosine triphosphate (ATP). Bone contains 85% of body phosphate. Twelve percent of serum phosphate is protein bound. The intracellular and extracellular fluid contains about the same phosphate concentration [12].

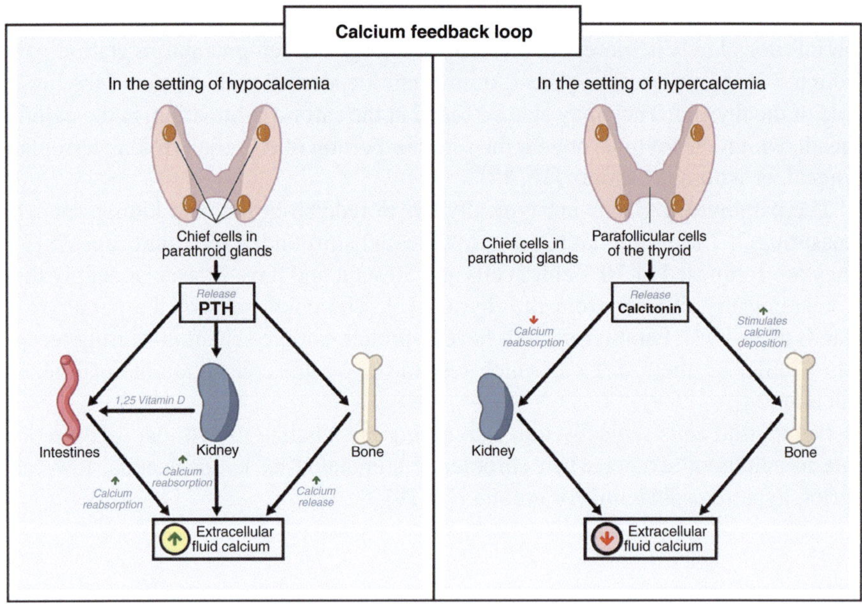

Fig. 2.1 Calcium/PTH feedback pathway. (Image courtesy of Sierra Finn, Chapel Hill, North Carolina, USA)

Regulation of Parathyroid Hormone in Response to Hypocalcemia

PTH is the peptide hormone that controls minute-to-minute ionized calcium levels in the extracellular fluid. PTH is an 84 amino acid protein that is released from the parathyroid glands when calcium is low. It exerts its effects through the interaction of its first 34 amino acids with the type 1 PTH/PTH-related peptide (PTHrP) receptor (PTHR1).

Although the major product of the chief cells of the parathyroid gland is the 84 amino acid peptide (1–84 PTH), there is considerable metabolism of this peptide, resulting in a heterogeneous assortment of circulating fragments [20]. PTH is cleaved in the liver and kidney to amino-terminal and carboxy-terminal. The amino- and carboxy-terminal fragments are present in circulation, but their clinical significance is unclear. In fact, only 5–30% of circulating PTH is the whole 84 amino acid fragment. Between 70% and 95% of circulating PTH is the carboxy-terminal fragment; the amino-terminal fragments comprise only a small percentage of circulating protein. PTH is rapidly metabolized by the liver and kidney and has a half-life of 2 min. The half-life is unaffected by serum levels of calcitriol or calcium.

Within seconds of detecting hypocalcemia by the CaSR on the parathyroid cells, the parathyroid glands release preformed PTH. PTH acts on the bone to cause calcium release and also acts on the kidney to increase calcium reabsorption and synthesis of the hormonally active 1,25-dihydroxy vitamin D (calcitriol). Calcitriol then acts on the intestine to increase the absorption of dietary calcium, as well as causing additional calcium influx from the bone and kidney. If hypocalcemia continues over the next 15–30 min, there is an increase in the net synthesis of PTH without a change in the mRNA due to decreased intracellular degradation of PTH. Within the next 12–24 h of hypocalcemia, there is an increase in the mRNA for PTH. If hypocalcemia occurs for days to weeks, the parathyroid gland cells begin to proliferate.

Increased calcitriol and ionized calcium then exert negative feedback on the parathyroid gland. Parathyroid cells respond to the absolute level of ionized calcium and the rate of fall of the calcium level. Less than 1% of the secreted hormone finds its way to the PTH receptor on the target organs.

Parathyroid Hormone Action on Bone

Skeletal release of calcium via osteoclasts occurs within 2–3 h of increased PTH release. Prolonged hyperparathyroidism causes increased number of osteoclasts, which erode bone matrix to mobilize calcium. This occurs predominantly in the metaphyses of the long bones. There is also increased activity of osteoblasts, which often results in new widely spaced delicate trabeculae [3]. In severe cases, the cortex may be thinned, and the marrow may contain increased fibrous tissue with foci of hemorrhage and cyst formation (osteitis fibrosa cystica).

Parathyroid Hormone Action on the Kidney

Almost all of the calcium filtered by the glomerulus is normally reabsorbed in the renal tubules. At least 65% is passively reabsorbed by the proximal convoluted and straight tubules through a paracellular route [21]. The remaining filtered calcium is absorbed more distally, 20% in the cortical thick ascending limb of the loop of Henle and 10% in the distal convoluted tubule and collecting tubules. The calcium transport into the cortical thick ascending limb of the loop of Henle is driven by the voltage gradient from active Na-K-Cl$_2$ reabsorption. Calcium absorption is inhibited by loop diuretics. The CaSR is also expressed in the cortical thick ascending limb, and it inhibits Na-K-Cl$_2$ reabsorption. Calcium absorption is subsequently inhibited when CaSR is stimulated by high serum calcium levels. Most of the action of PTH in the kidney is due to its impact on increasing absorption in the distal nephron. The kidney increases distal tubular calcium reabsorption in response to PTH within minutes. Renal synthesis of 1-alpha-hydroxylase and thus the production of calcitriol begin within days; this causes increased intestinal calcium absorption.

Parathyroid Hormone Action on the Intestine

Calcitriol increases intestinal calcium absorption by increasing the expression of gut lumen transport molecules. The greatest absorption is from the duodenum, but calcium is also absorbed through the entire small intestine and part of the colon.

Impact of Serum Phosphate

Hyperphosphatemia has a direct stimulatory effect on the parathyroid gland, resulting in increased PTH secretion in the short term and nodular hyperplasia of the parathyroid glands if the hyperphosphatemia is prolonged [22]. PTH also inhibits renal phosphate absorption and causes increased phosphaturia.

Clinical Evaluation

Historical Presentations

When first described in the 1920s, PHPT typically presented with severe symptoms of hypercalcemia with bone pain, spontaneous fractures, proximal muscle weakness with atrophy and hyperreflexia, gait disturbances, and nephrolithiasis [23–25]. Hyperparathyroid crisis, a discrete episode of life-threatening hypercalcemia, was also sometimes seen [25].

Current Presentation of Classic Primary Hyperparathyroidism

In the early 1970s, automated measurement of serum calcium became widespread in the United States and Europe. This allowed for routine biochemical screening of serum calcium and identifying a large number of patients without overt skeletal or renal complications [26]. In the United States and other Western countries today, the most common presentation of PHPT is a high serum calcium level identified by routine measurement in an asymptomatic individual [27, 28]. Subsequent workup will reveal concentrations of PTH elevated above the reference range, or PTH levels that are inappropriately normal in the context of hypercalcemia [29].

Overt symptoms now occur in less than 20% of patients diagnosed with PHPT [11, 30]. Nephrolithiasis is the most common overt complication of PHPT [31]. The renal stones are typically small and comprised of calcium oxalate or calcium phosphate. Renal stones and nephrocalcinosis will be seen on abdominal radiographs or renal ultrasound [24]. Even though the presentation is often asymptomatic, many PHPT patients still frequently demonstrate target organ involvement [31]. Although most asymptomatic patients are stable, progression may occur, and more than a third of patients develop nephrolithiasis, worsening hypercalcemia, or decreasing bone mineral density (BMD) at follow-up 15 years later [32]. Even mild PHPT is associated with an increased risk of vertebral, distal forearm, rib, and pelvic fractures [33].

Patients who do not have classical signs of PHPT may complain of fatigue, subjective weakness, polyuria, polydipsia, bone pain, joint pain, constipation, forgetfulness, and neuropsychiatric illness [11, 34]. There is debate about whether these symptoms can truly be attributed to PHPT, since they are common in the general population. Studies are mixed as to whether correction of PHPT resolves symptoms [35–37], though a meta-analysis suggested that parathyroidectomy yielded better quality of life and emotional well-being [38].

Normocalcemic Primary Hyperparathyroidism

Normocalcemic PHPT is now a well-recognized variant in the diagnostic spectrum of PHPT [7]. Patients present with consistently normal total and ionized calcium and elevated PTH without a clear cause for secondary elevation [6, 39]. In order to make the diagnosis, an isolated PTH level above the normal upper limit should be confirmed on several occasions over 3–6 months [7]. Disorders associated with secondary or compensatory elevations in PTH such as vitamin D deficiency, chronic kidney disease, and use of medications such as lithium, thiazide diuretics, and bone antiresorptive medication use should be excluded. Some patients with normocalcemic PHPT appear to remain stable over time without a decline in BMD. Other patients develop hypercalcemia, or other signs of PHPT with continued follow-up [40].

Laboratory Evaluation

Initial Laboratory Testing

Patients with classical hyperparathyroidism have hypercalcemia and either a PTH that is high or inappropriately normal in the setting of hypercalcemia [41]. They are often asymptomatic and referred for mild hypercalcemia on routine lab work. In severe, symptomatic PHPT, marked elevation of the serum calcium and PTH concentrations are common.

A panel of experts who have made major contributions to the understanding of asymptomatic PHPT meet regularly to make recommendations regarding the optimal management of the disease. Table 2.1 summarizes their most recent recommendations from the Fourth International Workshop, which convened in September 2013.

Table 2.1 Recommendations for the evaluation of patients with asymptomatic PHPT from the Fourth International Workshop [6]

		Notes
Recommended	Biochemistry panel	Calcium
		Phosphate
		Alkaline phosphatase
		BUN
		Creatinine
		25-Hydroxyvitamin D
	PTH	By second- or third-generation immunoassay
	BMD by DEXA	Lumbar spine
		Hip
		Distal 1/3 radius
	Vertebral spine assessment	X ray or VFA by DEXA
	24-hour urine	Calcium
		Creatinine
		Creatinine clearance
		Stone risk profile
	Abdominal imaging	X ray, ultrasound, or CT scan
Optional	HRpQCT	
	TBS by DEXA	
	Bone turnover markers	Bone-specific alkaline phosphatase activity
		Osteocalcin
		Procollagen type 1 N-propeptide
		Serum CTX or urinary CTX
	Fractional excretion of calcium on timed urine sample	
	DNA testing if genetic basis suspected	

Calcium

Corrected Calcium

Initial workup for hyperparathyroidism should include measurement of serum calcium and albumin. Calcium circulates in three distinct fractions. About 50% is the biologically important ionized fraction, 40% is protein-bound and is not filterable by the kidney, and 10% is complexed to anions. Most of the protein-bound calcium is bound to albumin, and the rest is complexed to globulins. In general, each 1 g/dL of albumin binds 0.2 mmol/L (0.8 mg/dL) of calcium [28]. The total serum calcium level should be adjusted for albumin according to the formula:

$$\text{Corrected calcium} = \text{total serum calcium in mg/dL} + 0.8 \times (4.0 \; \text{albumin in g/dL})$$

Ionized Calcium

Ionized calcium can be measured in addition to corrected calcium. Ionized calcium level is a more sensitive indicator of PHPT than corrected calcium [42]. Over 20% of patients with histologically proven parathyroid disease in one study had elevation of ionized calcium but not total calcium [43]. Direct measurement of ionized calcium can be useful in situations such as extreme hyper- or hypoalbuminemia, in the setting of changing serum pH, thrombocytosis, myeloma, and Waldenstrom's macroglobulinemia [29]. Measurement of ionized calcium was not recommended by the Fourth International Workshop for Management of Asymptomatic PHPT, because many facilities do not have sufficient capabilities to rely on an ionized free calcium concentration [6]. Direct measurement of ionized calcium is limited by difficulties in accurate analysis, lack of standardization, and need for special handling [44]. Patients with normocalcemic PHPT must also have normal ionized calcium concentrations [39].

Parathyroid Hormone Assays

First Generation Assays

First-generation PTH assays are radioimmunoassays. These assays used different polyclonal antibodies directed against predominantly the mid- or carboxy-terminal portion to the PTH molecule [45]. Therefore, these assays detected predominantly PTH fragments that lacked an intact amino terminus and therefore did not activate the PTH/PTHrP receptor or mediate the hormone's actions on calcium [46]. These assays have now largely been replaced by two site immunoassays, also known as sandwich assays.

Second- and Third-Generation Assays

Immunometric assays for PTH are referred to as second- and third-generation assays but may also be referred to as first- and second-generation immunometric assays. They are more sensitive and specific than the older radioimmunoassays [47]. Second-generation assays are also known as intact PTH assays and rely on the use of two antibodies. The traditional second-generation assays measure both intact PTH (1–84) and cross-react with large carboxy-terminal PTH fragments [7]. The third-generation assays (whole, bioactive, or biointact PTH assays) are more specific, because they use a labeled antibody directed at PTH (1–4), detect only PTH (1–84), and have less cross-reactivity with C-terminal fragments. These assays do react with a post-translational modified form of PTH, known as non-truncated amino-terminal PTH (N-PTH), representing up to 10% of PTH in normal individuals and 15% of patients with renal failure [7]. Second- and third-generation assays for PTH are equally helpful in diagnosing PHPT [6, 7]. The sensitivity of these assays for detecting PHPT ranges from 73% to 97% [7].

As measured by second- and third-generation assays, PTH concentrations are influenced by several conditions that interfere with the establishment of a reference interval [48]. PTH elevations have been described in older individuals, especially women, black people, people with lower calcium intake, and obese people [20]. Furthermore, 25-hydroxyvitamin D (vitamin D) deficiency frequently drives PTH elevation, and there is not yet a consensus on the optimal reference range for vitamin D [49–51]. An optimal reference interval for PTH in vitamin D replete individuals has yet to be established for second- and third-generation PTH assays using large population cohorts [7, 20]. The upper limit of the PTH reference interval is lower in individuals with vitamin D levels >20 ng/mL (50 nmol/L).

In the classic presentation of PHPT, PTH is high or inappropriately normal in the setting of hypercalcemia. When PTH is within the reference range in PHPT, it is more likely to be in the upper end of the reference range. In one large case series, only 1% of patients with PHPT had PTH levels within the lower half of the reference range [52]. PTH that is not suppressed in the setting of hypercalcemia is compatible with PHPT [7].

Measurement of Renal Function

Glomerular filtration rate (GFR) must be higher than 60 ml/min to substantiate the diagnosis of normocalcemic PHPT [39]. All glands are affected to a variable degree in patients with chronic renal failure. Surgical intervention requires inspection of all glands; therefore, localization is of limited value.

Serum Phosphate

Measurement of serum phosphate is recommended in the evaluation of PHPT [6]. In PHPT, serum phosphate levels may be low or low normal due to the phosphaturic effects of PTH [53]. In one series, there was no difference in serum phosphate levels between patients with and those without PHPT [54].

25-Hydroxyvitamin D (Vitamin D)

The vitamin D level should be measured in all patients evaluated for PHPT [6, 7, 20]. People from the same geographic region with PHPT appear to be more likely to have vitamin D deficiency than people without PHPT [27, 55]. The most likely cause of abnormally low vitamin D in PHPT is an increased metabolic clearance rate (24 hydroxylation) induced by calcitriol and possibly PTH [56]. After parathyroidectomy, vitamin D returns to concentrations found in the normal population [57].

There are consequences to low vitamin D levels in PHPT. PHPT appears to be more severe in patients with vitamin D deficiency, and low vitamin D levels are associated with larger parathyroid adenoma size [27, 58]. There is evidence that replacement of vitamin D to a level higher than 20 ng/mL in patients with PHPT and vitamin D insufficiency is associated with a decline in PTH as well as other markers of bone turnover, including alkaline phosphatase and urinary N-telopeptide [59, 60].

The diagnostic accuracy for PHPT is improved in a vitamin D replete population [61]. Despite this, the definition of normal vitamin D remains controversial. The Institute of Medicine (IOM) recommends a threshold for vitamin D of 20 ng/mL (50 nmol/L) [49, 50], but the Endocrine Society recommends a threshold of 30 ng/mL (75 nmol/L) [51]. Preoperative vitamin D deficiency is predictive of hungry bone syndrome postoperatively, and it is recommended that vitamin D be supplemented to a level greater than 20 mg/mL prior to parathyroidectomy [7, 62]. This should be done cautiously with low doses of up to 2000 units of cholecalciferol daily.

24-Hour Urine Calcium

A 24-hour urinalysis measuring urine creatinine and calcium should be performed to assess the urinary calcium excretion. This is important to evaluate the risk for developing nephrolithiasis and rule out other diagnostic considerations. This testing is ideally performed in the outpatient setting while the patient adheres to their regular diet and activities. Instructions for collecting a 24-hour urine sample vary by the laboratory, but typically the patient's first voided urine is discarded [63]. Then, all subsequent urine voided for the next 24 h, including the next morning's first voided urine, is collected in containers provided by the laboratory. A 24-hour urine collection can be inconvenient and difficult for some patients; therefore, it can be helpful to assess the accuracy of the urine collection. Urinary creatinine excretion is used to measure the adequacy of a 24-hour urine collection. Creatinine is a byproduct of muscle metabolism, so the excretion of creatinine is stable based on muscle mass. The average daily excretion of creatinine is 18–24 mg/kg for males and 15–20 mg/kg for females. A lower than expected creatinine excretion suggests an incomplete collection [63]. A urinary calcium to creatinine clearance ratio (UCCR) should be calculated as follows:

$$\text{Urinary calcium to creatinine clearance ratio} = \frac{\left(24 \ \text{hour urine calcium} \times \text{serum creatinine}\right)}{\left(\text{serum calcium} \times 24 \ \text{hour urine creatinine}\right)}$$

Patients with a UCCR less than 0.01 should be evaluated for familial hypocalciuric hypercalcemia [6, 7].

Biochemical Stone Risk Analysis

If a patient demonstrates marked hypercalciuria with 400 mg/day of urinary calcium excretion on the 24-hour urine calcium study, then a urinary biochemical stone risk profile should be obtained. This is available through many commercial laboratories. Patients with PHPT that experienced nephrolithiasis had higher urinary calcium excretion and 24-hour urine oxalate levels than patients that did not form stones. Hypercalciuria and relatively high oxaluria were associated with the stone formation in PHPT [64].

Markers of Bone Turnover

Increased bone turnover is characteristic of PHPT. Biochemical markers of bone formation, such as osteocalcin and alkaline phosphatase, and markers of bone resorption, such as deoxypyridinoline, N-telopeptide (NTX), and C-telopeptide (CTX), are typically markedly elevated in severe PHPT [24]. Patients with high bone turnover markers are more likely to have the skeletal disease. Alkaline phosphatase is significantly elevated in almost all patients with osteitis fibrosis cystica [65]. After parathyroidectomy, bone resorption markers rapidly improve, followed by a more gradual reduction in bone formation markers [66].

Tests of Low Clinical Utility

1,25-Dihydroxy Vitamin D (Calcitriol)

When measured in PHPT, calcitriol levels are typically at the upper limit of normal or occasionally mildly elevated [54]. High concentrations of calcitriol are associated with higher 24-hour urine calcium excretion and lower BMD [67]. Routine measurement of this active metabolite is not recommended since the additional information does not change management [6].

Laboratory Interpretation and Differential Diagnosis

Secondary Hyperparathyroidism

Secondary hyperparathyroidism (SHPT) is characterized by an increase in PTH that is an appropriate response to a stimulus. By definition, the serum calcium is normal, and the PTH is elevated. SHPT must be ruled out before a diagnosis of normocalcemic PHPT can be made.

Renal dysfunction can cause secondary elevation of PTH in normocalcemic individuals. PTH begins to rise when estimated GRF (eGFR) falls below 60 mL/min [7]. Long-standing chronic kidney disease is associated with several metabolic disturbances that lead to increased PTH secretion, including hyperphosphatemia, calcitriol deficiency, and hypocalcemia [22].

Vitamin D deficiency, increased urinary calcium excretion, and gastrointestinal malabsorption of calcium are also potential causes of SHPT. Vitamin D insufficiency or deficiency may cause secondary elevation of PTH in the setting of normal calcium concentrations. Vitamin D should be replaced until a level >30 ng/mL is achieved in patients with vitamin D deficiency and elevated PTH level before a diagnosis of normocalcemic hyperparathyroidism can be made [39]. Notably, it may take 6–12 months for PTH to decrease after vitamin D is replaced. Patients thought to have normocalcemic PHPT can develop hypercalcemia when 25-hydroxyvitamin D is increased above 30 ng/mL (75 nmol/L), thus making the diagnosis of hypercalcemic PHPT that was masked by 25-hydroxyvitamin D deficiency [7].

Hypercalciuria as a primary renal abnormality can be associated with normal serum calcium and a secondary increase in PTH levels [68].

Deficient calcium intake or gastrointestinal disorders associated with calcium malabsorption can also cause secondary elevations in PTH [69, 70]. These individuals will typically have a low-normal serum calcium concentration, vitamin D deficiency, and low urinary calcium excretion [39]. In general, malabsorption syndromes are clinically obvious. However, gluten enteropathy can cause calcium malabsorption in individuals with no symptoms of gastrointestinal disease.

A wide variety of secondary causes of PTH elevation can be mistaken for PHPT and especially normocalcemic PHPT. A thorough laboratory evaluation as described above is required to exclude these causes.

Medication Effects

The use of several medications is associated with elevated PTH, hypercalcemia, or both. The antiresorptive medications used to treat osteoporosis are associated with PTH elevation. Bisphosphonate treatment causes an early reduction in bone resorption. This induces a decrease in serum calcium, which leads to an increase in PTH [71]. This PTH elevation is a response to the change in serum calcium level and can occur even in the setting of hypercalcemia. The reduction in serum calcium occurs within days to weeks of the initiation of bisphosphonate treatment, earlier with intravenous therapy than with oral treatment. These changes may persist for weeks to months following the initiation of treatment [71]. Similarly, denosumab use causes PTH concentrations to be elevated for 3 months of the 6 months between doses [72].

Lithium can cause both transient and persistent hypercalcemia. Lithium decreases the sensitivity of the parathyroid gland to circulating calcium and lowers urinary calcium excretion [73]. This results in an increased calcium level and PTH in a majority of patients. This ultimately leads to parathyroid hyperplasia. After cessation of lithium, the patient should be monitored for 2–4 weeks to determine whether calcium metabolism has normalized [73]. If practical in light of any psychiatric comorbidities, discontinuation of lithium should be considered before making the diagnosis of PHPT [7].

Thiazide diuretics are some of the most frequently prescribed antihypertensive agents and are commonly associated with hypercalcemia. Thiazides exert their antihypertensive effects through an increase in sodium excretion by blocking the thiazide-sensitive NaCl transporter in the distal convoluted tubule, which causes increased renal tubular reabsorption of calcium and reduced urinary calcium excretion [74]. Thiazide-associated hypercalcemia occurs after an average of 5.2 years of treatment, and severe hypercalcemia is not usually observed despite continuation of thiazide [75]. About 20% of patients, who develop hypercalcemia while taking thiazide diuretics, are later found to have hyperparathyroidism, while hypercalcemia resolves in another 30% [75]. Prior to the diagnosis of PHPT, and especially in normocalcemic PHPT, thiazide diuretics should be discontinued, and diagnostic testing should be repeated when the patient has been off of thiazide treatment for several weeks [7].

Tertiary Hyperparathyroidism

Tertiary hyperparathyroidism (THPT) is characterized by excessive secretion of PTH causing hypercalcemia after long-standing SHPT. This typically occurs in individuals with chronic kidney disease and may occur after renal transplant. In these patients, long-standing hypocalcemia and hyperphosphatemia cause an increase in the number of cells secreting PTH [76]. The size of the parathyroid glands progressively increases as chronic kidney disease worsens and the glands may become autonomously functioning. These patients are most often identified by the persistence of hyperparathyroidism with hypercalcemia after renal transplantation [22].

Other rare causes of THPT include X-linked hypophosphatemic rickets, adult-onset (autosomal dominant) hypophosphatemic rickets, and oncogenic osteomalacia [22]. These diseases are typically treated chronically with high doses of oral phosphate. The increased phosphate transiently decreases ionized calcium and decreases the production of calcitriol. This can lead to increased secretion of PTH, which can become autonomous and eventually be associated with frank hypercalcemia and inappropriately elevated PTH [77–81].

Symptoms and signs of THPT may be similar to PHPT and are attributed to the level of PTH or degree of hypercalcemia. These symptoms can include bone pain, decreased bone mineral density, fractures, nephrolithiasis, soft tissue or vascular calcifications, muscle weakness, mental status changes, and impaired graft function in transplant patients [82]. There are no evidenced-based guidelines for when and how to treat THPT. Still, many clinicians intervene when the patient has long-term sustained hypercalcemia with PTH greater than nine times the upper limit of normal [22]. The decision to pursue parathyroidectomy should be deferred to at least 1 year after renal transplant. Subtotal parathyroidectomy is the treatment of choice because it decreases the risk of hypocalcemia and hyperphosphatemia postoperatively compared to total parathyroidectomy [83].

Familial Hypocalciuric Hypercalcemia

The key differential diagnosis in a patient with hypercalcemia and either a high PTH or PTH in the upper half of the reference interval is between PHPT and familial hypocalciuric hypercalcemia (FHH) [7]. FHH has been misdiagnosed as PHPT, because a significant number of these patients will have elevated PTH levels [84]. To rule out FHH, it is essential to measure the urinary calcium to creatinine clearance ratio (UCCR) [7]. A UCCR less than 0.01 is typically consistent with FHH. One caveat is that patients with vitamin D deficiency, renal insufficiency, or African origins may have low UCCR [85, 86]. In these patients and patients with UCCR between 0.01 and 0.02, genetic evaluation with mutational analysis for CaSR, GNA11, and APS2S1 genes can identify patients with FHH1, FHH2, and FHH3, respectively [87–89]. A UCCR greater than 0.02 is more consistent with a diagnosis of PHPT [90]. FHH is generally considered a benign condition due to a different calcium set point, and parathyroid surgery is not indicated in these patients. Although calcimimetics such as cinacalcet have not been approved for the treatment of THPT, a handful of small studies showed benefit with the improvement of serum calcium and a significant decrease in PTH [91–93].

Autoimmune Hypocalciuric Hypercalcemia

Anti-CaSR autoantibodies have been described in a handful of patients with PTH-dependent hypercalcemia. These patients tended to have decreased urinary calcium excretion and other autoimmune disorders and had either previously normal serum calcium levels or tested negative for the genetic mutations associated with FHH [94]. These patients are found to have blocking antibodies against the CaSR. Scant information is available to guide the diagnosis of this condition or the treatment of the associated hypercalcemia. The hypercalcemia does not respond to parathyroidectomy or bisphosphonate treatment but may respond to glucocorticoids [94–96].

Pseudohypoparathyroidism

Pseudohypoparathyroidism refers to a group of heterogeneous disorders whose common feature is renal resistance to PTH due to impaired activation of cAMP-dependent pathways via the Gsα protein [97]. Patients with pseudohypoparathyroidism present with hypocalcemia, hyperphosphatemia, and secondary hyperparathyroidism. They may have the physical findings of Albright hereditary osteodystrophy. Since PTH resistance only occurs in the kidney, these patients may develop osteitis fibrosa cystica and other PTH-mediated bone diseases. In the setting of prolonged hypocalcemia, people with pseudohypoparathyroidism can develop THPT requiring localization of the affected gland and potentially parathyroidectomy [98].

Genetic Evaluation for Primary Hyperparathyroidism

PHPT may occur as a sporadic disorder, a familial disorder that is a nonsyndromic isolated endocrinopathy, or a syndromic familial disorder. Syndromic forms of PHPT occur in MEN syndromes type 1 to 4 and hyperparathyroidism-jaw tumor syndrome. PHPT is the most common feature of MEN1 and occurs in approximately 90% of affected patients [99]. PHPT in patients with MEN1 occurs with an equal male to female ratio, at an earlier age (25 years compared to 55 years) and a more significant reduction in bone mineral density than in the general population [99–101]. It is helpful to know that the patient has a syndromic form of PHPT during clinical evaluation, because all four parathyroid glands may be affected, and imaging for localization is of little benefit [14, 99]. Inspection of all glands is necessary during surgery, even if localization studies show a unilateral abnormality.

Genetic evaluation should be sought in a patient who presents with typical familial forms of PHPT. Family history should be obtained in all patients with PHPT to determine whether first-degree relatives are affected. Patients who are less than 45 years old at the time of diagnosis [102] and have a multiglandular disease, parathyroid carcinoma, or atypical adenoma should be tested [7]. Mutational analysis should include evaluation for MEN1; CaSR; APS2S1; GNA11; CDKN-1A, CDKN-1B, CDKN-2B, and CDKN-2C; RET; and PTH in order of frequency of occurrence [7]. Genetic testing should use DNA obtained from non-tumor cells, including leukocytes, salivary cells, skin cells, or hair follicles, because DNA from parathyroid adenomas may contain multiple mutations [103]. Genetic testing should include informed consent from the patient with access to genetic counselors and occur at accredited centers [99].

If a germline mutation is identified, the patient should be started on an appropriate routine clinical, biochemical, and radiological screening for other diseases. First-degree relatives of a patient with a PHPT mutation should be identified and offered genetic counseling and genetic testing [7]. If the first-degree relative tests are negative for the causative mutation, they require no further follow-up.

Imaging Evaluation

PHPT is a biochemical diagnosis and should not be diagnosed using imaging studies [6]. Instead, imaging should be used to guide surgical decision-making and to localize abnormal glands.

Radiographic Findings of Hyperparathyroidism

Plain Radiography

The characteristic skeletal features of PHPT, as seen on plain radiographs, result from increased osteoclastic activity and bone resorption. A wide range of imaging findings may be present, including a "salt and pepper" appearance of the skull, tapering of the distal clavicle, subperiosteal resorption of the distal phalanges (typically bilateral and symmetric), bone cysts, and brown tumors (osteitis fibrosa cystica) [41]. Diffuse demineralization is often observed along with pathologic fractures, typically in the long bones of the extremities [24]. The cortex of long bones may be very thin and almost absent in some patients. Plain radiography is not sensitive for detecting bone loss due to hyperparathyroidism. Approximately 20–30% of bone mass must be depleted before osteoporosis can be detected on X-ray [104].

Dual-Energy X-ray Absorptiometry

Since routine measurement of serum calcium became widespread, it is rare for patients to have characteristic findings of hyperparathyroidism on plain radiography; however, evidence of such is more commonly seen on dual-energy X-ray absorptiometry (DEXA). This technique uses a fraction of the radiation dose of plain radiography. It allows calculation of BMD values (g/cm^2), which are compared against a reference population as T-scores or Z-scores [105, 106]. The BMD at the femoral neck, total hip, and L1–L4 vertebra are typically measured. Additionally, the distal 1/3 forearm BMD should be measured, if the hip or spine cannot be interpreted in the setting of hyperparathyroidism and in patients whose weight is over the limit of the DEXA table [107]. T-scores for the femoral neck and total hip are calculated against a white female reference population ages 20–29 years from the National Health and Nutritional Examination Survey III database. The device manufacturer database is used as the reference population for the lumbar spine measurements [107]. Z-scores are calculated to compare the patient' BMD against an age-, sex-, and ethnicity-matched reference population. The use of T-scores is preferred in postmenopausal women and men over age 50, while Z-scores are used in other populations. T-scores of −2.5 or less at the femoral neck meet the WHO international reference standard for osteoporosis.

PHPT has more catabolic impact on cortical bone than trabecular bone [31]. The densitometric profile of PHPT is reduced BMD at the distal 1/3 forearm, since it is composed primarily of cortical bone, while the lumbar spine shows relative preservation, as it is a predominantly trabecular site [11, 108]. DEXA of the distal 1/3 radius should be obtained in all patients with PHPT to evaluate for the catabolic effects of PTH in cortical bones (Fig. 2.2) [6]. In PHPT that is severe enough to

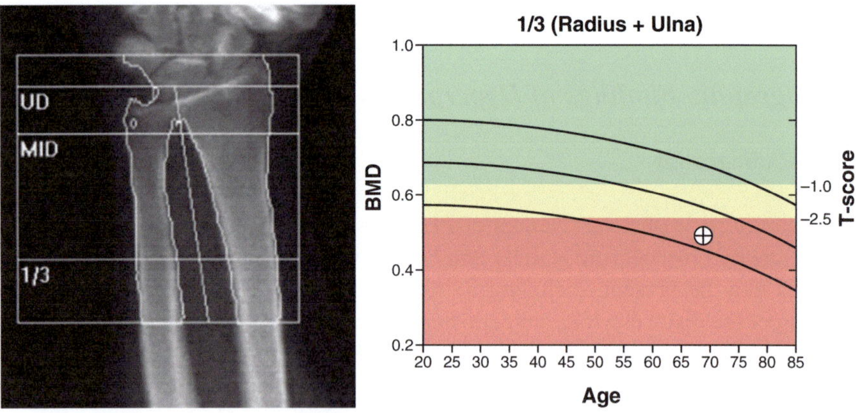

Fig. 2.2 DEXA scan in a 68-year-old female with primary hyperparathyroidism. Total T-score for the radius was −3.2 (indicated by the crosshair symbol in the graph) consistent with osteoporosis. (Image courtesy of Edgar Zamora, MD, Montefiore Medical Center, Bronx, NY)

cause osteitis fibrosa cystica, bone mineral density is often extremely low. In one case series of these patients, the mean T-scores by DEXA were −4.42 in the lumbar spine, −5.58 in the femoral neck, and −5.85 in the distal 1/3 radius [65].

Vertebral Fracture Assessment by DEXA

Vertebral fracture assessment (VFA) can be performed in patients undergoing DEXA at a fraction of the radiation dose of conventional radiography. VFA is indicated either in patients with a DEXA T-score of < -1.0 and one or more of the following conditions: (1) women $\geq$ age 70 or men $\geq$ age 80 years, (2) historical height loss greater than 4 cm, (3) self-reported but undocumented prior vertebral fracture, and (4) glucocorticoid therapy equivalent to ≥ 5 mg of prednisone or equivalent per day for 3 months or longer [109]. The spatial resolution of DEXA is much lower than that of plain radiography, and therefore, its utility for diagnosing mild vertebral fractures is limited [110]. Additionally, patients with multiple fractures are more easily identified than those with a single fracture [111]. In a systematic review, the sensitivity and specificity of VFA by DEXA on a per-vertebra basis ranged from 70% to 93% and from 96% to 100%, respectively [112].

Trabecular Bone Score by DEXA

One limitation of DEXA is the lack of information on bone microstructure, which is an essential determinant of bone strength. There is a significant overlap in density values between patients with and without fractures, and values in patients with degenerative sclerosis may be artifactually increased [110]. Trabecular bone score (TBS) is a post-processing technique based on textural analysis of grayscale pixel variations that can be applied to DEXA scans, providing a complementary measure of bone microarchitecture and strength. In essence, lower TBS values are associated with decreased bone strength, and differences are detectable in vertebral bodies that have similar densitometry values [113]. One large cohort study demonstrated that TBS values were not significantly affected by degenerative osteoarthrosis, as opposed to DEXA, where they may be artifactually increased [114]. In patients with PHPT, one study has correlated TBS values with parameters obtained from high-resolution peripheral quantitative CT (HRpQCT), where the authors found a positive association with volumetric density, cortical thickness, whole bone stiffness, trabecular number, and trabecular separation [115].

High-Resolution Peripheral Quantitative CT

HRpQCT is a three-dimensional imaging modality that permits noninvasive assessment of cortical and trabecular microarchitecture as well as volumetric mineral bone density of the distal radius and tibia [24, 116]. HRpQCT allows imaging of the appendicular skeleton but not the spine. This modality has a lower radiation dose than a traditional DEXA scan and can achieve spatial resolutions in the order of 130 to 160 µm (higher near the center of the field of view) [117–119]. Various morphometric measurements can be generated, including cortical thickness, trabecular number, trabecular separation, and cortical porosity [120]. These have been validated in several studies and highly correlated with metrics derived from µCT, a technique that can achieve higher spatial resolution but generally applied to ex vivo tissues [121–123]. One study using HRpQCT in postmenopausal women with PHPT showed decreased volumetric densities in trabecular and cortical bone of tibia and radius, with increased trabecular spacing and thinner cortices. Such changes were more profound in the radius [124]. In a separate study, PHPT resulted in abnormal cortical bone geometry and trabecular and cortical microarchitecture, as well as decreased volumetric density in the radius but not tibia [125]. Women with PHPT had improved cortical bone geometry and cortical and trabecular microarchitecture in both radius and tibia, as well as improvement in cancellous bone architecture 1 year following parathyroidectomy [126]. One limitation of HRpQCT is that the technique is susceptible to motion artifact and a typical scan takes approximately 3 min to complete [118]. The motion artifacts can confound the reproducibility and accuracy of morphometric measurements [127]. Although the use of HRpQCT is rapidly expanding in research settings, its use currently remains limited in clinical practice.

Gland Localization

Parathyroid Ultrasound

Neck ultrasound has become an important part of many endocrine and endocrine surgery practices. The use of point-of-care neck ultrasound in identifying parathyroid adenomas has enabled minimally invasive surgery as an outpatient procedure, which has shortened hospitalization and recovery times [128]. Neck ultrasound is an inexpensive and noninvasive approach to localizing a parathyroid adenoma, though the quality is operator-dependent.

Proper positioning is important for a neck ultrasound. The patient should lie on a firm table with pillows placed under the upper torso and shoulders to allow for full extension of the neck [14]. Patients with cervical spine diseases may not be able to fully extend their neck, which will impede the study [14]. A 3–5 cm linear 5–15 MHz multifrequency transducer should be applied to the anterior neck with ultrasound gel. Higher-frequency settings allow for finer discrimination, but higher frequencies attenuate more quickly. Lower-frequency settings are more effective at visualizing the deeper portions of the neck. The posterior margins of the thyroid capsule should be inspected first to identify lesions that could be consistent with an enlarged parathyroid gland. Parathyroid adenomas are inherently mobile, so it may be necessary to ask the patient to cough, Valsalva, swallow, take deep breaths, or turn their head from side to side to visualize the adenoma [14].

Due to their small size, normal parathyroid glands cannot usually be seen with current ultrasound equipment [14]. However, parathyroid adenomas may appear as a homogenous, hypoechoic, and hypervascular mass separate from and posterior to the thyroid on ultrasound [129]. Most parathyroid adenomas are located outside the posterior capsule of the thyroid gland [16, 17, 130]. The lesion lacks the echogenic fatty hilum that is typically seen in lymph nodes. A lesion along the posterior aspect of the thyroid gland in the context of hypercalcemia is likely a parathyroid adenoma. It is common to see the "the indentation sign" – an indentation made by the parathyroid adenoma on the posterior side of the thyroid gland [14]. There is usually an echogenic line of separation between the thyroid and the parathyroid gland, representing the fibro-fatty capsule. When seen on ultrasound, the parathyroid glands typically have variable shapes, allowing them to conform to the available space. In about 2–5% of cases, the parathyroid adenoma may be embedded in the thyroid gland, where it has the same appearance as a thyroid nodule [131]. The incidence of a parathyroid gland embedded in the thyroid may be as high as 15% in the setting of four gland hyperplasia [132]. The presence of a polar artery feeding a parathyroid adenoma can aid in detection and has been found in more than 80% of adenomas [133]. A "vascular arc" leading to the adenoma and diffuse blood flow within the adenoma have also been described [134].

In one surgical series, the sensitivity of high-resolution ultrasound for all patients with hyperparathyroidism was 57% [135]. In patients with primary hyperparathyroidism, the sensitivity of ultrasound for parathyroid localization was 66%. Specificity for parathyroid localization was 98% for all patients and was 98% and 100% for patients with primary and secondary or tertiary hyperparathyroidism, respectively [135]. In a meta-analysis, ultrasound had a sensitivity of 76.1% and a positive predictive value of 93.2% in localizing parathyroid adenomas [136]. The adenoma is unable to be visualized in about 10–20% of patients. This is usually due to posteriorly located glands, retropharyngeal superior adenomas, intrathoracic adenomas, or four gland hyperplasia [14].

SPECT-CT

In the 1990s, the chance observation that parathyroid tumors accumulate technetium 99m sestamibi due to richness in mitochondria led to the concept of presurgical localization of parathyroid adenomas and minimally invasive surgery [137]. Sestamibi imaging is most commonly used to localize a hyperfunctioning gland, either in the thyroid bed or in an ectopic location such as the neck or lower mediastinum. The most frequently used radiopharmaceutical is technetium 99m sestamibi (Cardiolite). It is a lipophilic isonitrile cation retained in the mitochondria of parathyroid adenomas due to their cellularity and vascularity. It is also used for cardiac stress tests [1]. The tracer is injected, and the patient imaged sequentially, first at 10–15 min and then at 1–3 h, normal thyroid tissue, and thyroid adenomas will be bright on early images and usually fade over 2 h, whereas parathyroid adenomas remain avid over time (Fig. 2.3). Atypical thyroid adenomas do not wash out and

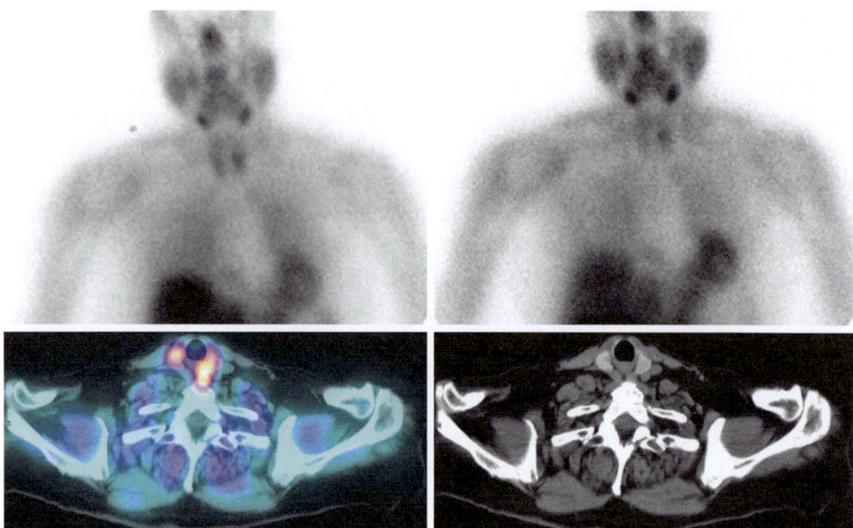

Fig. 2.3 Left superior parathyroid adenoma shows uptake which does not wash out (unlike thyroid uptake) and corresponds to soft tissue lesion posterior to thyroid on left. Persistent uptake is seen to a lesser degree in hypodense thyroid lesion on the right, possibly a thyroid adenoma

may produce a false positive result; more rarely, thyroid and parathyroid carcinomas may do so as well (though arguably a parathyroid carcinoma would be a true positive) [2]. Occasionally, the parathyroid adenoma may wash out on delayed images but is visible on early images [1].

Sensitivity is as high as 90% in solitary parathyroid adenomas, particularly if over 300–500 mg, but lower (50–60%) with multiple adenomas [1, 2]. Overall sensitivity is about 83%, similar to ultrasound (80%), although specificity is higher (87% versus 77%) [138]; the techniques are most useful in combination [139]. Patients who have normal vitamin D levels are more likely to have a scan successfully localizing the adenoma [58]. Patients with positive SPECT and negative ultrasound findings are more likely to have posteriorly located upper gland adenomas [140].

Planar gamma camera images showing a large field of view to find ectopic adenomas are often combined with SPECT or SPECT-CT, either for the early or delayed phases [2]. SPECT (with or without CT) is a technique where the camera slowly rotates around the patient and produces a three-dimensional image. It can be invaluable in localization but requires the patient to be able to hold still for 30–45 min.

Some centers use a subtraction technique where iodine-123 or Tc-99m pertechnetate images are obtained shortly after sestamibi injection and digitally subtracted; this can help differentiate parathyroid adenomas from thyroid adenomas (which will take up iodine) but can produce imaging artifacts due to patient movement and misalignment [1, 2].

In addition to presurgical imaging, the patient may be injected 2–4 h before surgery, and a small gamma probe is used intraoperatively to find the adenoma by the surgeon. This procedure is usually used if there is a solitary parathyroid adenoma and no thyroid adenoma; after removal, the parathyroid adenoma should be 20% higher than background thyroid activity [2].

There has been interest in tracers for positron emission tomography (PET) in recent years, (which has higher spatial resolution and often sensitivity), using choline, which is taken up more in highly proliferating cells. Recent meta-analyses showed a detection rate of 91–97% per patient and sensitivity 95% [141, 142], with choline tracers performing better than sestamibi everywhere they were compared, but the studies were heterogeneous with a lack of prospective trials or consistently applied reference standards [142]. At present, no choline tracer is FDA-approved for hyperparathyroidism.

4D Neck CT

Multiphasic CT of the neck has been increasingly used to detect and localize parathyroid adenomas within a given quadrant. It provides great anatomic detail and allows identification of adenomas both in eutopic and ectopic locations, as well as differentiation from mimics such as lymph nodes, thyroid nodules, and exophytic thyroid tissue. This technique is most widely used as a second-line investigation or in patients undergoing repeat surgery [143]. In one large study, 4D CT had an overall sensitivity of 79% compared with 58% for SPECT-CT. In a subset of patients with the single-gland disease, sensitivity was 93% for 4D CT compared with 75% for SPECT-CT [144].

The protocol typically includes a non-contrast scan followed by arterial and venous phases obtained 25 and 80 s after injection, respectively, acquired axially and reconstructed in sagittal and coronal planes (i.e., three dimensions) [143]. The "4D" designation refers to the dynamic perfusion information derived from the scan. The contrast-enhanced phases should cover from the angle of the mandible through the carina to allow detection of ectopic adenomas. The main disadvantage of 4D CT relative to SPECT-CT is its higher radiation dose. On 4D CT, the majority of adenomas demonstrate avid contrast enhancement on the arterial phase and rapid washout of contrast material (i.e., lower attenuation) on the venous phase (Fig. 2.4). Because of this washout, most parathyroid adenomas demonstrate lower attenuation than thyroid tissue or lymph nodes on the venous phase. However, approximately 22% of adenomas do not follow this pattern and may only be identified on the non-contrast scan, where they show low attenuation as opposed to the high-attenuating thyroid parenchyma [145]. A polar vessel sign is a characteristic finding that is present in about two-thirds of parathyroid adenomas, particularly those with more avid enhancement in the arterial phase [146].

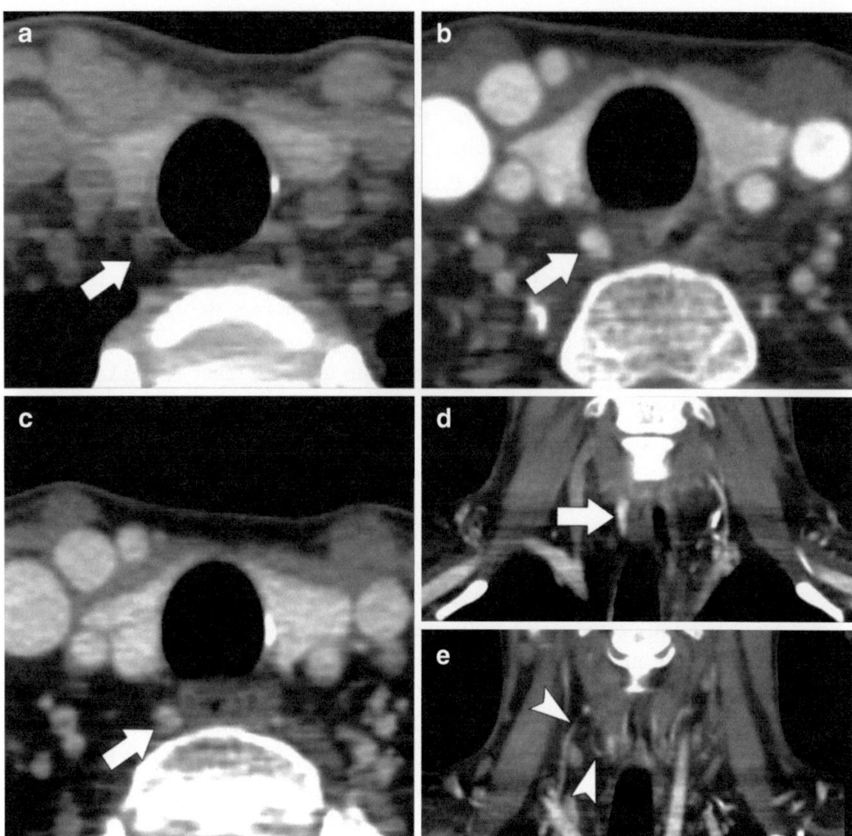

Fig. 2.4 4D CT in a 51-year-old female with PHPT and a parathyroid adenoma posterior to the right thyroid. Axial non-contrast CT (**a**) shows the adenoma (arrow) to have lower attenuation than the adjacent thyroid gland. Post-contrast CT 25 s (**b**) and 80 s (**c**) after the intravenous injection of iodinated contrast material show avid enhancement and rapid washout, respectively (arrows). Coronal CT reformats 25 s after injection (**d**) and (**e**) show that the adenoma has an ovoid shape (arrow in **d**) and a polar vessel (arrowheads in **e**)

Magnetic Resonance Imaging

Magnetic resonance imaging (MRI) does not play a major role in the workup of parathyroid adenomas in most clinical situations. The main advantage of MRI over CT and ultrasound is its higher soft tissue contrast, which generally allows better discrimination between tissues. Additionally, MRI does not require ionizing radiation. The major drawbacks are longer acquisition times and lower spatial resolution relative to CT and ultrasound. Parathyroid adenomas are typically hypointense on T1- and hyperintense on T2-weighted sequences [147, 148]. The addition of fat suppression techniques is crucial for both T2- and post-contrast T1-weighted sequences in order to discriminate the lesion from surrounding tissues because fat is intrinsically hyperintense. Similar to CT, parathyroid adenomas show avid enhancement on MRI following the intravenous administration of contrast material. In one study of 98 patients with surgical and pathological correlation, MRI had a sensitivity of 82% and a positive predictive value of 89% for detection parathyroid adenoma compared with a sensitivity of 85% and positive predictive value of 89% for technetium 99 m sestamibi scintigraphy [147]. One retrospective study using a dynamic contrast MRI technique in 30 patients with surgically proven parathyroid adenomas found a sensitivity/specificity of 88/90% and 91/95% for differentiating adenomas from lymph nodes and thyroid tissue, respectively [145].

Indications for Procedural Intervention (Surgery or Ablation)

Surgical management is recommended for any patient with symptomatic PHPT. Events that should prompt surgical referral include the occurrence of a fragility fracture and a kidney stone.

The Fourth International Workshop on PHPT identified several indications for parathyroidectomy in PHPT [6]. These recommendations are summarized in Table 2.2, and surgery should be recommended if one or more of the criteria are met. Surgery is recommended when serum calcium is >1 mg/dL (or 025 mM/L) above the upper limit of normal [6]. Decreased bone mineral density is a significant concern in patients with PHPT, both at diagnosis and as patients are being monitored. T-scores are used to assess bone mineral density for peri- and postmenopausal

Table 2.2 Indications for surgical management of asymptomatic primary hyperparathyroidism from the Fourth International Workshop [6]

Serum calcium	1.0 mg/dL (0.25 mmol/L) above the upper limit of normal
DEXA with T-score[a] < −2.5 at	Lumbar spine
	Total hip
	Femoral neck
	Distal 1/3 radius
Vertebral fracture by	X-ray
	CT
	MRI
	VFA
Renal	Creatinine clearance less than 60 ml/min
	24-hour urine calcium>400 mg/day (10 mmol/day) and increased stone risk by biochemical stone risk analysis
	Presence of nephrolithiasis or nephrocalcinosis by X-ray, ultrasound, or CT
Age	Less than 50 years

[a]T-score should be used in peri- or postmenopausal women and for men age 50 or older. In premenopausal women and men under age 50, then Z-score of <−2.5 is the recommended cut point at which surgery should be considered [107]

women and men over the age of 50. A T-score of -2.5 or less at the lumbar spine, femoral neck, total hip, or distal 1/3 radius is an indication for surgery. The International Society of Clinical Densitometry (ISCD) recommends the use of Z-scores instead of T-scores to assess the BMD of premenopausal women and men under the age of 50 [107]. Patients in this age group with Z-score of -2.5 or less are surgical candidates, although diagnosis of primary hyperparathyroidism under the age of 50 years is a surgical indication [6].

The workshop recognizes that the effects of elevated PTH may impact the proclivity for fracture in ways that cannot be predicted by DEXA alone. Clinicians may use TBS or HRpQCT to support a recommendation for surgery. If a vertebral fracture is present X-ray or VFA, then surgery is recommended.

Renal indications for parathyroidectomy include a decline in creatinine clearance to less than 60 ml/min. In clinical practice, this criterion is typically interpreted in the context of a patient's other comorbidities. For example, if a person has long-standing uncontrolled hypertension or diabetes, this may be a better explanation for the decline in renal function, and the elevated calcium and/or PTH may reflect SHPT or THPT instead of PHPT.

Patients should be evaluated for nephrolithiasis or nephrocalcinosis with renal imaging, which may include X-ray, ultrasound, or CT scan. If nephrolithiasis or nephrocalcinosis is seen, then surgery should be recommended. If the patient demonstrates marked hypercalciuria with more than 400 mg/day of urinary calcium, then a complete urinary biochemical stone profile should be considered. If the urinary biochemical stone profile indicates an increased risk of stone formation, then a criterion for surgery is met.

Conclusions

The parathyroid glands are an important part of the feedback system that regulates serum calcium and phosphorus levels, both of which control many biological processes. The parathyroid glands may become autonomously overactive, resulting in hypercalcemia. PTH may also be appropriately elevated due to other causes, such as renal dysfunction, hypocalcemia, vitamin D deficiency, and hyperphosphatemia. PHPT is the most common cause of hypercalcemia in the outpatient setting, typically occurring in asymptomatic patients. PHPT may be due to a single parathyroid adenoma, multiple parathyroid adenomas, multiple parathyroid adenomas, four-gland hyperplasia, and very rarely parathyroid carcinoma or ectopic PTH secretion. Hyperparathyroidism may occur as part of genetic syndromes, which may cause the involvement of more than one gland. Hyperparathyroidism may decrease bone mineral density and cause nephrolithiasis, and if there is evidence of end organ damage, localization of the offending gland and surgical removal are typically indicated. Imaging studies help localize a parathyroid adenoma, guide surgery, and lead to advancements in minimally invasive resection. Parathyroid ultrasound and SPECT CT are the most commonly used methods to identify an enlarged parathyroid gland, but 4D neck CT is a promising technique being used with increased frequency.

Acknowledgments Paul Guido, MD – Division of Endocrinology and Metabolism, Department of Internal Medicine, University of North Carolina at Chapel Hill, Chapel Hill, North Carolina, USA.

Nitya Kumar, MD – Division of Endocrinology and Metabolism, Department of Internal Medicine, Duke University, Durham, North Carolina, USA.

References

1. Ziessman H. Endocrine system. Nuclear medicine: the requisites. 4th ed. Philadelphia: Elsevier Mosby; 2015. p. 66–97.
2. Mettler F, Guiberteau M. Essentials of nuclear medicine and molecular imaging. Elsevier; 2019. p. 85–115.
3. Kumar V, Abbas AK, Aster JC. Robbins and Cotran pathologic basis of disease. 9th ed. Philadelphia: Elsevier/Saunders; 2015. p 1126–9.
4. Brewer K, Costa-Guda J, Arnold A. Molecular genetic insights into sporadic primary hyperparathyroidism. Endocr Relat Cancer. 2019;26(2):R53–72.
5. Arnold A, Staunton CE, Kim HG, Gaz RD, Kronenberg HM. Monoclonality and abnormal parathyroid hormone genes in parathyroid adenomas. N Engl J Med. 1988;318(11):658–62.
6. Bilezikian JP, Brandi ML, Eastell R, Silverberg SJ, Udelsman R, Marcocci C, et al. Guidelines for the management of asymptomatic primary hyperparathyroidism: summary statement from the Fourth International Workshop. J Clin Endocrinol Metab. 2014;99(10):3561–9.
7. Eastell R, Brandi ML, Costa AG, D'Amour P, Shoback DM, Thakker RV. Diagnosis of asymptomatic primary hyperparathyroidism: proceedings of the Fourth International Workshop. J Clin Endocrinol Metab. 2014;99(10):3570–9.
8. Shepard MM, Smith JW 3rd. Hypercalcemia. Am J Med Sci. 2007;334(5):381–5.
9. Yu N, Donnan PT, Murphy MJ, Leese GP. Epidemiology of primary hyperparathyroidism in Tayside, Scotland, UK. Clin Endocrinol. 2009;71(4):485–93.
10. Yeh MW, Ituarte PH, Zhou HC, Nishimoto S, Liu IL, Harari A, et al. Incidence and prevalence of primary hyperparathyroidism in a racially mixed population. J Clin Endocrinol Metab. 2013;98(3):1122–9.
11. Silverberg SJ, Shane E, Jacobs TP, Siris E, Bilezikian JP. A 10-year prospective study of primary hyperparathyroidism with or without parathyroid surgery. N Engl J Med. 1999;341(17):1249–55.
12. Melmed S, Auchus RJ, Goldfine AB, Koenig RJ, Rosen CJ. Williams textbook of endocrinology. 14th ed. Philadelphia: Elsevier, Inc; 2019. p 1331.
13. Bandeira FA, Oliveira RI, Griz LH, Caldas G, Bandeira C. Differences in accuracy of 99mTc-sestamibi scanning between severe and mild forms of primary hyperparathyroidism. J Nucl Med Technol. 2008;36(1):30–5.
14. Abraham D. Ultrasonography of the parathyroid glands. In: Duick D, Levine R, Lupo M, editors. Thyroid and parathyroid ultrasound and ultrasound-guided FNA. Cham: Springer Nature; 2018. p. 263–8.
15. Moore KL, Agur AMR, Dalley AF. Essential clinical anatomy. 4th ed. Baltimore: Lippincott Williams & Wilkins; 2011. p 620–1.
16. Lappas D, Noussios G, Anagnostis P, Adamidou F, Chatzigeorgiou A, Skandalakis P. Location, number and morphology of parathyroid glands: results from a large anatomical series. Anat Sci Int. 2012;87(3):160–4.

17. Schneider R, Waldmann J, Ramaswamy A, Fernandez ED, Bartsch DK, Schlosser K. Frequency of ectopic and supernumerary intrathymic parathyroid glands in patients with renal hyperparathyroidism: analysis of 461 patients undergoing initial parathyroidectomy with bilateral cervical thymectomy. World J Surg. 2011;35(6):1260–5.
18. Brown EM. Role of the calcium-sensing receptor in extracellular calcium homeostasis. Best Pract Res Clin Endocrinol Metab. 2013;27(3):333–43.
19. Wang Q, Palnitkar S, Parfitt AM. The basal rate of cell proliferation in normal human parathyroid tissue: implications for the pathogenesis of hyperparathyroidism. Clin Endocrinol. 1997;46(3):343–9.
20. Eastell R, Arnold A, Brandi ML, Brown EM, D'Amour P, Hanley DA, et al. Diagnosis of asymptomatic primary hyperparathyroidism: proceedings of the third international workshop. J Clin Endocrinol Metab. 2009;94(2):340–50.
21. Friedman PA, Gesek FA. Calcium transport in renal epithelial cells. Am J Phys. 1993;264(2 Pt 2):F181–98.
22. Jamal SA, Miller PD. Secondary and tertiary hyperparathyroidism. J Clin Densitom. 2013;16(1):64–8.
23. Albright F, Aub JC, Bauer W. Hyperparathyroidism: a common and polymorphic condition as illustrated by seventeen proved cases from one clinic. JAMA. 1934;102:1276–87.
24. Bandeira F, Cusano NE, Silva BC, Cassibba S, Almeida CB, Machado VC, et al. Bone disease in primary hyperparathyroidism. Arq Bras Endocrinol Metabol. 2014;58(5):553–61.
25. Turken SA, Cafferty M, Silverberg SJ, De La Cruz L, Cimino C, Lange DJ, et al. Neuromuscular involvement in mild, asymptomatic primary hyperparathyroidism. Am J Med. 1989;87(5):553–7.
26. Adami S, Marcocci C, Gatti D. Epidemiology of primary hyperparathyroidism in Europe. J Bone Miner Res. 2002;17(Suppl 2):N18–23.
27. Silverberg SJ. Vitamin D deficiency and primary hyperparathyroidism. J Bone Miner Res. 2007;22(Suppl 2):V100–4.
28. Bushinsky DA, Monk RD. Electrolyte quintet: calcium. Lancet. 1998;352(9124):306–11.
29. Sociedade Brasileira de Endocrinologia e M, Bandeira F, Griz L, Chaves N, Carvalho NC, Borges LM, et al. Diagnosis and management of primary hyperparathyroidism--a scientific statement from the Department of Bone Metabolism, the Brazilian Society for Endocrinology and Metabolism. Arq Bras Endocrinol Metabol. 2013;57(6):406–24.
30. Wermers RA, Khosla S, Atkinson EJ, Hodgson SF, O'Fallon WM, Melton LJ 3rd. The rise and fall of primary hyperparathyroidism: a population-based study in Rochester, Minnesota, 1965-1992. Ann Intern Med. 1997;126(6):433–40.
31. Silverberg SJ, Clarke BL, Peacock M, Bandeira F, Boutroy S, Cusano NE, et al. Current issues in the presentation of asymptomatic primary hyperparathyroidism: proceedings of the Fourth International Workshop. J Clin Endocrinol Metab. 2014;99(10):3580–94.
32. Rubin MR, Bilezikian JP, McMahon DJ, Jacobs T, Shane E, Siris E, et al. The natural history of primary hyperparathyroidism with or without parathyroid surgery after 15 years. J Clin Endocrinol Metab. 2008;93(9):3462–70.
33. Khosla S, Melton LJ 3rd, Wermers RA, Crowson CS, O'Fallon W, Riggs B. Primary hyperparathyroidism and the risk of fracture: a population-based study. J Bone Miner Res. 1999;14(10):1700–7.
34. Walgenbach S, Hommel G, Junginger T. Outcome after surgery for primary hyperparathyroidism: ten-year prospective follow-up study. World J Surg. 2000;24(5):564–9; discussion 9–70
35. Rao DS, Phillips ER, Divine GW, Talpos GB. Randomized controlled clinical trial of surgery versus no surgery in patients with mild asymptomatic primary hyperparathyroidism. J Clin Endocrinol Metab. 2004;89(11):5415–22.
36. Ambrogini E, Cetani F, Cianferotti L, Vignali E, Banti C, Viccica G, et al. Surgery or surveillance for mild asymptomatic primary hyperparathyroidism: a prospective, randomized clinical trial. J Clin Endocrinol Metab. 2007;92(8):3114–21.

37. Bollerslev J, Jansson S, Mollerup CL, Nordenstrom J, Lundgren E, Torring O, et al. Medical observation, compared with parathyroidectomy, for asymptomatic primary hyperparathyroidism: a prospective, randomized trial. J Clin Endocrinol Metab. 2007;92(5):1687–92.
38. Cheng SP, Lee JJ, Liu TP, Yang PS, Liu SC, Hsu YC, et al. Quality of life after surgery or surveillance for asymptomatic primary hyperparathyroidism: a meta-analysis of randomized controlled trials. Medicine (Baltimore). 2015;94(23):e931.
39. Cusano NE, Silverberg SJ, Bilezikian JP. Normocalcemic primary hyperparathyroidism. J Clin Densitom. 2013;16(1):33–9.
40. Lowe H, McMahon DJ, Rubin MR, Bilezikian JP, Silverberg SJ. Normocalcemic primary hyperparathyroidism: further characterization of a new clinical phenotype. J Clin Endocrinol Metab. 2007;92(8):3001–5.
41. Bilezikian JP, Bandeira L, Khan A, Cusano NE. Hyperparathyroidism. Lancet. 2018;391(10116):168–78.
42. Tee MC, Holmes DT, Wiseman SM. Ionized vs serum calcium in the diagnosis and management of primary hyperparathyroidism: which is superior? Am J Surg. 2013;205(5):591–6; discussion 6
43. Ong GS, Walsh JP, Stuckey BG, Brown SJ, Rossi E, Ng JL, et al. The importance of measuring ionized calcium in characterizing calcium status and diagnosing primary hyperparathyroidism. J Clin Endocrinol Metab. 2012;97(9):3138–45.
44. Calvi LM, Bushinsky DA. When is it appropriate to order an ionized calcium? J Am Soc Nephrol. 2008;19(7):1257–60.
45. Berson SA, Yalow RS, Aurbach GD, Potts JT. Immunoassay of bovine and human parathyroid hormone. Proc Natl Acad Sci U S A. 1963;49(5):613–7.
46. Gao P, D'Amour P. Evolution of the parathyroid hormone (PTH) assay--importance of circulating PTH immunoheterogeneity and of its regulation. Clin Lab. 2005;51(1–2):21–9.
47. Ekins R. More sensitive immunoassays. Nature. 1980;284(5751):14–5.
48. Aloia JF, Feuerman M, Yeh JK. Reference range for serum parathyroid hormone. Endocr Pract. 2006;12(2):137–44.
49. Ross AC, Manson JE, Abrams SA, Aloia JF, Brannon PM, Clinton SK, et al. The 2011 report on dietary reference intakes for calcium and vitamin D from the Institute of Medicine: what clinicians need to know. J Clin Endocrinol Metab. 2011;96(1):53–8.
50. Medicine Io. Dietary reference intakes for calcium and vitamin D. Washington, DC: The National Academies Press; 2011.
51. Holick MF, Binkley NC, Bischoff-Ferrari HA, Gordon CM, Hanley DA, Heaney RP, et al. Evaluation, treatment, and prevention of vitamin D deficiency: an Endocrine Society clinical practice guideline. J Clin Endocrinol Metab. 2011;96(7):1911–30.
52. Wallace LB, Parikh RT, Ross LV, Mazzaglia PJ, Foley C, Shin JJ, et al. The phenotype of primary hyperparathyroidism with normal parathyroid hormone levels: how low can parathyroid hormone go? Surgery. 2011;150(6):1102–12.
53. Al-Azem H, Khan A. Primary hyperparathyroidism. CMAJ. 2011;183(10):E685–9.
54. Priya G, Jyotsna VP, Gupta N, Chumber S, Bal CS, Karak AK, et al. Clinical and laboratory profile of primary hyperparathyroidism in India. Postgrad Med J. 2008;84(987):34–9.
55. Boudou P, Ibrahim F, Cormier C, Sarfati E, Souberbielle JC. A very high incidence of low 25 hydroxy-vitamin D serum concentration in a French population of patients with primary hyperparathyroidism. J Endocrinol Investig. 2006;29(6):511–5.
56. Bollerslev J, Marcocci C, Sosa M, Nordenstrom J, Bouillon R, Mosekilde L. Current evidence for recommendation of surgery, medical treatment and vitamin D repletion in mild primary hyperparathyroidism. Eur J Endocrinol. 2011;165(6):851–64.
57. Amstrup AK, Rejnmark L, Vestergaard P, Sikjaer T, Rolighed L, Heickendorff L, et al. Vitamin D status, physical performance and body mass in patients surgically cured for primary hyperparathyroidism compared with healthy controls - a cross-sectional study. Clin Endocrinol. 2011;74(1):130–6.

58. Kandil E, Tufaro AP, Carson KA, Lin F, Somervell H, Farrag T, et al. Correlation of plasma 25-hydroxyvitamin D levels with severity of primary hyperparathyroidism and likelihood of parathyroid adenoma localization on sestamibi scan. Arch Otolaryngol Head Neck Surg. 2008;134(10):1071–5.
59. Grey A, Lucas J, Horne A, Gamble G, Davidson JS, Reid IR. Vitamin D repletion in patients with primary hyperparathyroidism and coexistent vitamin D insufficiency. J Clin Endocrinol Metab. 2005;90(4):2122–6.
60. Walker MD, Cong E, Lee JA, Kepley A, Zhang C, McMahon DJ, et al. Vitamin D in primary hyperparathyroidism: effects on clinical, biochemical, and densitometric presentation. J Clin Endocrinol Metab. 2015;100(9):3443–51.
61. Fillee C, Keller T, Mourad M, Brinkmann T, Ketelslegers JM. Impact of vitamin D-related serum PTH reference values on the diagnosis of mild primary hyperparathyroidism, using bivariate calcium/PTH reference regions. Clin Endocrinol. 2012;76(6):785–9.
62. Brasier AR, Nussbaum SR. Hungry bone syndrome: clinical and biochemical predictors of its occurrence after parathyroid surgery. Am J Med. 1988;84(4):654–60.
63. Corder CJ, Leslie SW. 24-hour urine collection. Treasure Island: StatPearls; 2020.
64. Corbetta S, Baccarelli A, Aroldi A, Vicentini L, Fogazzi GB, Eller-Vainicher C, et al. Risk factors associated to kidney stones in primary hyperparathyroidism. J Endocrinol Investig. 2005;28(2):122–8.
65. Franca TC, Griz L, Pinho J, Diniz ET, Andrade LD, Lucena CS, et al. Bisphosphonates can reduce bone hunger after parathyroidectomy in patients with primary hyperparathyroidism and osteitis fibrosa cystica. Rev Bras Reumatol. 2011;51(2):131–7.
66. Costa AG, Bilezikian JP. Bone turnover markers in primary hyperparathyroidism. J Clin Densitom. 2013;16(1):22–7.
67. Moosgaard B, Christensen SE, Vestergaard P, Heickendorff L, Christiansen P, Mosekilde L. Vitamin D metabolites and skeletal consequences in primary hyperparathyroidism. Clin Endocrinol. 2008;68(5):707–15.
68. Coe FL, Canterbury JM, Firpo JJ, Reiss E. Evidence for secondary hyperparathyroidism in idiopathic hypercalciuria. J Clin Invest. 1973;52(1):134–42.
69. Balsa JA, Botella-Carretero JI, Peromingo R, Zamarron I, Arrieta F, Munoz-Malo T, et al. Role of calcium malabsorption in the development of secondary hyperparathyroidism after biliopancreatic diversion. J Endocrinol Investig. 2008;31(10):845–50.
70. Selby PL, Davies M, Adams JE, Mawer EB. Bone loss in celiac disease is related to secondary hyperparathyroidism. J Bone Miner Res. 1999;14(4):652–7.
71. Vasikaran SD. Bisphosphonates: an overview with special reference to alendronate. Ann Clin Biochem. 2001;38(Pt 6):608–23.
72. Makras P, Polyzos SA, Papatheodorou A, Kokkoris P, Chatzifotiadis D, Anastasilakis AD. Parathyroid hormone changes following denosumab treatment in postmenopausal osteoporosis. Clin Endocrinol. 2013;79(4):499–503.
73. Mallette LE, Eichhorn E. Effects of lithium carbonate on human calcium metabolism. Arch Intern Med. 1986;146(4):770–6.
74. Grieff M, Bushinsky DA. Diuretics and disorders of calcium homeostasis. Semin Nephrol. 2011;31(6):535–41.
75. Griebeler ML, Kearns AE, Ryu E, Thapa P, Hathcock MA, Melton LJ 3rd, et al. Thiazide-associated hypercalcemia: incidence and association with primary hyperparathyroidism over two decades. J Clin Endocrinol Metab. 2016;101(3):1166–73.
76. Brown EM, Hebert SC. A cloned Ca(2+)-sensing receptor: a mediator of direct effects of extracellular Ca2+ on renal function? J Am Soc Nephrol. 1995;6(6):1530–40.
77. Sato K, Obara T, Yamazaki K, Kanbe M, Nakajima K, Yamada A, et al. Somatic mutations of the MEN1 gene and microsatellite instability in a case of tertiary hyperparathyroidism occurring during high phosphate therapy for acquired, hypophosphatemic osteomalacia. J Clin Endocrinol Metab. 2001;86(11):5564–71.

78. Rivkees SA, el-Hajj-Fuleihan G, Brown EM, Crawford JD. Tertiary hyperparathyroidism during high phosphate therapy of familial hypophosphatemic rickets. J Clin Endocrinol Metab. 1992;75(6):1514–8.
79. Knudtzon J, Halse J, Monn E, Nesland A, Nordal KP, Paus P, et al. Autonomous hyperparathyroidism in X-linked hypophosphataemia. Clin Endocrinol. 1995;42(2):199–203.
80. Makitie O, Kooh SW, Sochett E. Prolonged high-dose phosphate treatment: a risk factor for tertiary hyperparathyroidism in X-linked hypophosphatemic rickets. Clin Endocrinol. 2003;58(2):163–8.
81. Huang QL, Feig DS, Blackstein ME. Development of tertiary hyperparathyroidism after phosphate supplementation in oncogenic osteomalacia. J Endocrinol Investig. 2000;23(4):263–7.
82. Gilat H, Feinmesser R, Vinkler Y, Morgenstern S, Shvero J, Bachar G, et al. Clinical and operative management of persistent hyperparathyroidism after renal transplantation: a single-center experience. Head Neck. 2007;29(11):996–1001.
83. Hsieh TM, Sun CK, Chen YT, Chou FF. Total parathyroidectomy versus subtotal parathyroidectomy in the treatment of tertiary hyperparathyroidism. Am Surg. 2012;78(5):600–6.
84. Eldeiry LS, Ruan DT, Brown EM, Gaglia JL, Garber JR. Primary hyperparathyroidism and familial hypocalciuric hypercalcemia: relationships and clinical implications. Endocr Pract. 2012;18(3):412–7.
85. Jayasena CN, Mahmud M, Palazzo F, Donaldson M, Meeran K, Dhillo WS. Utility of the urine calcium-to-creatinine ratio to diagnose primary hyperparathyroidism in asymptomatic hypercalcaemic patients with vitamin D deficiency. Ann Clin Biochem. 2011;48(Pt 2):126–9.
86. Taha W, Singh N, Flack JM, Abou-Samra AB. Low urine calcium excretion in African American patients with primary hyperparathyroidism. Endocr Pract. 2011;17(6):867–72.
87. Nesbit MA, Hannan FM, Howles SA, Babinsky VN, Head RA, Cranston T, et al. Mutations affecting G-protein subunit alpha11 in hypercalcemia and hypocalcemia. N Engl J Med. 2013;368(26):2476–86.
88. Hannan FM, Nesbit MA, Zhang C, Cranston T, Curley AJ, Harding B, et al. Identification of 70 calcium-sensing receptor mutations in hyper- and hypo-calcaemic patients: evidence for clustering of extracellular domain mutations at calcium-binding sites. Hum Mol Genet. 2012;21(12):2768–78.
89. Nesbit MA, Hannan FM, Howles SA, Reed AA, Cranston T, Thakker CE, et al. Mutations in AP2S1 cause familial hypocalciuric hypercalcemia type 3. Nat Genet. 2013;45(1):93–7.
90. Christensen SE, Nissen PH, Vestergaard P, Heickendorff L, Brixen K, Mosekilde L. Discriminative power of three indices of renal calcium excretion for the distinction between familial hypocalciuric hypercalcaemia and primary hyperparathyroidism: a follow-up study on methods. Clin Endocrinol. 2008;69(5):713–20.
91. Serra AL, Schwarz AA, Wick FH, Marti HP, Wuthrich RP. Successful treatment of hypercalcemia with cinacalcet in renal transplant recipients with persistent hyperparathyroidism. Nephrol Dial Transplant. 2005;20(7):1315–9.
92. Serra AL, Savoca R, Huber AR, Hepp U, Delsignore A, Hersberger M, et al. Effective control of persistent hyperparathyroidism with cinacalcet in renal allograft recipients. Nephrol Dial Transplant. 2007;22(2):577–83.
93. Kruse AE, Eisenberger U, Frey FJ, Mohaupt MG. The calcimimetic cinacalcet normalizes serum calcium in renal transplant patients with persistent hyperparathyroidism. Nephrol Dial Transplant. 2005;20(7):1311–4.
94. Pallais JC, Kemp EH, Bergwitz C, Kantham L, Slovik DM, Weetman AP, et al. Autoimmune hypocalciuric hypercalcemia unresponsive to glucocorticoid therapy in a patient with blocking autoantibodies against the calcium-sensing receptor. J Clin Endocrinol Metab. 2011;96(3):672–80.
95. Pallais JC, Kifor O, Chen YB, Slovik D, Brown EM. Acquired hypocalciuric hypercalcemia due to autoantibodies against the calcium-sensing receptor. N Engl J Med. 2004;351(4):362–9.

96. Kifor O, Moore FD Jr, Delaney M, Garber J, Hendy GN, Butters R, et al. A syndrome of hypocalciuric hypercalcemia caused by autoantibodies directed at the calcium-sensing receptor. J Clin Endocrinol Metab. 2003;88(1):60–72.
97. Mantovani G. Clinical review: Pseudohypoparathyroidism: diagnosis and treatment. J Clin Endocrinol Metab. 2011;96(10):3020–30.
98. Neary NM, El-Maouche D, Hopkins R, Libutti SK, Moses AM, Weinstein LS. Development and treatment of tertiary hyperparathyroidism in patients with pseudohypoparathyroidism type 1B. J Clin Endocrinol Metab. 2012;97(9):3025–30.
99. Thakker RV, Newey PJ, Walls GV, Bilezikian J, Dralle H, Ebeling PR, et al. Clinical practice guidelines for multiple endocrine neoplasia type 1 (MEN1). J Clin Endocrinol Metab. 2012;97(9):2990–3011.
100. Eller-Vainicher C, Chiodini I, Battista C, Viti R, Mascia ML, Massironi S, et al. Sporadic and MEN1-related primary hyperparathyroidism: differences in clinical expression and severity. J Bone Miner Res. 2009;24(8):1404–10.
101. Machens A, Schaaf L, Karges W, Frank-Raue K, Bartsch DK, Rothmund M, et al. Age-related penetrance of endocrine tumours in multiple endocrine neoplasia type 1 (MEN1): a multicentre study of 258 gene carriers. Clin Endocrinol. 2007;67(4):613–22.
102. El Lakis M, Nockel P, Gaitanidis A, Guan B, Agarwal S, Welch J, et al. Probability of positive genetic testing results in patients with family history of primary hyperparathyroidism. J Am Coll Surg. 2018;226(5):933–8.
103. Newey PJ, Nesbit MA, Rimmer AJ, Attar M, Head RT, Christie PT, et al. Whole-exome sequencing studies of nonhereditary (sporadic) parathyroid adenomas. J Clin Endocrinol Metab. 2012;97(10):E1995–2005.
104. Licata AA, Williams SE. A DXA primer for the practicing clinician: a case-based manual for understanding and interpreting bone densitometry. New York: Springer; 2014. xix, 167 pages p.
105. El Maghraoui A, Roux C. DXA scanning in clinical practice. QJM. 2008;101(8):605–17.
106. Lorente-Ramos R, Azpeitia-Arman J, Munoz-Hernandez A, Garcia-Gomez JM, Diez-Martinez P, Grande-Barez M. Dual-energy x-ray absorptiometry in the diagnosis of osteoporosis: a practical guide. AJR Am J Roentgenol. 2011;196(4):897–904.
107. Shuhart CR, Yeap SS, Anderson PA, Jankowski LG, Lewiecki EM, Morse LR, et al. Executive summary of the 2019 ISCD position development conference on monitoring treatment, DXA cross-calibration and least significant change, spinal cord injury, peri-prosthetic and orthopedic bone health, transgender medicine, and pediatrics. J Clin Densitom. 2019;22(4):453–71.
108. Silverberg SJ, Shane E, de la Cruz L, Dempster DW, Feldman F, Seldin D, et al. Skeletal disease in primary hyperparathyroidism. J Bone Miner Res. 1989;4(3):283–91.
109. Laster A. A basic primer on vertebral fracture assessment (VFA): the International Society for Clinical Densitometry; 2012. Available from: https://www.iscd.org/publications/osteoflash/a-basic-primer-on-vertebral-fracture-assessment-vfa/.
110. Lewiecki EM, Laster AJ. Clinical review: clinical applications of vertebral fracture assessment by dual-energy x-ray absorptiometry. J Clin Endocrinol Metab. 2006;91(11):4215–22.
111. Kaptoge S, Armbrecht G, Felsenberg D, Lunt M, O'Neill TW, Silman AJ, et al. When should the doctor order a spine X-ray? Identifying vertebral fractures for osteoporosis care: results from the European Prospective Osteoporosis Study (EPOS). J Bone Miner Res. 2004;19(12):1982–93.
112. Lee JH, Lee YK, Oh SH, Ahn J, Lee YE, Pyo JH, et al. A systematic review of diagnostic accuracy of vertebral fracture assessment (VFA) in postmenopausal women and elderly men. Osteoporos Int. 2016;27(5):1691–9.
113. Silva BC, Leslie WD, Resch H, Lamy O, Lesnyak O, Binkley N, et al. Trabecular bone score: a noninvasive analytical method based upon the DXA image. J Bone Miner Res. 2014;29(3):518–30.

114. Dufour R, Winzenrieth R, Heraud A, Hans D, Mehsen N. Generation and validation of a normative, age-specific reference curve for lumbar spine trabecular bone score (TBS) in French women. Osteoporos Int. 2013;24(11):2837–46.
115. Silva BC, Boutroy S, Zhang C, McMahon DJ, Zhou B, Wang J, et al. Trabecular bone score (TBS)--a novel method to evaluate bone microarchitectural texture in patients with primary hyperparathyroidism. J Clin Endocrinol Metab. 2013;98(5):1963–70.
116. Cheung AM, Adachi JD, Hanley DA, Kendler DL, Davison KS, Josse R, et al. High-resolution peripheral quantitative computed tomography for the assessment of bone strength and structure: a review by the Canadian Bone Strength Working Group. Curr Osteoporos Rep. 2013;11(2):136–46.
117. Burghardt AJ, Pialat JB, Kazakia GJ, Boutroy S, Engelke K, Patsch JM, et al. Multicenter precision of cortical and trabecular bone quality measures assessed by high-resolution peripheral quantitative computed tomography. J Bone Miner Res. 2013;28(3):524–36.
118. Tjong W, Kazakia GJ, Burghardt AJ, Majumdar S. The effect of voxel size on high-resolution peripheral computed tomography measurements of trabecular and cortical bone microstructure. Med Phys. 2012;39(4):1893–903.
119. Whittier DE, Boyd SK, Burghardt AJ, Paccou J, Ghasem-Zadeh A, Chapurlat R, et al. Guidelines for the assessment of bone density and microarchitecture in vivo using high-resolution peripheral quantitative computed tomography. Osteoporos Int. 2020;31(9):1607–27.
120. Krug R, Burghardt AJ, Majumdar S, Link TM. High-resolution imaging techniques for the assessment of osteoporosis. Radiol Clin N Am. 2010;48(3):601–21.
121. Liu XS, Zhang XH, Sekhon KK, Adams MF, McMahon DJ, Bilezikian JP, et al. High-resolution peripheral quantitative computed tomography can assess microstructural and mechanical properties of human distal tibial bone. J Bone Miner Res. 2010;25(4):746–56.
122. Burghardt AJ, Kazakia GJ, Majumdar S. A local adaptive threshold strategy for high resolution peripheral quantitative computed tomography of trabecular bone. Ann Biomed Eng. 2007;35(10):1678–86.
123. MacNeil JA, Boyd SK. Accuracy of high-resolution peripheral quantitative computed tomography for measurement of bone quality. Med Eng Phys. 2007;29(10):1096–105.
124. Stein EM, Silva BC, Boutroy S, Zhou B, Wang J, Udesky J, et al. Primary hyperparathyroidism is associated with abnormal cortical and trabecular microstructure and reduced bone stiffness in postmenopausal women. J Bone Miner Res. 2013;28(5):1029–40.
125. Hansen S, Beck Jensen JE, Rasmussen L, Hauge EM, Brixen K. Effects on bone geometry, density, and microarchitecture in the distal radius but not the tibia in women with primary hyperparathyroidism: a case-control study using HR-pQCT. J Bone Miner Res. 2010;25(9):1941–7.
126. Hansen S, Hauge EM, Rasmussen L, Jensen JE, Brixen K. Parathyroidectomy improves bone geometry and microarchitecture in female patients with primary hyperparathyroidism: a one-year prospective controlled study using high-resolution peripheral quantitative computed tomography. J Bone Miner Res. 2012;27(5):1150–8.
127. Pialat JB, Burghardt AJ, Sode M, Link TM, Majumdar S. Visual grading of motion induced image degradation in high resolution peripheral computed tomography: impact of image quality on measures of bone density and micro-architecture. Bone. 2012;50(1):111–8.
128. Kebebew E, Clark OH. Parathyroid adenoma, hyperplasia, and carcinoma: localization, technical details of primary neck exploration, and treatment of hypercalcemic crisis. Surg Oncol Clin N Am. 1998;7(4):721–48.
129. Kamaya A, Quon A, Jeffrey RB. Sonography of the abnormal parathyroid gland. Ultrasound Q. 2006;22(4):253–62.
130. Alveryd A. Parathyroid glands in thyroid surgery. I. Anatomy of parathyroid glands. II. Postoperative hypoparathyroidism--identification and autotransplantation of parathyroid glands. Acta Chir Scand. 1968;389:1–120.

131. Andre V, Andre M, Le Dreff P, Granier H, Forlodou P, Garcia JF. [Intrathyroid parathyroid adenoma]. J Radiol. 1999;80(6):591–2.
132. McIntyre RC Jr, Eisenach JH, Pearlman NW, Ridgeway CE, Liechty RD. Intrathyroidal parathyroid glands can be a cause of failed cervical exploration for hyperparathyroidism. Am J Surg. 1997;174(6):750–3; discussion 3–4
133. Lane MJ, Desser TS, Weigel RJ, Jeffrey RB Jr. Use of color and power Doppler sonography to identify feeding arteries associated with parathyroid adenomas. AJR Am J Roentgenol. 1998;171(3):819–23.
134. Wolf RJ, Cronan JJ, Monchik JM. Color Doppler sonography: an adjunctive technique in assessment of parathyroid adenomas. J Ultrasound Med. 1994;13(4):303–8.
135. Purcell GP, Dirbas FM, Jeffrey RB, Lane MJ, Desser T, McDougall IR, et al. Parathyroid localization with high-resolution ultrasound and technetium Tc 99m sestamibi. Arch Surg. 1999;134(8):824–8; discussion 8–30
136. Cheung K, Wang TS, Farrokhyar F, Roman SA, Sosa JA. A meta-analysis of preoperative localization techniques for patients with primary hyperparathyroidism. Ann Surg Oncol. 2012;19(2):577–83.
137. Udelsman R, Donovan PI. Open minimally invasive parathyroid surgery. World J Surg. 2004;28(12):1224–6.
138. Nafisi Moghadam R, Amlelshahbaz AP, Namiranian N, Sobhan-Ardekani M, Emami-Meybodi M, Dehghan A, et al. Comparative diagnostic performance of ultrasonography and 99mTc-Sestamibi scintigraphy for parathyroid adenoma in primary hyperparathyroidism; systematic review and meta-analysis. Asian Pac J Cancer Prev. 2017;18(12):3195–200.
139. Frank E, Ale-Salvo D, Park J, Liu Y, Simental A Jr, Inman JC. Preoperative imaging for parathyroid localization in patients with concurrent thyroid disease: a systematic review. Head Neck. 2018;40(7):1577–87.
140. Harari A, Mitmaker E, Grogan RH, Lee J, Shen W, Gosnell J, et al. Primary hyperparathyroidism patients with positive preoperative sestamibi scan and negative ultrasound are more likely to have posteriorly located upper gland adenomas (PLUGs). Ann Surg Oncol. 2011;18(6):1717–22.
141. Treglia G, Piccardo A, Imperiale A, Strobel K, Kaufmann PA, Prior JO, et al. Diagnostic performance of choline PET for detection of hyperfunctioning parathyroid glands in hyperparathyroidism: a systematic review and meta-analysis. Eur J Nucl Med Mol Imaging. 2019;46(3):751–65.
142. Broos WAM, van der Zant FM, Knol RJJ, Wondergem M. Choline PET/CT in parathyroid imaging: a systematic review. Nucl Med Commun. 2019;40(2):96–105.
143. Hoang JK, Sung WK, Bahl M, Phillips CD. How to perform parathyroid 4D CT: tips and traps for technique and interpretation. Radiology. 2014;270(1):15–24.
144. Yeh R, Tay YD, Tabacco G, Dercle L, Kuo JH, Bandeira L, et al. Diagnostic performance of 4D CT and Sestamibi SPECT/CT in localizing parathyroid adenomas in primary hyperparathyroidism. Radiology. 2019;291(2):469–76.
145. Bahl M, Sepahdari AR, Sosa JA, Hoang JK. Parathyroid adenomas and hyperplasia on four-dimensional CT scans: three patterns of enhancement relative to the thyroid gland justify a three-phase protocol. Radiology. 2015;277(2):454–62.
146. Bahl M, Muzaffar M, Vij G, Sosa JA, Choudhury KR, Hoang JK. Prevalence of the polar vessel sign in parathyroid adenomas on the arterial phase of 4D CT. AJNR Am J Neuroradiol. 2014;35(3):578–81.
147. Gotway MB, Reddy GP, Webb WR, Morita ET, Clark OH, Higgins CB. Comparison between MR imaging and 99mTc MIBI scintigraphy in the evaluation of recurrent of persistent hyperparathyroidism. Radiology. 2001;218(3):783–90.
148. Grayev AM, Gentry LR, Hartman MJ, Chen H, Perlman SB, Reeder SB. Presurgical localization of parathyroid adenomas with magnetic resonance imaging at 3.0 T: an adjunct method to supplement traditional imaging. Ann Surg Oncol. 2012;19(3):981–9.

Chapter 3
Clinical, Laboratory, and Radiological Diagnosis of Hyperandrogenism

Diana Soliman, Ali Qamar, and Lauren M. B. Burke

Introduction

Hyperandrogenism is characterized by high levels of androgens in women. Two main natural androgens are testosterone and dihydrotestosterone (DHT). The most common signs of androgen excess are hirsutism, acne, and alopecia. It is important to recognize and treat androgen excess disorders as long-standing hyperandrogenism is associated with dyslipidemia, hypertension, and impaired glucose tolerance [1].

Etiology

Hyperandrogenism is typically caused by excess production of sex hormones by the adrenal glands, ovaries, or both. Excess androgen production can be due to organ dysfunction, hyperplasia, or neoplasm. Rarely, it can be caused by a defect in the androgen receptor in target cells or abnormalities in the peripheral metabolism of steroids. Other causes of androgen excess include medications, hypothyroidism, hyperprolactinemia, and Cushing's syndrome.

D. Soliman (✉) · A. Qamar
Division of Endocrinology, Diabetes and Metabolism, Duke University School of Medicine, Durham, NC, USA
e-mail: diana.botros@duke.edu; ali.qamar@duke.edu

L. M. B. Burke
Department of Radiology, Division of Abdominal Imaging, University of North Carolina School of Medicine, Chapel Hill, NC, USA
e-mail: lauren_burke@med.unc.edu

© The Author(s), under exclusive license to Springer Nature Switzerland AG 2022

H. Yu et al. (eds.), *Diagnosis and Management of Endocrine Disorders in Interventional Radiology*, https://doi.org/10.1007/978-3-030-87189-5_3

Epidemiology

Hyperandrogenism affects between 5% and 10% of women of reproductive age. The most common cause of hyperandrogenism is polycystic ovarian syndrome (PCOS). In patients with androgen excess, the prevalence is about 72–82% for PCOS, 7–16% for idiopathic hyperandrogenism, 5–8% for idiopathic hirsutism, 1.5–4% for 21-hydroxylase-deficient nonclassic congenital adrenal hyperplasia (NCCAH), 3% for hyperandrogenic insulin-resistant acanthosis nigricans (HAIR-AN) syndrome, and 0.2% for androgen-secreting tumors [2, 3]. Androgen-secreting tumors can originate from the ovaries or adrenal glands.

Pathophysiology

Androgen production occurs in the endocrine glands and peripheral tissues. The endocrine glands responsible for androgen production are the adrenal glands and ovaries. The peripheral tissues involved in androgen production are the liver, gut, fat, and, most importantly, skin.

Androgen Production by Endocrine Glands

The androgens secreted by the endocrine glands are dehydroepiandrosterone sulfate (DHEAS), dehydroepiandrosterone (DHEA), androstenedione, testosterone, and androstenediol [4]. Androstenediol is rarely measured in clinical practice. Testosterone has the most significant androgenic effect, but DHEAS, DHEA, and androstenedione are precursors to testosterone. Androstenedione is produced in the ovaries and adrenal glands, and it is a direct precursor to testosterone. DHEAS (made in the adrenal glands) and DHEA (made in the ovaries and adrenal glands) are converted to androstenedione, which is then converted to testosterone. Since DHEAS is made only in the adrenal glands, it becomes an important marker of adrenal androgen production.

Androgen Production in Peripheral Tissues

Testosterone is converted to dihydrotestosterone (DHT), a potent androgen, by the enzyme 5-alpha-reductase present in the liver, hair follicles, and other androgen target cells. Testosterone can also be converted to estradiol by aromatase in adipose tissue.

Clinical Evaluation

Hyperandrogenism can lead to hirsutism, which is the excessive growth of terminal (coarse, thick) hair in a male-like pattern, including the upper lip, chin, sideburns, earlobes, tip of the nose, back, chest, areole, axillae, lower abdomen, pubic triangle, and anterior thighs. There are scoring systems available for quantifying hirsutism, such as the Ferriman and Gallwey scale shown in Fig. 3.1 [5]. Not all patients with hirsutism have hyperandrogenism, and conversely, not all patients with androgen excess are found to have hirsutism. Familial, genetic, and ethnic differences can influence the degree of hirsutism.

Acne, androgenic alopecia, and ovulatory dysfunction are also commonly found in women with androgen excess. Though acne is common in adolescents, resistant acne that persists into adulthood and is associated with hirsutism or ovulatory dysfunction raises concern for hyperandrogenism. Androgenic alopecia is male-pattern temporal balding. Ovulatory dysfunction occurs to varying degrees in women with hyperandrogenism and can include oligomenorrhea, amenorrhea, menorrhagia, metrorrhagia, pelvic pain, premenstrual dysphoric syndrome, or infertility.

Virilization is a rare clinical finding of hyperandrogenism and occurs as a result of severe androgen excess. In addition to hirsutism, acne, and androgenic alopecia, virilization includes deepening of the voice, decreased breast size, increased muscle mass, clitoral enlargement, and amenorrhea. Virilization is usually caused by an

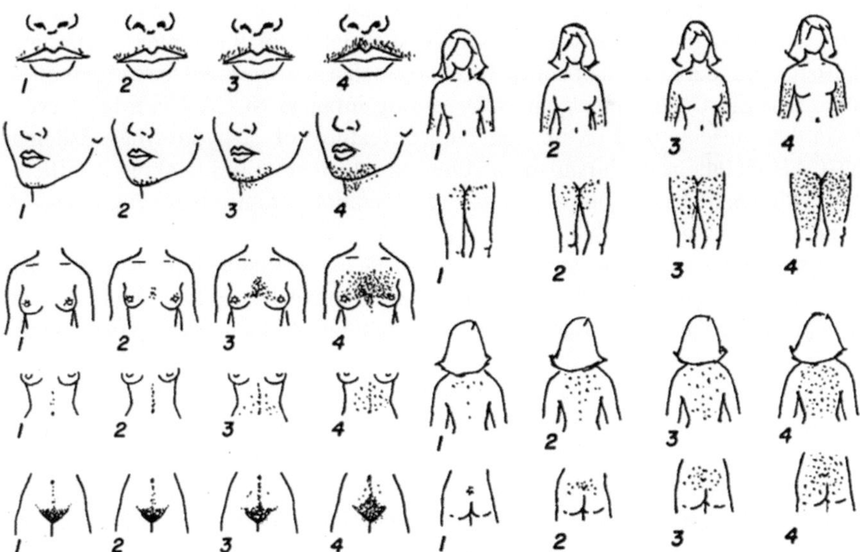

Fig. 3.1 Hirsutism scoring standards showing a spectrum from minimal hirsutism (grade 1) to frank virilization (grade 4). The scores in each of these body regions are summed, and a total score of 8 or more indicates hirsutism. (Reprinted from Hatch et al. [5] with permission from Elsevier)

androgen-producing tumor but can also be caused by congenital adrenal hyperplasia (CAH) or ovarian hyperthecosis (a severe PCOS variant).

A thorough history and physical exam are essential for the diagnosis of hyperandrogenism. In patients with suspected androgen excess, androgenic drugs should first be excluded. Medications that are associated with hyperandrogenism include exogenous androgens, anabolic steroids, danazol, and valproic acid. Patients should specifically be asked about topical androgen use by themselves and their partners. Medications that can cause hypertrichosis (excessive growth of androgen-independent hair) include phenytoin, penicillamine, diazoxide, minoxidil, and cyclosporine. The onset and progression of androgen excess symptoms should be identified, as severe, rapid, and progressive symptoms raise concern for an adrenal or ovarian androgen-secreting tumor. On physical exam, the provider should determine if signs of hyperandrogenism are present. When evaluating for hirsutism, one should keep in mind that ethnic and genetic factors can contribute to idiopathic hirsutism.

The diagnosis of PCOS is made if other disorders that can mimic PCOS (thyroid disease, hyperprolactinemia, NCCAH) have been ruled out and two out of the three following criteria are met: (1) clinical or biochemical androgen excess, (2) ovulatory dysfunction, or (3) polycystic ovaries on ultrasound [6]. Polycystic ovaries are the result of increased androgen levels leading to inhibition of follicular development. PCOS is frequently associated with obesity, insulin resistance, dyslipidemia, and obstructive sleep apnea. Clinical signs of insulin resistance include acanthosis nigricans and skin tags.

CAHs are autosomal recessive disorders and are most commonly caused by a deficiency of 21-hydroxylase. A deficiency of this enzyme results in impaired cortisol synthesis that leads to corticotropin stimulation of the adrenal cortex and subsequent accumulation of cortisol precursors that are converted to sex hormones. While classic CAH typically presents during infancy, NCCAH is a less severe form that presents later in life. The clinical features of 21-hydroxylase-deficient NCCAH include acne, hirsutism, and menstrual irregularities, making it difficult to distinguish based on a clinical presentation from other etiologies of hyperandrogenism.

In Cushing's syndrome, signs of androgen excess, including hirsutism and virilization, typically occur with adrenocortical carcinomas because these tumors tend to secrete large amounts of androgen precursors with cortisol. Hyperprolactinemia can lead to menstrual cycle dysfunction due to inhibition of gonadotropin-releasing hormone (GnRH). It can also cause hirsutism and acne, possibly due to prolactin increasing the adrenal androgens and dehydroepiandrosterone sulfate [7]. Hyperandrogenic insulin-resistant acanthosis nigricans (HAIR-AN) syndrome is characterized by hyperinsulinemia, acanthosis nigricans, and hyperandrogenism, including hirsutism, acne, menstrual irregularities, androgenic alopecia, and changes in muscle mass.

Laboratory Evaluation

In the evaluation of androgen excess, the most useful initial test is a *serum total testosterone level*. Eighty percent of testosterone is bound to sex hormone-binding globulin (SHBG), 19% is bound to albumin, and 1% is free. Decreases in SHBG, which is made by the liver, increases the fraction of testosterone available to androgen-sensitive hair and thereby promotes hirsutism. Conditions that decrease SHBG include obesity, acromegaly, hypothyroidism, and liver disease. In clinical practice, we measure total testosterone, but this correlates well with non-SHBG-bound testosterone, allowing providers to predict bioavailable testosterone from the total testosterone level [8]. In patients with normal total testosterone levels, assessment of plasma free testosterone levels may help detect subtle hyperandrogenemia [1].

Women with normal testosterone levels and cyclic menses likely have idiopathic hirsutism, and no further workup is needed. Idiopathic hirsutism is thought to be caused by increased activity of 5-alpha-reductase, which leads to increased conversion of testosterone to DHT. For women with confirmed or suspected androgen excess, the following tests should be added as clinically indicated: serum prolactin, TSH, FSH, LH, 17-hydroxyprogesterone, and DHEAS (Table 3.1) [9]. In anovulatory women with elevated testosterone levels, it is recommended to obtain serum TSH and prolactin. In PCOS, testosterone is mildly elevated or at the upper limit of normal. Some but not all patients with PCOS have an elevated LH/FSH ratio, and this is not required for the diagnosis. In PCOS, DHEAS can be mildly elevated, but it is not recommended to check a DHEAS level unless there is a concern for an androgen-producing tumor. Patients presenting with hyperandrogenism should be screened for NCCAH due to 21-hydroxylase deficiency with a 17-hydroxyprogesterone level. It is recommended to check early morning 17-hydroxyprogesterone levels in the follicular phase or on a random day for those with amenorrhea or infrequent menses [10]. If the 17-hydroxyprogesterone level is over 2 ng/mL, further evaluation should be conducted with a cosyntropin stimulation test. Androgen-producing tumors are suspected when the total testosterone level in a female is persistently

Table 3.1 Laboratory evaluation of hyperandrogenism

	Total testosterone	DHEAS	
Idiopathic hirsutism	Normal	Normal	
PCOS	High-normal or high	Normal or high	Can have elevated LH/FSH ratio
Nonclassic adrenal hyperplasia	High	Normal	Elevated serum 17-hydroxyprogesterone
Adrenal androgen-producing tumor	Very high	Very high	
Ovarian androgen-producing tumor	Very high	Normal	

greater than 200 ng/dL [11]. When the testosterone level is very high, and DHEAS is greater than 7000 ng/mL, then it is likely an androgen-producing adrenal tumor is present. If there is a concern for the HAIR-AN syndrome, basal insulin level and its response to an oral glucose load should be measured. Patients with the HAIR-AN syndrome will have basal insulin greater than 80 μU/mL if fasting or above 500 μU/mL after glucose administration [11].

Imaging Evaluation

Imaging is typically reserved for patients with very high testosterone levels (e.g., >150 ng/dL), clitoromegaly, rapidly progressive hirsutism, or severe hirsutism. A wide range of pathologies can account for elevated androgen levels, prohibiting a single imaging test as the test of choice for all cases.

Given that PCOS accounts for more than 80% of patients with androgen excess, the initial test of choice is a pelvic endovaginal ultrasound. In the setting of PCOS, endovaginal ultrasound demonstrates enlarged ovaries (volume > 10 cm^3) with multiple small follicles (≥12 follicles, measuring 2–9 mm in size) as shown in Fig. 3.2 [12]. Prominent central stroma within the ovary was historically described in patients with PCOS. However, this has failed to be a reproducible finding as there is no standardized method to measure stromal volume. While findings are typically bilateral, only unilateral findings are needed to be considered positive. It is important to note that patients with PCOS may have normal-appearing ovaries on ultrasound. Conversely, imaging findings alone cannot diagnose PCOS; the Rotterdam criteria requires two of three criteria to be met for diagnosis [13]. The Rotterdam criteria includes clinical or biochemical hyperandrogenism, oligo or anovulation, and polycystic ovaries.

Additional ovarian pathologies such as fibrothecomas, luteomas of pregnancy, Sertoli-Leydig tumors, and massive ovarian edema, each have their own radiologic presentation on pelvic ultrasound but can all be evaluated with endovaginal

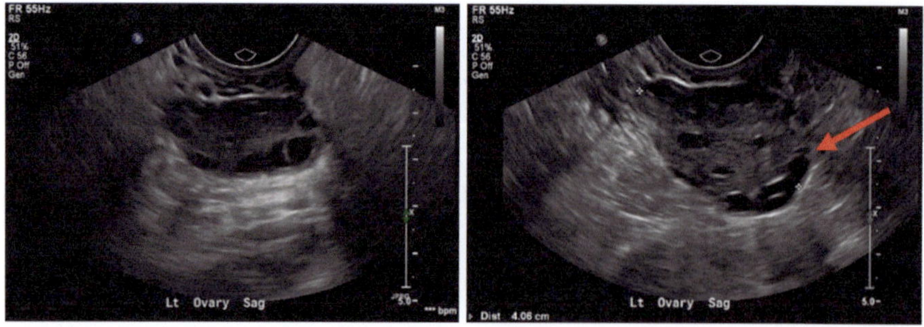

Fig. 3.2 Selected ultrasound images of a left ovary demonstrating an enlarged ovary with multiple small follicles, compatible with imaging findings of PCOS

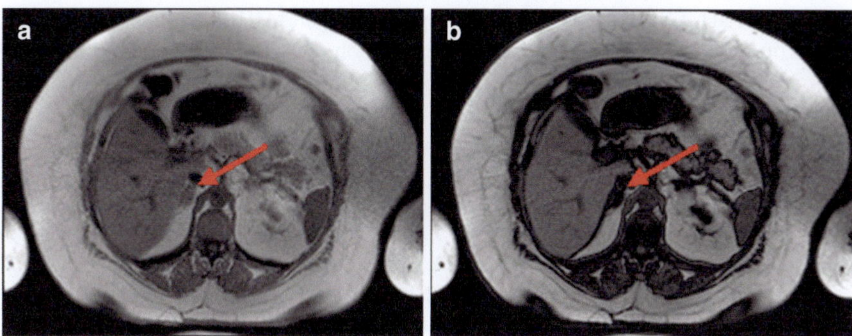

Fig. 3.3 In-phase (**a**) and out-of-phase (**b**) MR imaging of a 45-year female which demonstrates loss of signal on out-of-phase imaging within a small right adrenal lesion, compatible with an adrenal adenoma

ultrasound. In cases where endovaginal ultrasound is limited, magnetic resonance imaging (MRI) of the pelvis may be helpful for further evaluation. CT has a limited role in the diagnosis of primary ovarian pathology [14].

Although less common, significantly elevated DHEAS levels and abnormal 24-hour urine-free cortisol levels can suggest underlying adrenal pathology [11]. Such pathologies include adrenal hyperplasia, adrenal adenomas, and adrenal cortical carcinoma. All adrenal pathologies can be imaged using multiphase CT or MRI cross-sectional imaging of the abdomen. Adrenal hyperplasia typically appears as thickened (over 10 mm) adrenal limbs, occasionally with a micronodular appearance. Adrenal adenomas present as discrete adrenal nodules which demonstrate characteristic low signal on noncontrast CT (>10 HU), rapid washout (>60% absolute washout) on 15-min delayed phase CT imaging, or intravoxel fat (seen as a signal loss) on out-of-phase imaging on MRI (Fig. 3.3). The dreaded but rare adrenal cortical carcinoma presents as a large adrenal mass (>6 cm) with necrosis and venous invasion as common secondary findings.

Finally, pituitary tumors should be imaged using an MRI of the brain with high-resolution imaging of the pituitary gland as these micro- and macroadenomas of the pituitary may be subtle. Thyroid ultrasound can be utilized in patients who have suspected thyroid hypoplasia or agenesis.

Conclusion

In summary, symptoms of hyperandrogenism include hirsutism, alopecia, ovulatory dysfunction, and virilization in severe cases. The most common cause of androgen excess is PCOS, but idiopathic hirsutism, NCCAH, and androgen-secreting tumors should also be considered. A thorough history and physical exam are essential. Patients should be asked about medications as well as the onset and progression of symptoms. Initial laboratory evaluation should include total testosterone, but prolactin, TSH, FSH, LH, 17-hydroxyprogesterone, and DHEAS can be considered based on the patient's presentation. Depending on the suspected etiology, imaging may include pelvic endovaginal ultrasound, abdominal CT, or abdominal MRI.

References

1. Goodman NF, Bledsoe MB, Cobin RH, Futterweit W, Goldzieher JW, Petak SM, et al. American Association of Clinical Endocrinologists medical guidelines for the clinical practice for the diagnosis and treatment of hyperandrogenic disorders. Endocr Pract Off J Am Coll Endocrinol Am Assoc Clin Endocrinol. 2001;7(2):120–34.
2. Azziz R, Sanchez LA, Knochenhauer ES, Moran C, Lazenby J, Stephens KC, et al. Androgen excess in women: experience with over 1000 consecutive patients. J Clin Endocrinol Metab. 2004;89(2):453–62.
3. Carmina E, Rosato F, Jannì A, Rizzo M, Longo RA. Extensive clinical experience: relative prevalence of different androgen excess disorders in 950 women referred because of clinical hyperandrogenism. J Clin Endocrinol Metab. 2006;91(1):2–6.
4. Stanczyk FZ. Diagnosis of hyperandrogenism: biochemical criteria. Best Pract Res Clin Endocrinol Metab. 2006;20(2):177–91.
5. Hatch R, Rosenfield RL, Kim MH, Tredway D. Hirsutism: implications, etiology, and management. Am J Obstet Gynecol. 1981;140(7):815–30.
6. Legro RS, Arslanian SA, Ehrmann DA, Hoeger KM, Murad MH, Pasquali R, et al. Diagnosis and treatment of polycystic ovary syndrome: an Endocrine Society clinical practice guideline. J Clin Endocrinol Metab. 2013;98(12):4565–92.
7. Majumdar A, Mangal NS. Hyperprolactinemia. J Hum Reprod Sci. 2013;6(3):168–75.
8. Schwartz U, Moltz L, Brotherton J, Hammerstein J. The diagnostic value of plasma free testosterone in non-tumorous and tumorous hyperandrogenism. Fertil Steril. 1983;40(1):66–72.
9. Williams R. In: Melmed S, Polonsky KS, Larsen PR, Kronenberg H, editors. Williams textbook of endocrinology. 13th ed. Philadelphia: Elsevier; 2016. p. 615–38.
10. Martin KA, Anderson RR, Chang RJ, Ehrmann DA, Lobo RA, Murad MH, et al. Evaluation and treatment of hirsutism in premenopausal women: an Endocrine Society clinical practice guideline. J Clin Endocrinol Metab. 2018;103(4):1233–57.
11. Practice Committee of the American Society for Reproductive Medicine. The evaluation and treatment of androgen excess. Fertil Steril. 2006;86(5 Suppl 1):S241–7.
12. Lee TT, Rausch ME. Polycystic ovarian syndrome: role of imaging in diagnosis. Radiogr Rev Publ Radiol Soc N Am Inc. 2012;32(6):1643–57.
13. Rotterdam ESHRE/ASRM-Sponsored PCOS Consensus Workshop Group. Revised 2003 consensus on diagnostic criteria and long-term health risks related to polycystic ovary syndrome. Fertil Steril. 2004;81(1):19–25.
14. Jeong YY, Outwater EK, Kang HK. Imaging evaluation of ovarian masses. Radiogr Rev Publ Radiol Soc N Am Inc. 2000;20(5):1445–70.

Chapter 4
Clinical, Laboratory, and Radiological Diagnosis of Hypercortisolism

Paul A. Guido and Carlos A. Zamora

Introduction

Hypercortisolism and its associated clinical findings, otherwise known as Cushing's syndrome, is a classical endocrine condition of hormone excess. There are many physical findings of hypercortisolism that clinicians should recognize as a reason to evaluate for the condition. The state of excess cortisol can lead to significant morbidity and mortality if untreated. The diagnosis can be quite challenging due to confounders and multiple different etiologies. Furthermore, the treatment paradigms of the various causes differ greatly and range from the cessation of offending medications to pituitary or adrenal surgery. Therefore, accurate diagnosis of the cause of hypercortisolism is important and requires collaboration among endocrinologists, diagnostic radiologists, and interventional radiologists to recommend appropriate medical or surgical therapy. In this chapter, we will review the clinical, laboratory, and radiological diagnosis of hypercortisolism.

Etiology

The physical manifestations of hypercortisolism can be similar for all different etiologies of Cushing's syndrome. The etiologies are separated by whether the

P. A. Guido (✉)
Department of Endocrinology, University of North Carolina, Chapel Hill, NC, USA
e-mail: Paul.guido@tuhs.temple.edu

C. A. Zamora
Division of Neuroradiology, Department of Radiology, University of North Carolina at Chapel Hill, Chapel Hill, NC, USA
e-mail: carlos_zamora@med.unc.edu

© The Author(s), under exclusive license to Springer Nature Switzerland AG 2022

H. Yu et al. (eds.), *Diagnosis and Management of Endocrine Disorders in Interventional Radiology*, https://doi.org/10.1007/978-3-030-87189-5_4

hypercortisolism is due to exogenous or endogenous sources of corticosteroids. By far, the most common etiology is exogenous corticosteroid administration. Overt symptoms of hypercortisolism can manifest quickly due to high doses of high-potency systemic glucocorticoids. On the other hand, the indolent subclinical disease may manifest due to low doses of oral corticosteroids or even due to topical steroids administered chronically. Millions of patients receive corticosteroids for autoimmune disease, dermatologic problems, transplants, and malignancies. The clinician must be diligent in excluding all prescribed and unprescribed oral, injectable, inhaled, or topical forms of corticosteroid before working up endogenous hypercortisolism.

Endogenous causes of hypercortisolism are much less common than exogenous sources. The overall incidence of endogenous hypercortisolism has been reported between 1.8 and 2.3 per million annually based on different population studies [1–3]. Endogenous hypercortisolism can be further characterized as adrenocorticotropic hormone (ACTH) dependent or independent. The pathophysiologic details of the various etiologies will be further discussed in later sections. ACTH-dependent causes include ACTH-producing pituitary adenoma (Cushing's disease), which is the most common (66–80% of cases) [4]. Other ACTH-dependent causes include ectopic ACTH syndromes, where the source of the ACTH is outside the pituitary. These are often due to neuroendocrine malignancies such as carcinoid tumors or small cell lung cancer. Very rarely can a tumor produce ectopic (non-hypothalamic) corticotrophin-releasing hormone (CRH), which leads to excess pituitary production of ACTH.

ACTH-independent causes of hypercortisolism are responsible for 20–30% of cases [4, 5]. Most common are unilateral benign adrenal adenomas that produce cortisol, followed by unilateral malignant adrenocortical carcinomas that produce cortisol and precursor hormones. The bilateral adrenal disease that is ACTH independent is rare and comprises bilateral macronodular adrenal hyperplasia and primary pigmented nodular adrenal disease.

Epidemiology

Endogenous hypercortisolism is estimated to have an incidence of 1.8–2.3 per million annually. The majority (74–81%) of cases are found in women, and the median age of presentation is 39–44 [1–4]. Mortalities in cohort studies range from 11% to 15%, and meta-analyses show a standardized mortality ratio (SMR) of 1.84 in patients with pituitary disease compared with 1.90 in patients with the adrenal disease [6]. In patients with adrenocortical carcinoma, SMR is 48.00. In patients with hypercortisolism due to ectopic ACTH syndromes, SMR is 13.33 [7]. Mortality is predominantly driven by cardiovascular disease and infections in nonmalignant causes of hypercortisolism. Specific morbidity will be discussed in the clinical evaluation section. Patients presenting with certain comorbidities, such as diabetes or osteoporosis, are more likely to have hypercortisolism [8, 9]. However, the constellation of symptoms and comorbidities, which is described further in this chapter, is required to consider screening, as there is no single condition or recommended universal screening guidelines [10].

Pathophysiology

To understand how the different etiologies of hypercortisolism arise, it is important to examine them in the context of the hypothalamic-pituitary-adrenal (HPA) axis (Fig. 4.1). The paraventricular nuclei of the hypothalamus secrete corticotrophin-releasing hormone (CRH) in response to systemic cortisol levels, various physiological stressors, and the circadian rhythm. CRH and vasopressin, which is also secreted from the hypothalamus, act upon the corticotroph cells of the anterior pituitary, resulting in the release of ACTH. Production of ACTH is diurnal, with a peak in the morning, around 8:00 am and nadir around midnight. ACTH then acts upon the cortex of the adrenal gland to cause the synthesis of corticosteroids. Cortisol then acts upon the glucocorticoid receptor in tissues throughout the body. Negative feedback from cortisol occurs at both the hypothalamus and the anterior pituitary, reducing, first, release of ACTH, and, second, synthesis of CRH. The balance between all components of this neuroendocrine system is highly regulated and excessive hormone at each level can contribute to hypercortisolism.

Pituitary Corticotroph Adenomas: Cushing's Disease

This ACTH-dependent process is almost always caused by a pituitary microadenoma (<10 mm) that produces ACTH with incomplete resistance to cortisol negative feedback. Macroadenomas (>10 mm) are less common (7% of Cushing's disease in a single-center study) [11]. All corticotroph adenomas form in the anterior pituitary gland and are typically driven by somatic mutations in tumor suppressor genes or glucocorticoid receptor pathways. Much less common (about 5% of adenomas) are germline mutations inherited in familial syndromes such as multiple endocrine neoplasia type 1 [12, 13]. The clonal proliferation of corticotroph cells leads to the development of the tumor and subsequent elevation in plasma ACTH levels. It is important to note that the degree of ACTH elevation does not necessarily correlate to the severity of the disease. In fact, ACTH levels can be in the normal range but are considered "inappropriately normal" in the context of systemic hypercortisolemia [14]. This is due to the incomplete resistance to cortisol feedback in the adenoma. ACTH produced by the adenoma then acts physiologically on both adrenal glands to cause excess endogenous hypercortisolism. This can lead to adrenal hyperplasia. The disease can be subclinical to overt in severity.

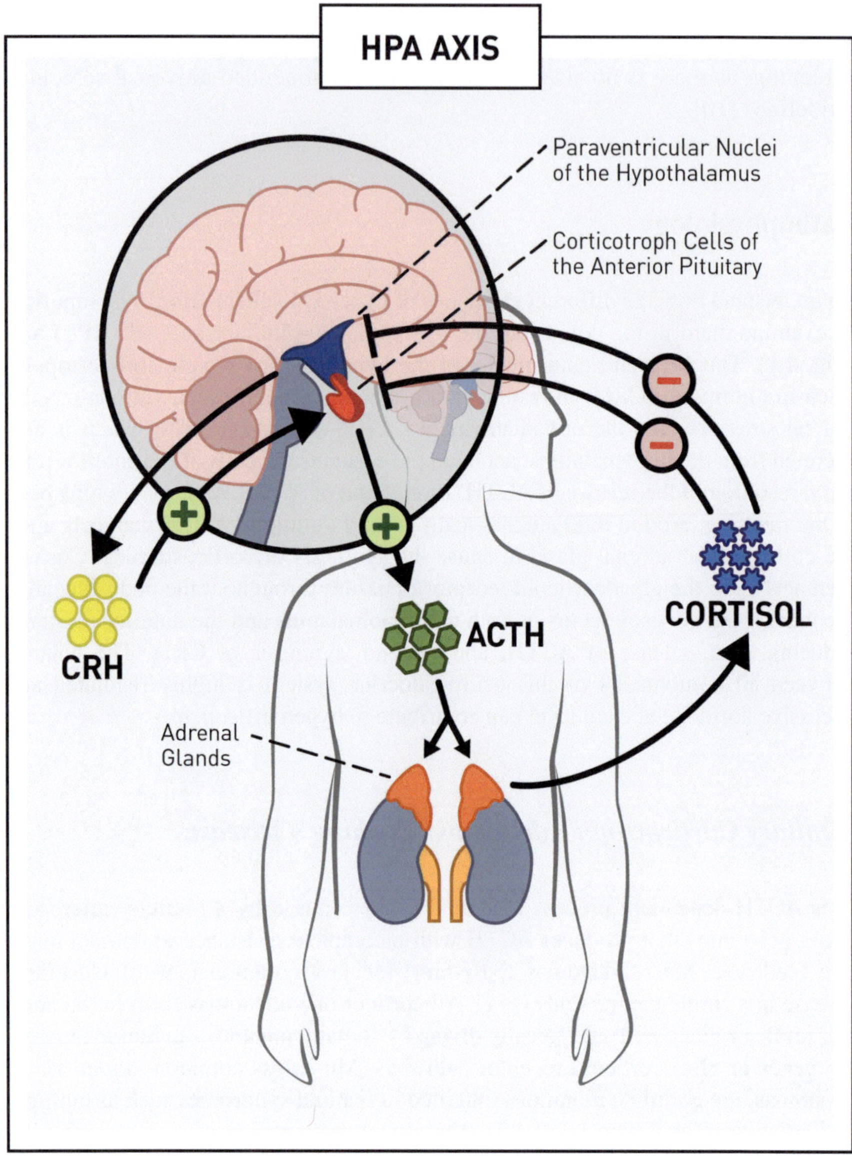

Fig. 4.1 Cartoon representation of positive (+) and negative (−) feedback within the hypothalamic-pituitary-adrenal axis. Corticotropin-releasing hormone from the hypothalamic paraventricular nuclei acts upon the corticotroph cells of the anterior pituitary to cause production of adrenocorticotropic hormone (ACTH). ACTH acts upon the adrenal cortex to cause production of cortisol. Cortisol exerts negative feedback on the hypothalamus and pituitary. (Illustration courtesy of Sierra Finn, Chapel Hill, NC)

Ectopic ACTH Syndrome

This ACTH-dependent process is typically caused by neuroendocrine tumors located outside of the pituitary. These are either well-differentiated neuroendocrine tumors, such as bronchial carcinoid, gastrointestinal carcinoid, and islet cell tumors, or poorly differentiated tumors such as small cell lung carcinoma, medullary thyroid carcinoma, or pheochromocytoma [15, 16]. A key concept for these tumors is that they tend to produce ACTH and its precursors at higher levels than found in pituitary sources, and the ACTH is fully resistant to cortisol negative feedback. The elevated levels of ACTH act on the adrenal glands to produce endogenous hypercortisolemia. This leads to more aggressive disease and is typically more clinically apparent.

Unilateral Adrenal Adenoma

This is an ACTH-independent process. A benign tumor forms in the adrenal cortex and produces cortisol without signaling from pituitary ACTH. The autonomously produced cortisol will then cause negative feedback on the normal HPA axis and result in atrophy of the pituitary corticotroph cells and the contralateral adrenal gland. In contrast to adrenocortical carcinoma, adrenal adenomas typically produce mature glucocorticoid products instead of precursors. In patients with unilateral disease, somatic mutations are often found in cell cycle proteins or, less frequently, transmembrane signaling receptors that respond to other hormonal pathways [17, 18]. The disease can be subclinical to overt in severity.

Adrenocortical Carcinoma

This is an ACTH-independent process. A malignant tumor forms in the adrenal cortex and often produces a state of hormonal excess. This frequently involves the production of cortisol, androgens, aldosterone, and immature precursors. Hormonal excess is found in approximately 60% of cases [19, 20]. These tumors can often present with mass effect or symptoms from metastatic disease. Adrenocortical carcinomas can be associated with inheritable syndromes such as Li-Fraumeni, Beckwith Wiedemann, or multiple endocrine neoplasia type 1. Sporadic mutations cause most cases and involve multiple mutations, often including TP53 [21]. They are aggressive tumors with a poor prognosis due to both the excess hormonal state and the spread of malignancy with associated complications.

Bilateral Adrenal Nodular Disease

These are ACTH-independent processes. They are separated into macronodular and micronodular diseases based on the appearance of the adrenal glands on cross-sectional imaging or pathology. Macronodular (bilateral macronodular adrenal hyperplasia [BMAH]) disease has nodules greater than 1 cm in diameter. The large adrenal glands secrete cortisol or multiple adrenal hormones and precursors autonomously and lead to Cushing's syndrome. BMAH can be associated with several inheritable conditions such as McCune-Albright syndrome, multiple endocrine neoplasia type 1, adenomatous polyposis coli, or familial inheritance of BMAH alone [22]. Somatic mutations during embryogenesis can lead to BMAH and often involve the cyclic AMP/protein kinase A pathway or transmembrane peptide hormone receptors that respond to vasopressin or gastrointestinal inhibitory peptide [23]. The disease can be overt or subclinical. Micronodular (primary pigmented nodular adrenal disease [PPNAD]) disease has innumerable small nodules less than 1 cm that are darkly colored on pathology. The normal adrenal glands can also produce cortisol autonomously. This disease is the most frequent manifestation of the Carney complex (spotty skin pigmentation, endocrine tumors including PPNAD, pituitary tumors, or thyroid tumors, testicular tumors, breast tumors, and cardiac myxomas). The disease is due to a mutation in the PRKARA1 tumor suppressor gene [24]. Hypercortisolism can be subclinical or overt.

Clinical Evaluation

Clinical suspicion of hypercortisolism remains an exercise in understanding the constellation of symptoms that can manifest. Since the incidence of obesity and metabolic syndrome has drastically increased since Harvey Cushing, the classical description of the patient with a moon-shaped face, obesity, and hirsutism is no longer specific. Many of the signs and symptoms overlap with other conditions, and hypercortisolism can be subclinical in nature. As a result, the workup can be a challenging task and requires a firm understanding of the laboratory evaluation as well. Severe disease is often unmistakable and progresses quickly. As discussed previously, the clinician should first exclude all exogenous sources of glucocorticoids, including topical preparations, as these are responsible for most hypercortisolism cases. It is also important to consider states of physiologic hypercortisolism. This is sometimes referenced as pseudo-Cushing's and can be found in patients with chronic alcoholism, severely uncontrolled diabetes, and extreme physical or psychological stress. Once these are excluded, the clinician can utilize the constellation of features of hypercortisolism and their probabilities to consider further workup. A cartoon representation of a patient with manifestations of hypercortisolism is seen in Fig. 4.2. As reported in the guidelines for the diagnosis of Cushing's syndrome by the Endocrine Society, laboratory screening should be considered for patients

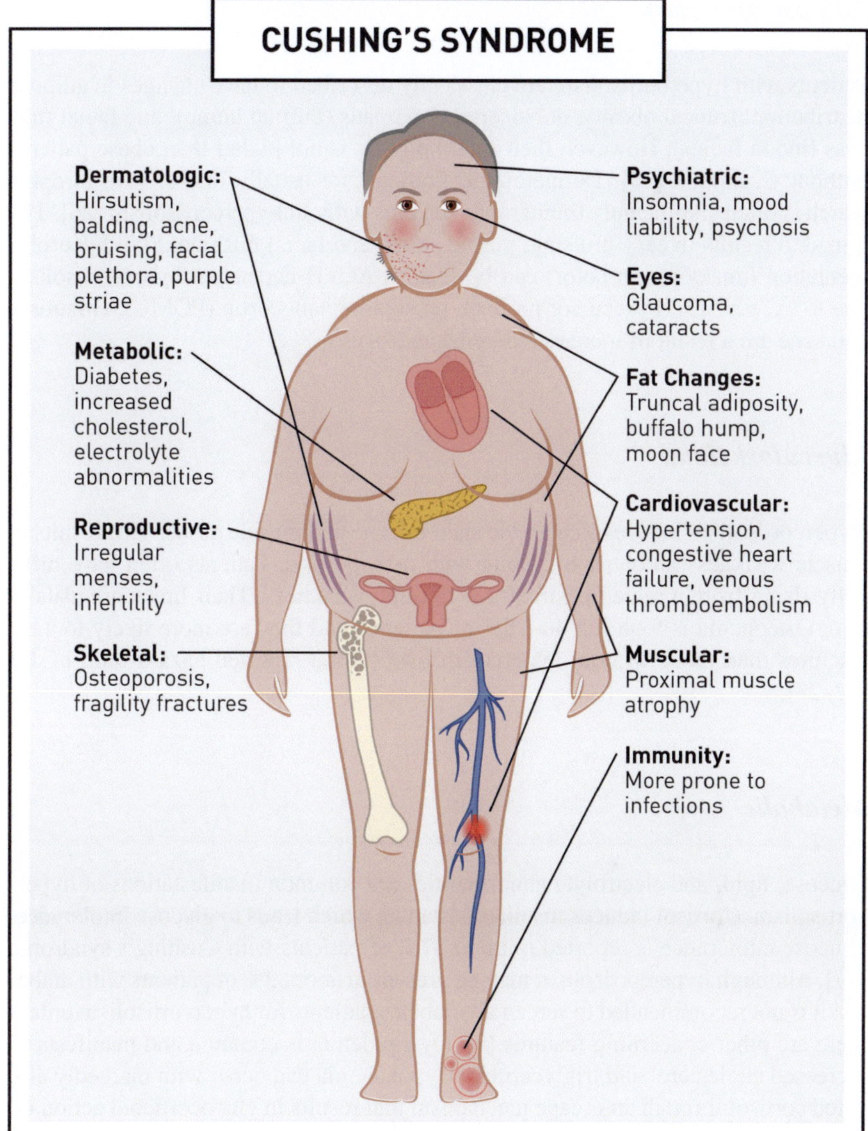

Fig. 4.2 Cartoon representation of the clinical manifestations of hypercortisolism. (Illustration courtesy of Sierra Finn, Chapel Hill, NC)

with multiple or progression of the following exam features: easy bruising, facial plethora, proximal muscle weakness, purple striae greater than one centimeter wide, or in children with weight gain and decreasing growth velocity. The guidelines also recommend screening for patients with unusually severe osteoporosis, hypertension, or those with adrenal incidentalomas [10].

Adipose and Skin

Patients with hypercortisolism are classically described to have changes in adipose distribution: truncal obesity, dorsocervical fat pads (buffalo hump), and facial fullness (moon facies). However, their total body fat is not higher than obese patients without Cushing's [25]. Dermatologic findings are usually due to skin atrophy, which is often significantly thinner than patients without hypercortisolism [26]. The thin skin results in easy bruising, purple striae, and facial flushing. Skin hyperpigmentation (dusky tan in color) can be seen in ACTH-dependent hypercortisolism due to excess ACTH precursor product, pro-opiomelanocortin (POMC). Hirsutism and acne are a result of increased adrenal androgens.

Musculoskeletal

Hypercortisolism induces a catabolic state in bone and muscle tissue. This results in muscle weakness and atrophy, along with osteoporosis. Patients often have difficulty rising from a seated position due to thigh weakness. Their limbs are usually thin. Osteopenia is found in 40–78% of patients, and they are more likely to have fractures than those without hypercortisolism with a reported hazard ratio of 1.4 [27, 28].

Metabolic

Glucose, lipid, and electrolyte abnormalities are common manifestations of hypercortisolism. Cortisol induces insulin resistance, which leads to glucose intolerance. Glucose intolerance is reported in up to 87% of patients with Cushing's syndrome [27]. Although hypercortisolism may be present in about 2% of patients with diabetes, it is not recommended to screen all diabetes patients for hypercortisolism unless there are other concerning features [8]. Dyslipidemia is common and manifests as increased cholesterol and triglycerides. Hypokalemia can occur with markedly elevated cortisol through an escape mechanism that results in glucocorticoid action on the mineralocorticoid receptor.

Cardiovascular

Hypertension is the predominant cardiovascular abnormality, found in up to 85% of patients with hypercortisolism [29]. In conjunction with the metabolic syndrome discussed previously, this leads to high cardiovascular risk for patients with

Cushing's syndrome. There is a demonstrated increase in atherosclerotic and car-diomyopathic disease. Hypercortisolism can also lead to an increased risk of venous thromboembolism due to the induction of a hypercoagulable state. Between 1.9% and 2.5% of patients with hypercortisolism are reported to have unprovoked venous thromboembolism [30].

Reproductive

Elevated cortisol exerts negative feedback on the hypothalamic-pituitary-gonadal axis leading to hypogonadotropic hypogonadism. In women, this leads to irregular menstrual cycles and infertility. In men, this leads to decreased testosterone levels and sperm counts. Both genders can have diminished libido. Etiologies that produce excess adrenal androgens, such as adrenocortical carcinoma, can also result in virilization.

Immune

Endogenous cortisol can lead to immune suppression in a similar fashion as exog-enous corticosteroids when used for rheumatologic and inflammatory conditions. This raises the risk for infection, which is the cause of death in 21% of patients with Cushing's disease [31]. Opportunistic infections can occur in more severe hypercor-tisolism, but typical bacterial infections are more common [32].

Psychiatric

Chronic hypercortisolism leads to neuropsychiatric changes due to the effect of cortisol on the central nervous system. Depression is common, reported in up to 81% of patients. Anxiety is found in 66% of patients, along with irritability, insom-nia, and cognitive impairments. The constellation can lead to suicidal thoughts, and suicide was attempted in 5% of patients [33].

Laboratory Evaluation

Laboratory evaluation of hypercortisolism is a multistep process. The first and most important task is to establish the diagnosis of hypercortisolism. The second task is to determine if the hypercortisolemia is ACTH dependent or independent. The third task is to determine the etiology. The decision to start a laboratory workup is dependent on the constellation of possible clinical findings as previously described. The Endocrine Society guidelines recommend three screening tests: (1) a 24-hour urine free cortisol collection, (2) a low-dose dexamethasone suppression test, and (3) a midnight salivary free cortisol [10]. Each test has benefits and limitations, and the clinician must understand both to make the diagnosis accurately. One test alone should not be used to make the diagnosis; if a screening test is positive, a second test should be performed. If there is high clinical suspicion, but the test is negative, the clinician should consider a different screening test.

Diagnosing Hypercortisolemia: 24-Hour Urine Free Cortisol

The 24-hour urine free cortisol collection is a simple test that measures cortisol in the urine that is not bound to cortisol-binding globulin. This is important because medications and physiologic states affect cortisol-binding globulin and, therefore, total serum cortisol levels. These include exogenous estrogens and pregnancy. This test is not affected by either. Since the sample is collected for 24 h, the test is less affected by variation in cortisol levels throughout the day. A value above the upper limit of normal should be considered a positive result. In patients with true hypercortisolism, the 24-hour urinary free cortisol has a likelihood ratio of 10.6 of a positive result and 0.16 of a negative result [34]. Negative results are typically found in patients with mild subclinical hypercortisolism. The confounders of this test include the following: dependence on patients collecting an adequate sample, renal failure, and high urine volumes. A concomitantly collected 24-hour urine creatinine can help delineate errors in the collection.

Diagnosing Hypercortisolemia: Low-Dose Dexamethasone Suppression Test

The patient is instructed to take 1 mg of dexamethasone orally at 23:00, followed by the collection of serum cortisol level at 08:00. An alternative form of the test utilizes 0.5 mg of dexamethasone every 6 h for 48 h. This dynamic test relies upon negative feedback from the high-potency glucocorticoid on the HPA axis. Normal patients will suppress their cortisol levels upon dexamethasone administration. There is considerable literature dedicated to the cutoff value for the serum cortisol level. The Endocrine Society recommends a cutoff value of less than 1.8 µg/dL to maintain optimal sensitivity of greater than 95% [10]. Patients with true hypercortisolism had a likelihood ratio of 11.6 for a positive result and 0.09 for a negative result using a 1 mg overnight dexamethasone suppression test [34]. This test is confounded by changes in cortisol-binding globulin such as pregnancy or exogenous estrogen, as well as medications that alter dexamethasone metabolism via the CYP3A4 pathway. Some examples include antiepileptics, like phenobarbital, phenytoin, or carbamazepine; antimicrobials like rifampin, rifapentine, itraconazole, or ritonavir; or others such as cimetidine, fluoxetine, or diltiazem. Some clinicians will measure a dexamethasone level to confirm that the patient did indeed take the medication, though this is not available at all labs. The low-dose dexamethasone suppression test is the preferred test for the evaluation of adrenal incidentaloma due to its high sensitivity.

Diagnosing Hypercortisolemia: Late Night Salivary Free Cortisol

The patient is instructed to collect a saliva sample at midnight. Like the 24-hour urine collection test, salivary cortisol is not bound to cortisol-binding globulin and is therefore unaffected by conditions that alter cortisol-binding globulin concentration, such as pregnancy or estrogen use. This test utilizes the diurnal variation in cortisol to screen for abnormalities. Patients with hypercortisolism first lose the late-night nadir in cortisol levels. Patients with true hypercortisolism had a likelihood ratio of 8.8 for a positive result and 0.07 for a negative result [34]. The Endocrine Society guidelines recommend a cutoff of less than 145 ng/dL for a normal result [10]. Confounders for this test include tobacco, licorice, or disruptions to a normal sleep-wake cycle such as night shift workers.

Determining ACTH Status

Once hypercortisolism is confirmed with at least two screening tests as above, the next step is to determine the ACTH status. Serum ACTH levels that are suppressed less than 10 pg/mL suggest an ACTH-independent cause of hypercortisolemia. ACTH levels greater than 20 pg/mL suggest an ACTH-dependent cause of hypercortisolemia. Values between 10 and 20 pg/mL are indeterminate, and the use of a CRH stimulation test can help determine the ACTH status [35]. Pituitary adenomas respond to stimulation and will increase ACTH and cortisol compared to ACTH-independent etiologies. CRH is injected intravenously, and cortisol and ACTH levels are collected at 15-min intervals. Cutoff levels are different at various centers. For all tests, it is important to note that ACTH is very unstable and must be collected and transported quickly to the lab on ice.

Determining the Etiology

Once the ACTH-dependent or independent status is determined, there are several methods to differentiate the etiologies. Most depend on adrenal or pituitary imaging studies, as discussed in the imaging section. For ACTH-independent etiologies, abdominal computed tomography (CT) is frequently used to look for adrenal adenomas, adrenocortical carcinoma, or bilateral nodular disease. Occasionally, adrenal venous sampling is required for a definitive diagnosis, as discussed in a later chapter. For ACTH-dependent etiologies, the first step is typically pituitary magnetic resonance imaging (MRI). If the tumor is smaller than 6 mm, neurointerventional radiologists often perform inferior petrosal sinus sampling (IPSS), which is the gold standard for determining whether an ACTH-dependent hypercortisolemia is due to a pituitary or ectopic lesion [36]. IPSS is discussed in detail in a later chapter. If IPSS is unavailable or nondiagnostic, there are two laboratory tests that can help differentiate pituitary from ectopic ACTH etiologies. The CRH stimulation test, as mentioned previously, will cause an elevation in ACTH and cortisol in pituitary adenomas, but not in ectopic ACTH syndromes as the tumors lack CRH receptors and have suppressed the normal pituitary response to CRH. This test is 86% sensitive and 90% specific [37]. The high-dose dexamethasone suppression test is conducted by collecting a baseline 08:00 cortisol, having the patient take 8 mg of dexamethasone at 23:00, and collecting cortisol levels the next day at 08:00. Suppression of cortisol by >50% is due to a pituitary adenoma. Less than 50% suppression is likely due to an ectopic ACTH syndrome. This test is 88% sensitive and 57% specific [38].

Imaging Evaluation

ACTH-Secreting Pituitary Adenomas

MRI is the mainstay modality for evaluating pituitary adenomas due to its better soft tissue contrast compared with CT. Typical protocols include a combination of T1- and T2-weighted sequences with sagittal and coronal acquisitions through the pituitary gland using thin slices ($\leq$3 mm) with a small field of view. Although signal intensity is variable, ACTH-secreting adenomas are generally iso- to mildly hyperintense on T2- and hypointense on noncontrast T1-weighted sequences relative to the cerebral cortex. Hemorrhagic adenomas may contain fluid-blood levels or areas of intrinsic T1 hyperintensity due to methemoglobin.

While small adenomas can be challenging to visualize, coronal images may show a more pronounced convex margin on the side of the lesion and deviation of the pituitary infundibulum to the contralateral side [39]. Intravenous administration of gadolinium is necessary to characterize the tumor and delineate its extent. Most adenomas enhance less avidly than the pituitary parenchyma and, therefore, will appear relatively hypointense on post-contrast T1-weighted sequences [40]. However, some pituitary microadenomas (<1 cm) are not seen on routine imaging and may only be identified utilizing dynamic MRI protocols. These are achieved by acquiring serial coronal images through the pituitary gland in 10- to 15-s intervals following the intravenous injection of gadolinium. In the early phases of a dynamic scan, a pituitary adenoma usually appears hypointense compared to the avidly enhancing normal pituitary gland. In the later phases, there is a progressive enhancement of the adenoma, which tends to "blend in" and approximate the signal intensity of the pituitary gland (Fig. 4.3).

One small retrospective study was able to identify microadenomas in 96% (23 of 24) of patients with mild Cushing's disease utilizing dynamic MRI, compared to 15% (3 of 20) on non-dynamic sequences [41]. In a different study, dynamic MRI had higher sensitivity compared with non-dynamic MRI (67% vs. 52%, respectively) but lower specificity (80% vs. 100%, respectively) [42]. A more recent study that evaluated different MRI techniques for detecting microadenomas in patients with Cushing's disease found that adding a 3D post-contrast non-dynamic T1 sequence resulted in a higher sensitivity than adding routine dynamic scans alone (54% vs. 47%, respectively) [43]. On the downside, there was a trade-off for lower specificity (66% for 3D vs. 77% for dynamic MRI); however, the change in diagnostic accuracy was minimal (54 vs. 53%, respectively).

Some institutions employ heavily T2-weighted high-resolution MRI sequences such as constructive interference in steady state (CISS) or fast imaging employing steady-state acquisition (FIESTA) after injecting gadolinium, which can be

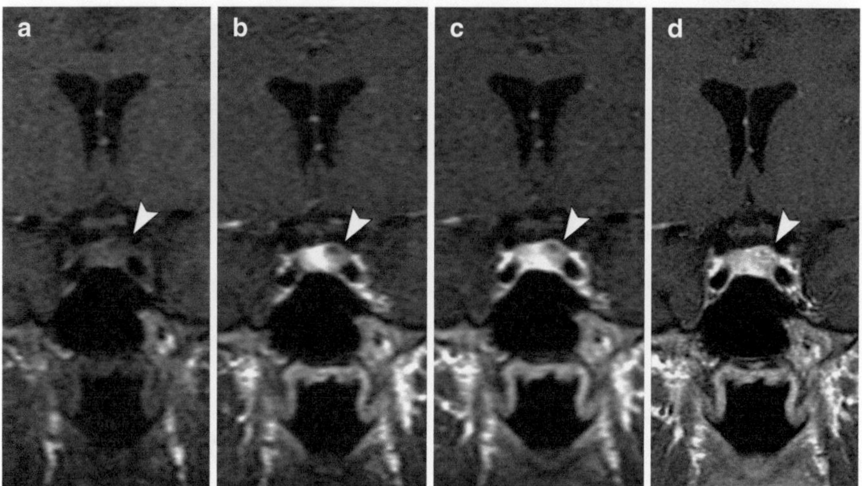

Fig. 4.3 Coronal dynamic pituitary protocol MRI with noncontrast (**a**) and serial post-contrast (**b–d**) T1-weighted sequences after gadolinium injection. There is a microadenoma within the left pituitary gland (arrowheads), which appears hypointense on the early phases and blends in with the surrounding parenchyma on the later sequences. Note more pronounced convexity of the upper left pituitary contour and mild deviation of the infundibulum to the right

done at 0.7 mm slice thickness or less. However, like other 3D sequences, CISS and FIESTA are sensitive to motion artifact. A recent study comparing a 3D post-contrast T1 sequence with CISS found similar sensitivities between the two techniques with an increased detection rate when they were used in conjunction (Fig. 4.4) [44].

The presence of cavernous sinus invasion by a pituitary adenoma is associated with decreased rates of hormonal remission and need for further intervention [45]. MRI has been utilized preoperatively to predict cavernous sinus invasion with variable results. Knosp et al. developed the most widely utilized classification system, which describes the extent of invasion using the cavernous internal carotid arteries (ICAs) as a landmark [46]. Grading is assessed on coronal post-contrast T1 images and ranges from grade 0, where there is no extension beyond the medial margin of the ICA, to grade 3, where the tumor extends beyond the lateral margin, and grade 4, where there is complete carotid encasement [47]. The rate of cavernous sinus invasion of grade 3 lesions ranges between 38% and 65%, and the most

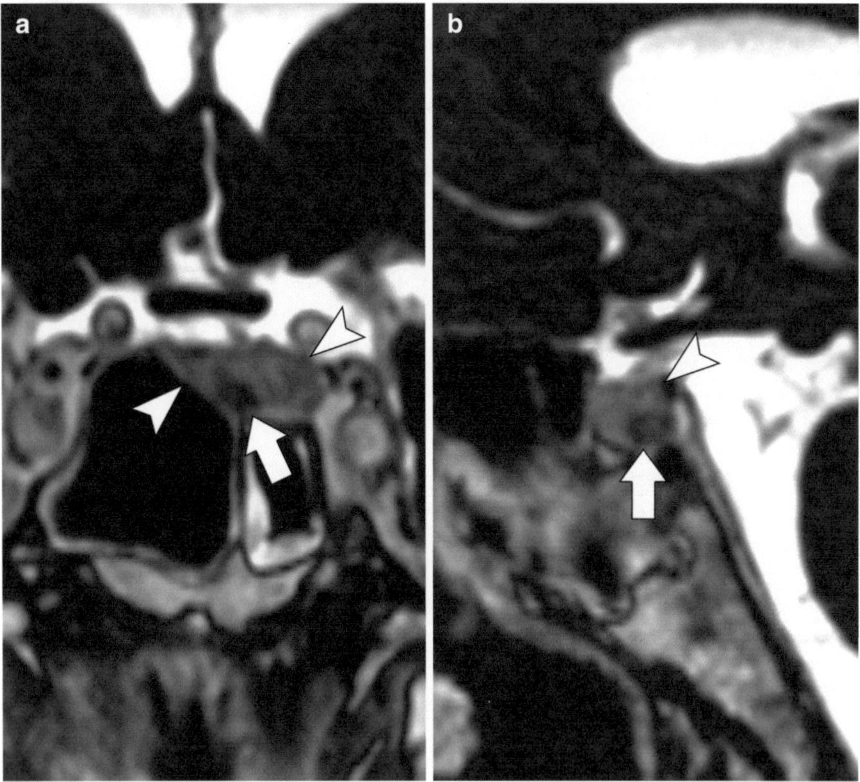

Fig. 4.4 Coronal (**a**) and sagittal (**b**) post-contrast CISS sequences through the pituitary gland demonstrate a hypoenhancing microadenoma (arrows) surrounded by the avidly enhancing pituitary parenchyma (arrowheads). Note deviation of the infundibulum to the left

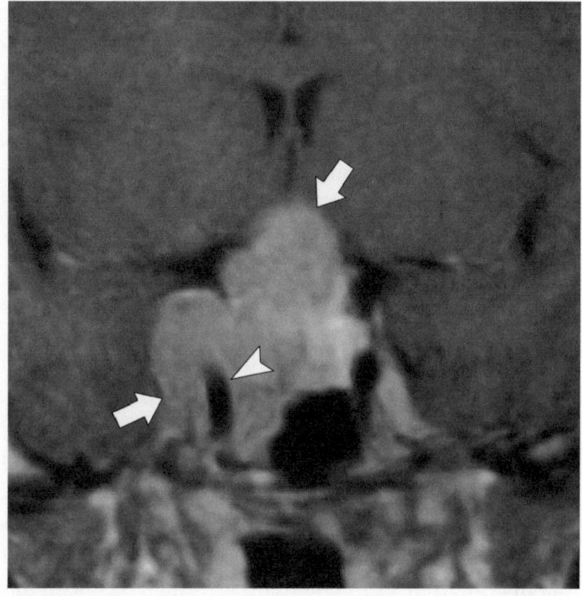

Fig. 4.5 Coronal post-contrast T1-weighted image demonstrates a macroadenoma (arrows) with cavernous sinus invasion completely encasing the right internal carotid artery (arrowhead)

predictive finding is complete carotid encasement (grade 4) with 100% invasion rate (Fig. 4.5) [47–49]. The rate of cavernous sinus invasion for grade 1 and 2 lesions is 2% and 10%, respectively [47].

Ectopic ACTH Syndrome

Ectopic ACTH production accounts for 20% of ACTH-dependent hypercortisolism and is most commonly secondary to small cell carcinoma of the lung and bronchial carcinoid tumors [50]. In patients with ACTH-dependent hypercortisolism who have a negative or equivocal MRI and non-localizing inferior petrosal sinus sampling, imaging evaluation of the neck, chest, and abdomen is indicated utilizing CT or MRI [51]. If a lesion remains undetected, one can proceed with nuclear medicine studies, such as somatostatin analogue scans or F-18 fluorodeoxyglucose (FDG) positron emission tomography (PET).

Thoracic Sources of Ectopic ACTH Production

Because thoracic tumors represent the most common etiology of ectopic ACTH syndrome, the most appropriate initial investigation is a chest CT. In a study evaluating 383 patients with ectopic ACTH syndrome, 23% were secondary to bronchial carcinoid, and 22% were due to small cell lung cancer, followed by 13% of patients with gastroenterohepatic neuroendocrine tumors [52].

Bronchial carcinoid tumors are neuroendocrine neoplasms, ranging from low-grade typical lesions to more aggressive high-grade neoplasms. They most commonly occur in association with a segmental or larger caliber bronchus but may also occur peripherally [53]. Carcinoid tumors present as hilar or perihilar masses that are usually round, well-circumscribed, and slightly lobulated. Foci of calcification or ossification are common [54]. Because carcinoids are highly vascular tumors, most lesions show avid and homogeneous contrast enhancement following the intravenous administration of iodinated contrast material [54]. FDG-PET is based on the evaluation of glucose metabolism and has shown some utility in detecting bronchial carcinoids that are not seen on conventional chest CT (Fig. 4.6). A meta-analysis showed a pooled sensitivity of 71% of FDG-PET to detect bronchial carcinoids [55]. However, because the majority of these tumors have a low metabolic rate, they may be more difficult to visualize than lung malignancies, which usually show very avid FDG uptake. Therefore, the absence of an FDG-avid lesion cannot reliably exclude the presence of a bronchial carcinoid [56]. Because carcinoid tumors are rich in somatostatin receptors, they may be imaged utilizing different radiotracers. Gallium (Ga)-68 DOTA-peptide, a somatostatin analogue, can be used in conjunction with PET and has shown much higher affinity to somatostatin receptors than Indium 111 pentetreotide, which has been the gold standard for over two decades [57]. Ga-68 DOTA-peptide has higher sensitivity for the detection of primary pulmonary carcinoids compared with F-18 FDG-PET (90% vs. 71%, respectively) [55].

Small cell lung cancer typically presents as a hilar mass with bulky mediastinal adenopathy. Although the size of the primary tumor may be relatively small, these

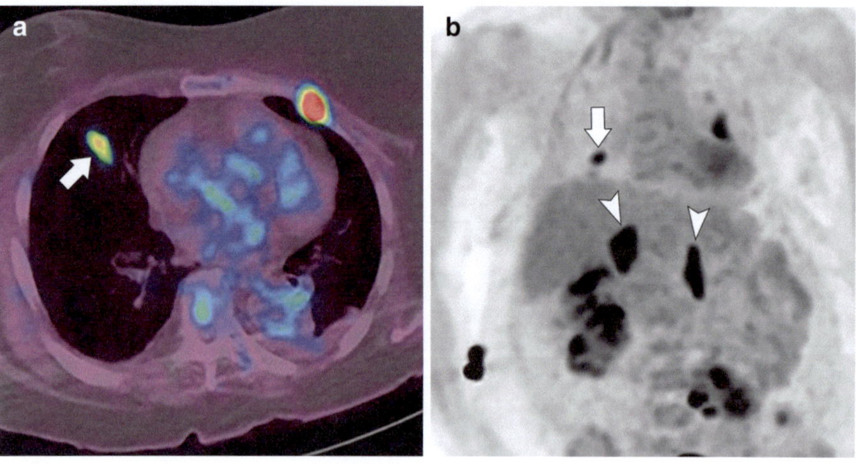

Fig. 4.6 Axial fused F-18 FDG-PET/CT (**a**) demonstrates avid uptake in a right bronchial carcinoid (arrow). A separate focus of uptake in the left anterior chest corresponds to a rib fracture. Frontal view from whole-body F-18 FDG-PET (**b**) shows the right bronchial carcinoid (arrow) and increased uptake in the adrenal glands (arrowheads) due to overstimulation. (Image courtesy of Edgar Zamora, MD, Montefiore Medical Center, The Bronx, NY)

tumors have a rapid doubling time and vascular invasion is common [58]. Lesions are usually lobulated and are less likely to show the characteristic spiculation that is commonly seen in primary lung malignancies [59]. CT has traditionally been used for lesion identification and to characterize the extent of intrathoracic disease; however, more recent studies have shown FDG-PET to be highly sensitive and more accurate in determining the stage and treatment response [60].

Abdominal Sources of Ectopic ACTH Production

Thirteen percent of ectopic ACTH production cases are secondary to gastroenterohepatic neuroectodermal tumors, most commonly pancreatic islet cell tumors, intestinal carcinoids, and pheochromocytomas [52]. After ruling out an ectopic thoracic source, the presence of abdominal lesions can be initially investigated with contrast-enhanced CT or MRI. Pancreatic neuroendocrine tumors are typically round and well-circumscribed and, due to a rich capillary network, show avid contrast enhancement on both CT and MRI. Contrast enhancement is usually homogeneous but may be ring-like or heterogeneous, particularly in larger lesions [61]. Although protocols vary by institution, a typical approach on CT is to image the abdomen in both arterial and venous phases (20–25 and 55–70 s after intravenous contrast injection, respectively) as the lesion may be detectable in one phase but not the other [61, 62].

The small intestine is the most common location for gastrointestinal carcinoids, which are most frequently located in the distal ileum [63]. Like their bronchial counterparts, small intestine carcinoids are highly vascular masses that show avid contrast enhancement, and calcification is common. Because they are generally small, the sensitivity of conventional CT or MRI for detection of a primary lesion is low. However, studies have shown improved detection with multiphasic CT utilizing neutral oral contrast (e.g., water or low-attenuation barium sulfate suspension) [64]. Gastrointestinal carcinoids most commonly metastasize to the liver and lymph nodes. Mesenteric metastases can have a desmoplastic reaction resulting in a spiculated, "spoke-like" appearance of the mesenteric vessels [65]. As mentioned in the preceding section, the use of FDG-PET may be limited due to the low metabolic activity of most carcinoids, while somatostatin receptor scintigraphy is more sensitive [66].

ACTH-Independent Hypercortisolism

Abdominal imaging is indicated in patients with ACTH-independent hypercortisolism to evaluate a possible adrenal source [51]. CT is highly accurate for the detection and characterization of adrenal lesions and is usually the first imaging modality; however, MRI may also be utilized. Adrenal adenomas are typically round and well-circumscribed. Functioning lesions resulting in Cushing's syndrome are typically larger than 2 cm and readily identifiable [67]. Approximately 70% of adrenal adenomas are rich in lipids leading to low attenuation on noncontrast CT. An attenuation value of less than 10 Hounsfield units on noncontrast CT has demonstrated a sensitivity of 71% and specificity of 98% for diagnosis of an adenoma [68]. Those that are lipid poor (and which therefore do not have low attenuation on noncontrast CT) can be investigated with contrast-enhanced CT using venous (60–75 s) and delayed (15 min) scans, although protocols vary by institution [69]. Because of their rich vascularity, adrenal adenomas demonstrate rapid washin and rapid washout of contrast material, compared with non-adenomatous lesions which tend to wash out more slowly [67]. The diagnosis of adrenal adenomas on MRI is based on the "chemical shift" phenomenon. Because of slight differences in the magnetic resonant frequencies of water and fat molecules, lipid-rich adenomas demonstrate decreased signal intensity on out-of-phase MRI sequences [69]. Notably, the majority of adrenal adenomas are nonfunctioning. The distinction between functioning and nonfunctioning lesions cannot be made on imaging findings alone and may necessitate adrenal venous sampling [70]. In patients with primary pigmented nodular adrenal disease, the adrenal glands typically show multiple small nodules with interposed atrophy of the adrenal cortex, although findings can also be normal on CT. In macronodular adrenal hyperplasia, the glands appear massively enlarged and distorted with multiple nodules of varying sizes (Fig. 4.7) [71].

Adrenal cortical carcinomas are aggressive malignancies that may result in ACTH-independent hypercortisolism or primary aldosteronism. The majority are large at presentation and commonly present with necrosis, hemorrhage, and heterogeneous contrast enhancement [72]. Calcification is seen in 24% of patients [73]. Signal intensities on MRI are variable and depend on the extent of hemorrhage, necrosis, and calcification [74].

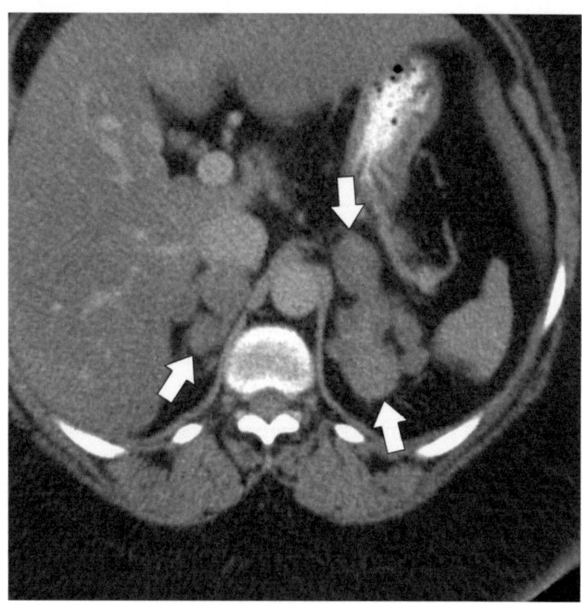

Fig. 4.7 Axial post-contrast CT demonstrates marked enlargement of the adrenal glands with nodules of varying sizes (arrows) in a patient with hypercortisolism secondary to ACTH-independent macronodular adrenal hyperplasia. (Image courtesy of Israel Saramago, MD, UNC Health, Chapel Hill, NC)

References

1. Lindholm J, Juul S, Jørgensen JO, Astrup J, Bjerre P, Feldt-Rasmussen U, Hagen C, Jørgensen J, Kosteljanetz M, Kristensen L, Laurberg P, Schmidt K, Weeke J. Incidence and late prognosis of Cushing's syndrome: a population-based study. J Clin Endocrinol Metab. 2001;86(1):117–23.
2. Bolland MJ, Holdaway IM, Berkeley JE, Lim S, Dransfield WJ, Conaglen JV, Croxson MS, Gamble GD, Hunt PJ, Toomath RJ. Mortality and morbidity in Cushing's syndrome in New Zealand. Clin Endocrinol. 2011;75(4):436–42.
3. Steffensen C, Bak AM, Rubeck KZ, Jørgensen JO. Epidemiology of Cushing's syndrome. Neuroendocrinology. 2010;92(Suppl 1):1–5.
4. Valassi E, Santos A, Yaneva M, Tóth M, Strasburger CJ, Chanson P, Wass JA, Chabre O, Pfeifer M, Feelders RA, Tsagarakis S, Trainer PJ, Franz H, Zopf K, Zacharieva S, Lamberts SW, Tabarin A, Webb SM, ERCUSYN Study Group. The European Registry on Cushing's syndrome: 2-year experience. Baseline demographic and clinical characteristics. Eur J Endocrinol. 2011;165(3):383–92.
5. Porterfield JR, Thompson GB, Young WF Jr, Chow JT, Fryrear RS, van Heerden JA, Farley DR, Atkinson JL, Meyer FB, Abboud CF, Nippoldt TB, Natt N, Erickson D, Vella A, Carpenter PC, Richards M, Carney JA, Larson D, Schleck C, Churchward M, Grant CS. Surgery for Cushing's syndrome: an historical review and recent ten-year experience. World J Surg. 2008;32(5):659–77.
6. Graversen D, Vestergaard P, Stochholm K, Gravholt CH, Jørgensen JO. Mortality in Cushing's syndrome: a systematic review and meta-analysis. Eur J Intern Med. 2012;23(3):278–82.
7. Yaneva M, Kalinov K, Zacharieva S. Mortality in Cushing's syndrome: data from 386 patients from a single tertiary referral center. Eur J Endocrinol. 2013;169(5):621–7.
8. Catargi B, Rigalleau V, Poussin A, Ronci-Chaix N, Bex V, Vergnot V, Gin H, Roger P, Tabarin A. Occult Cushing's syndrome in type-2 diabetes. J Clin Endocrinol Metab. 2003;88(12):5808–13.
9. Chiodini I, Mascia ML, Muscarella S, Battista C, Minisola S, Arosio M, Santini SA, Guglielmi G, Carnevale V, Scillitani A. Subclinical hypercortisolism among outpatients referred for osteoporosis. Ann Intern Med. 2007;147(8):541–8.
10. Nieman LK, Biller BM, Findling JW, Newell-Price J, Savage MO, Stewart PM, Montori VM. The diagnosis of Cushing's syndrome: an Endocrine Society clinical practice guideline. J Clin Endocrinol Metab. 2008;93(5):1526–40.
11. Katznelson L, Bogan JS, Trob JR, Schoenfeld DA, Hedley-Whyte ET, Hsu DW, Zervas NT, Swearingen B, Sleeper M, Klibanski A. Biochemical assessment of Cushing's disease in patients with corticotroph macroadenomas. J Clin Endocrinol Metab. 1998;83(5):1619–23.
12. Zhou Y, Zhang X, Klibanski A. Genetic and epigenetic mutations of tumor suppressive genes in sporadic pituitary adenoma. Mol Cell Endocrinol. 2014;386(1–2):16–33.
13. Huizenga NA, de Lange P, Koper JW, Clayton RN, Farrell WE, van der Lely AJ, Brinkmann AO, de Jong FH, Lamberts SW. Human adrenocorticotropin-secreting pituitary adenomas show frequent loss of heterozygosity at the glucocorticoid receptor gene locus. J Clin Endocrinol Metab. 1998;83(3):917–21.
14. Raff H, Findling JW. A physiologic approach to diagnosis of the Cushing syndrome. Ann Intern Med. 2003;138(12):980–91.
15. Aniszewski JP, Young WF Jr, Thompson GB, Grant CS, van Heerden JA. Cushing syndrome due to ectopic adrenocorticotropic hormone secretion. World J Surg. 2001;25(7):934–40.
16. de Keyzer Y, Lenne F, Auzan C, Jégou S, René P, Vaudry H, Kuhn JM, Luton JP, Clauser E, Bertagna X. The pituitary V3 vasopressin receptor and the corticotroph phenotype in ectopic ACTH syndrome. J Clin Invest. 1996;97(5):1311–8.
17. Zilbermint M, Stratakis CA. Protein kinase A defects and cortisol-producing adrenal tumors. Curr Opin Endocrinol Diabetes Obes. 2015;22(3):157–62.

18. Bourdeau I, Lampron A, Costa MH, Tadjine M, Lacroix A. Adrenocorticotropic hormone-independent Cushing's syndrome. Curr Opin Endocrinol Diabetes Obes. 2007;14(3):219–25.
19. Allolio B, Fassnacht M. Clinical review: adrenocortical carcinoma: clinical update. J Clin Endocrinol Metab. 2006;91(6):2027–37.
20. Luton JP, Cerdas S, Billaud L, Thomas G, Guilhaume B, Bertagna X, Laudat MH, Louvel A, Chapuis Y, Blondeau P, et al. Clinical features of adrenocortical carcinoma, prognostic factors, and the effect of mitotane therapy. N Engl J Med. 1990;322(17):1195–201.
21. Koch CA, Pacak K, Chrousos GP. The molecular pathogenesis of hereditary and sporadic adrenocortical and adrenomedullary tumors. J Clin Endocrinol Metab. 2002;87(12):5367–84.
22. Hsiao HP, Kirschner LS, Bourdeau I, Keil MF, Boikos SA, Verma S, Robinson-White AJ, Nesterova M, Lacroix A, Stratakis CA. Clinical and genetic heterogeneity, overlap with other tumor syndromes, and atypical glucocorticoid hormone secretion in adrenocorticotropin-independent macronodular adrenal hyperplasia compared with other adrenocortical tumors. J Clin Endocrinol Metab. 2009;94(8):2930–7.
23. De Venanzi A, Alencar GA, Bourdeau I, Fragoso MC, Lacroix A. Primary bilateral macronodular adrenal hyperplasia. Curr Opin Endocrinol Diabetes Obes. 2014;21(3):177–84.
24. Stratakis CA, Kirschner LS, Carney JA. Clinical and molecular features of the Carney complex: diagnostic criteria and recommendations for patient evaluation. J Clin Endocrinol Metab. 2001;86(9):4041–6.
25. Wajchenberg BL, Bosco A, Marone MM, Levin S, Rocha M, Lerário AC, Nery M, Goldman J, Liberman B. Estimation of body fat and lean tissue distribution by dual energy X-ray absorptiometry and abdominal body fat evaluation by computed tomography in Cushing's disease. J Clin Endocrinol Metab. 1995;80(9):2791–4.
26. Corenblum B, Kwan T, Gee S, Wong NC. Bedside assessment of skin-fold thickness. A useful measurement for distinguishing Cushing's disease from other causes of hirsutism and oligomenorrhea. Arch Intern Med. 1994;154(7):777–81.
27. Pivonello R, Isidori AM, De Martino MC, Newell-Price J, Biller BM, Colao A. Complications of Cushing's syndrome: state of the art. Lancet Diabetes Endocrinol. 2016;4(7):611–29.
28. Dekkers OM, Horváth-Puhó E, Jørgensen JO, Cannegieter SC, Ehrenstein V, Vandenbroucke JP, Pereira AM, Sørensen HT. Multisystem morbidity and mortality in Cushing's syndrome: a cohort study. J Clin Endocrinol Metab. 2013;98(6):2277–84.
29. Mancini T, Kola B, Mantero F, Boscaro M, Arnaldi G. High cardiovascular risk in patients with Cushing's syndrome according to 1999 WHO/ISH guidelines. Clin Endocrinol. 2004;61(6):768–77.
30. Van Zaane B, Nur E, Squizzato A, Dekkers OM, Twickler MT, Fliers E, Gerdes VE, Büller HR, Brandjes DP. Hypercoagulable state in Cushing's syndrome: a systematic review. J Clin Endocrinol Metab. 2009;94(8):2743–50.
31. Ntali G, Asimakopoulou A, Siamatras T, Komninos J, Vassiliadi D, Tzanela M, Tsagarakis S, Grossman AB, Wass JA, Karavitaki N. Mortality in Cushing's syndrome: systematic analysis of a large series with prolonged follow-up. Eur J Endocrinol. 2013;169(5):715–23.
32. Sarlis NJ, Chanock SJ, Nieman LK. Cortisolemic indices predict severe infections in Cushing syndrome due to ectopic production of adrenocorticotropin. J Clin Endocrinol Metab. 2000;85(1):42–7.
33. Pivonello R, Simeoli C, De Martino MC, Cozzolino A, De Leo M, Iacuaniello D, Pivonello C, Negri M, Pellecchia MT, Iasevoli F, Colao A. Neuropsychiatric disorders in Cushing's syndrome. Front Neurosci. 2015;9:129.
34. Elamin MB, Murad MH, Mullan R, Erickson D, Harris K, Nadeem S, Ennis R, Erwin PJ, Montori VM. Accuracy of diagnostic tests for Cushing's syndrome: a systematic review and metaanalyses. J Clin Endocrinol Metab. 2008;93(5):1553–62.
35. Arnaldi G, Angeli A, Atkinson AB, Bertagna X, Cavagnini F, Chrousos GP, Fava GA, Findling JW, Gaillard RC, Grossman AB, Kola B, Lacroix A, Mancini T, Mantero F, Newell-Price J, Nieman LK, Sonino N, Vance ML, Giustina A, Boscaro M. Diagnosis and complications of Cushing's syndrome: a consensus statement. J Clin Endocrinol Metab. 2003;88(12):5593–602.

36. Lacroix A, Feelders RA, Stratakis CA, Nieman LK. Cushing's syndrome. Lancet. 2015;386(9996):913–27.
37. Reimondo G, Paccotti P, Minetto M, Termine A, Stura G, Bergui M, Angeli A, Terzolo M. The corticotrophin-releasing hormone test is the most reliable noninvasive method to differentiate pituitary from ectopic ACTH secretion in Cushing's syndrome. Clin Endocrinol. 2003;58(6):718–24.
38. Dichek HL, Nieman LK, Oldfield EH, Pass HI, Malley JD, Cutler GB Jr. A comparison of the standard high dose dexamethasone suppression test and the overnight 8-mg dexamethasone suppression test for the differential diagnosis of adrenocorticotropin-dependent Cushing's syndrome. J Clin Endocrinol Metab. 1994;78(2):418–22.
39. Peck WW, Dillon WP, Norman D, Newton TH, Wilson CB. High-resolution MR imaging of pituitary microadenomas at 1.5 T: experience with Cushing disease. AJR Am J Roentgenol. 1989;152(1):145–51.
40. Sakamoto Y, Takahashi M, Korogi Y, Bussaka H, Ushio Y. Normal and abnormal pituitary glands: gadopentetate dimeglumine-enhanced MR imaging. Radiology. 1991;178(2):441–5.
41. Friedman TC, Zuckerbraun E, Lee ML, Kabil MS, Shahinian H. Dynamic pituitary MRI has high sensitivity and specificity for the diagnosis of mild Cushing's syndrome and should be part of the initial workup. Horm Metab Res. 2007;39(6):451–6.
42. Tabarin A, Laurent F, Catargi B, Olivier-Puel F, Lescene R, Berge J, et al. Comparative evaluation of conventional and dynamic magnetic resonance imaging of the pituitary gland for the diagnosis of Cushing's disease. Clin Endocrinol. 1998;49(3):293–300.
43. Grober Y, Grober H, Wintermark M, Jane JA, Oldfield EH. Comparison of MRI techniques for detecting microadenomas in Cushing's disease. J Neurosurg. 2018;128(4):1051–7.
44. Lang M, Habboub G, Moon D, Bandyopadhyay A, Silva D, Kennedy L, et al. Comparison of constructive interference in steady-state and T1-weighted MRI sequence at detecting pituitary adenomas in Cushing's disease patients. J Neurol Surg B Skull Base. 2018;79(6):593–8.
45. Ajlan A, Achrol AS, Albakr A, Feroze AH, Westbroek EM, Hwang P, et al. Cavernous sinus involvement by pituitary adenomas: clinical implications and outcomes of endoscopic endonasal resection. J Neurol Surg B Skull Base. 2017;78(3):273–82.
46. Knosp E, Steiner E, Kitz K, Matula C. Pituitary adenomas with invasion of the cavernous sinus space: a magnetic resonance imaging classification compared with surgical findings. Neurosurgery. 1993;33(4):610–7; discussion 7–8
47. Micko AS, Wohrer A, Wolfsberger S, Knosp E. Invasion of the cavernous sinus space in pituitary adenomas: endoscopic verification and its correlation with an MRI-based classification. J Neurosurg. 2015;122(4):803–11.
48. Buchy M, Lapras V, Rabilloud M, Vasiljevic A, Borson-Chazot F, Jouanneau E, et al. Predicting early post-operative remission in pituitary adenomas: evaluation of the modified knosp classification. Pituitary. 2019;22(5):467–75.
49. Cottier JP, Destrieux C, Brunereau L, Bertrand P, Moreau L, Jan M, et al. Cavernous sinus invasion by pituitary adenoma: MR imaging. Radiology. 2000;215(2):463–9.
50. Newell-Price J, Bertagna X, Grossman AB, Nieman LK. Cushing's syndrome. Lancet. 2006;367(9522):1605–17.
51. Wagner-Bartak NA, Baiomy A, Habra MA, Mukhi SV, Morani AC, Korivi BR, et al. Cushing syndrome: diagnostic workup and imaging features, with clinical and pathologic correlation. AJR Am J Roentgenol. 2017;209(1):19–32.
52. Ejaz S, Vassilopoulou-Sellin R, Busaidy NL, Hu MI, Waguespack SG, Jimenez C, et al. Cushing syndrome secondary to ectopic adrenocorticotropic hormone secretion: the University of Texas MD Anderson Cancer Center Experience. Cancer. 2011;117(19):4381–9.
53. Zwiebel BR, Austin JH, Grimes MM. Bronchial carcinoid tumors: assessment with CT of location and intratumoral calcification in 31 patients. Radiology. 1991;179(2):483–6.
54. Jeung MY, Gasser B, Gangi A, Charneau D, Ducroq X, Kessler R, et al. Bronchial carcinoid tumors of the thorax: spectrum of radiologic findings. Radiographics. 2002;22(2):351–65.

55. Jiang Y, Hou G, Cheng W. The utility of 18F-FDG and 68Ga-DOTA-peptide PET/CT in the evaluation of primary pulmonary carcinoid: a systematic review and meta-analysis. Medicine (Baltimore). 2019;98(10):e14769.
56. Tatci E, Ozmen O, Gokcek A, Biner IU, Ozaydin E, Kaya S, et al. 18F-FDG PET/CT rarely provides additional information other than primary tumor detection in patients with pulmonary carcinoid tumors. Ann Thorac Med. 2014;9(4):227–31.
57. Deppen SA, Liu E, Blume JD, Clanton J, Shi C, Jones-Jackson LB, et al. Safety and efficacy of 68Ga-DOTATATE PET/CT for diagnosis, staging, and treatment management of neuroendocrine tumors. J Nucl Med. 2016;57(5):708–14.
58. Carter BW, Glisson BS, Truong MT, Erasmus JJ. Small cell lung carcinoma: staging, imaging, and treatment considerations. Radiographics. 2014;34(6):1707–21.
59. Lee D, Rho JY, Kang S, Yoo KJ, Choi HJ. CT findings of small cell lung carcinoma: can recognizable features be found? Medicine (Baltimore). 2016;95(47):e5426.
60. Kut V, Spies W, Spies S, Gooding W, Argiris A. Staging and monitoring of small cell lung cancer using [18F]fluoro-2-deoxy-D-glucose-positron emission tomography (FDG-PET). Am J Clin Oncol. 2007;30(1):45–50.
61. Lewis RB, Lattin GE Jr, Paal E. Pancreatic endocrine tumors: radiologic-clinicopathologic correlation. Radiographics. 2010;30(6):1445–64.
62. Tamm EP, Bhosale P, Lee JH, Rohren EM. State-of-the-art imaging of pancreatic neuroendocrine tumors. Surg Oncol Clin N Am. 2016;25(2):375–400.
63. Levy AD, Sobin LH. From the archives of the AFIP: gastrointestinal carcinoids: imaging features with clinicopathologic comparison. Radiographics. 2007;27(1):237–57.
64. Ganeshan D, Bhosale P, Yang T, Kundra V. Imaging features of carcinoid tumors of the gastrointestinal tract. AJR Am J Roentgenol. 2013;201(4):773–86.
65. Giambelluca D, Cannella R, Midiri M, Salvaggio G. The "spoke wheel" sign in mesenteric carcinoid. Abdom Radiol (NY). 2019;44(5):1949–50.
66. Evangelista L, Ravelli I, Bignotto A, Cecchin D, Zucchetta P. Ga-68 DOTA-peptides and F-18 FDG PET/CT in patients with neuroendocrine tumor: a review. Clin Imaging. 2020;67:113–6.
67. Lattin GE Jr, Sturgill ED, Tujo CA, Marko J, Sanchez-Maldonado KW, Craig WD, et al. From the radiologic pathology archives: adrenal tumors and tumor-like conditions in the adult: radiologic-pathologic correlation. Radiographics. 2014;34(3):805–29.
68. Boland GW, Lee MJ, Gazelle GS, Halpern EF, McNicholas MM, Mueller PR. Characterization of adrenal masses using unenhanced CT: an analysis of the CT literature. AJR Am J Roentgenol. 1998;171(1):201–4.
69. Blake MA, Cronin CG, Boland GW. Adrenal imaging. AJR Am J Roentgenol. 2010;194(6):1450–60.
70. Papakokkinou E, Jakobsson H, Sakinis A, Muth A, Wangberg B, Ehn O, et al. Adrenal venous sampling in patients with ACTH-independent hypercortisolism. Endocrine. 2019;66(2):338–48.
71. Rockall AG, Babar SA, Sohaib SA, Isidori AM, Diaz-Cano S, Monson JP, et al. CT and MR imaging of the adrenal glands in ACTH-independent Cushing syndrome. Radiographics. 2004;24(2):435–52.
72. Bharwani N, Rockall AG, Sahdev A, Gueorguiev M, Drake W, Grossman AB, et al. Adrenocortical carcinoma: the range of appearances on CT and MRI. AJR Am J Roentgenol. 2011;196(6):W706–14.
73. Fishman EK, Deutch BM, Hartman DS, Goldman SM, Zerhouni EA, Siegelman SS. Primary adrenocortical carcinoma: CT evaluation with clinical correlation. AJR Am J Roentgenol. 1987;148(3):531–5.
74. Elsayes KM, Mukundan G, Narra VR, Lewis JS Jr, Shirkhoda A, Farooki A, et al. Adrenal masses: MR imaging features with pathologic correlation. Radiographics. 2004;24(Suppl 1):S73–86.

Chapter 5
Clinical, Laboratory, and Radiological Diagnosis of Pancreatic Islet Cell Tumors

Jashalynn German, Lauren M. B. Burke, and Jennifer V. Rowell

Introduction

Neuroendocrine tumors (NETs) include a diverse group of tumors that stem from a lineage of sensory/neural and secretory cells. There is heterogeneity among specific tumor types, but they share certain biological characteristics. NETs are predominately located within the bronchopulmonary and gastrointestinal systems [1]. For the scope of this chapter, we will focus on a subset of NETs that derive from the pancreas. Pancreatic endocrine tumors (PETs) may also be referred to as pancreatic neuroendocrine tumors, as pancreatic islet cell tumors, and, historically, as islet of Langerhans tumors [2].

The diagnosis of PETs is based on clinical presentation, laboratory data, and, often, a variety of imaging findings, all of which may vary based on the specific neoplasm. PETs may range in presentation from nonfunctioning to hormone-secreting tumors or aggressive debilitating malignancies [2]. Nonfunctioning tumors may be discovered incidentally on imaging, and patients may be without noticeable symptoms, while other patients may present with nonspecific symptoms such as abdominal pain, which may be due to local compression/mass effect secondary to primary tumor growth, vascular invasion, or metastatic disease [3]. Functional PETs may present with a specific pattern of syndromes due to ectopic release of hormones, including insulinomas, gastrinomas, VIPomas, etc. [4–7]. This chapter will discuss these functional PETs in more detail (Table 5.1).

J. German (✉) · J. V. Rowell
Department of Medicine, Division of Endocrinology, Metabolism and Nutrition, Duke University, Durham, NC, USA
e-mail: Jashalynn.german@duke.edu; Jennifer.rowell@duke.edu

L. M. B. Burke
Department of Radiology, Division of Abdominal Imaging, University of North Carolina School of Medicine, Chapel Hill, NC, USA
e-mail: Lauren_burke@med.unc.edu

© The Author(s), under exclusive license to Springer Nature Switzerland AG 2022

H. Yu et al. (eds.), *Diagnosis and Management of Endocrine Disorders in Interventional Radiology*, https://doi.org/10.1007/978-3-030-87189-5_5

Table 5.1 Tumor characteristics

Tumor name (associated hormone)	Estimated incidence	Clinical presentation characteristics	Laboratory data	Tumor characteristics
Gastrinoma (gastrin)	1–3 per million population	Recurrent peptic ulcer disease, severe gastroesophageal reflux, diarrhea	Fasting gastrin levels >500 pg/mL or >fivefold the upper limit OR gastrin level rising above 200 pg/mL or doubling from baseline after secretin administration	MEN1 frequently associated with multiple tumors, high risk of malignancy (approx. half are metastasized at time of diagnosis)
Glucagonoma (glucagon)	Less than 0.1 per million population	Necrolytic migratory erythema, new-onset diabetes mellitus or worsening glycemia, higher risk for acute deep venous thrombosis and pulmonary embolism	Plasma glucagon levels >500 pg/mL or 10–20-fold from normal reference ranges	Typically a solitary tumor with a relatively larger size than other panNets, and approximately 50–80% are metastatic at diagnosis
Insulinoma (insulin)	1–2 per million population	Whipple's triad: • Confirmatory fasting hypoglycemia • Neuroglycopenic symptoms and/or autonomic nervous system dysfunction • Improvement in symptoms with resolution of hypoglycemia	All of the following: • Plasma glucose less than 55 mg/dl • Insulin $\geq$3.0 µU/m • C-peptide $\geq$0.6 ng/mL • Proinsulin $\geq$5.0 pmol/L • Negative insulin antibodies • Negative oral hypoglycemic agent screen	Solitary neoplasms or multiple pancreatic tumors which may be benign or malignant in nature
Somatostatinoma (somatostatin)	Less than 0.1 per million population	Abdominal pain, triad of glucose intolerance/diabetes mellitus, cholelithiasis, and steatorrhea	Elevated fasting plasma levels of somatostatin (usually exceeding 30 pg/mL)	Larger primary tumors (median size pancreatic tumor 4.25 cm) and >70% are malignant with the majority having metastasis at time of diagnosis

Table 5.1   (continued)

Tumor name (associated hormone)	Estimated incidence	Clinical presentation characteristics	Laboratory data	Tumor characteristics
VIPoma (vasoactive intestinal peptide)	0.1 per million population	Recurrent episodes of facial flushing, severe secretory watery diarrhea, hypokalemia, and hypochlorhydria or achlorhydria	VIP levels higher than 500 pg/mL	More than 60% of VIPomas are malignant, with up to 60% having metastasized to lymph nodes, liver, kidneys, or bone

Etiology/Physiology

Historically, gastroenteropancreatic NETs were classified based on embryologic origin, with tumors of the pancreas considered to arise from the foregut along with tumors of the pulmonary tree, stomach, gallbladder, and duodenum [8]. The pancreas has exocrine and endocrine functions. The majority of the gland is made up of acinar cells, involved in exocrine function pathways, and, to a lesser extent, areas of secretory tissue formally called islet of Langerhans cells. These specialized secretory cells arise from endoderm and neuroectodermal precursors [9]. PETs originate from these heterogeneous populations of cells, with shared characteristics including amine and neuropeptide hormone production and secretion in dense-core vesicles [10].

Gastroenteropancreatic endocrine cells have characteristic neuroendocrine markers, including synaptophysin, the most sensitive, and chromogranin A, the most specific marker [11]. In addition, there are additional markers such as CDX2, Islet 1 (ISL-1), which are specific to endocrine cell subtypes and are beneficial in instances of metastatic disease from an unknown primary site [12]. PETs may present sporadically or in association with hereditary genetic mutations that predispose patients to well-differentiated NETs such as multiple endocrine neoplasia syndrome 1 (MEN1), neurofibromatosis 1, and von Hippel-Lindau disease [1].

The World Health Organization (WHO) has released guidance on the classification of NETs based on histologic features. The grading of NETs is based on mitotic counts and the Ki-67 labeling index. The American Joint Committee on Cancer (AJCC) staging of gastroenteropancreatic NETs uses a TNM system based on primary tumor characteristics. The TNM system involves assessing the primary tumor size (<2 cm, 2–4 cm, >4 cm), presence of invasion of adjacent organs, involvement of regional lymph nodes, and distant metastasis (hepatic vs. extrahepatic) [13].

Epidemiology

The incidence of all NET is estimated to have increased from 3.6- to 4.8-fold over the past four decades [14–16]. The incidence of gastroenteropancreatic NET has increased over recent years, now annually, approximating 5.25 per 100,000 [17]. The current incidence of PETs is estimated to be 0.32–0.8 per 100,000 cases [18]. Rising incidence is related to advances in imaging technology and an aging population [19, 20].

According to the Surveillance, Epidemiology, and End Results (SEER) database, from 1973 to 2000, most PETs diagnosed were nonfunctional tumors (90.8%). Nonfunctional PETs include tumors that do not produce hormones, tumors that produce hormones at a low enough level to not cause classic syndromes, or tumors that produce hormones but do not cause symptoms. Examples include pancreatic polypeptide, chromogranin A, ghrelin, calcitonin, or neurotensin. Chromogranin A is detectable in the plasma of patients with a range of neuroendocrine neoplasms, including nonfunctional PETs. Patients who present with PETs in the setting of genetic mutations such as MEN1 are more likely to present at younger ages and are more likely to have multifocal tumors. Sporadic cases commonly present with solitary masses during the 5th decade of life [21].

Insulinoma

Etiology/Pathophysiology

Insulinomas are PETs that secrete excessive amounts of insulin, a peptide hormone that has effects on glucose metabolism, including inhibition of glycogenolysis and gluconeogenesis, increased glucose transport into fat and muscle, increased glycolysis in fat and muscle, and stimulation of glycogen synthesis [22]. Evolving research has brought new histological data on the origin of insulinomas. It is believed that these tumors arise from cells of the ductular/acinar system of the pancreas rather than from neoplastic proliferation of islet cells, as previously thought [23]. Presenting symptoms are related to severe hypoglycemia due to loss of homeostasis of the pathways mentioned above.

Epidemiology

Insulinomas are one of the most common types of functional PETs, with an annual incidence of 1–2 per million [18]. Insulinomas can present as solitary neoplasms or multiple pancreatic tumors, which may be benign or malignant in nature, defined as the presence of metastases. The majority of insulinomas are sporadic and are usually diagnosed after the 5th decade of life, while the minority of insulinomas related to MEN1 syndrome (10%) tend to occur before the 4th decade of life [24, 25].

Clinical Evaluation

Patients with insulinomas often present with Whipple's triad, consisting of (1) laboratory proven hypoglycemia, (2) neuroglycopenic symptoms (e.g., vision changes, confusion, coma, or seizure) and autonomic dysfunction (e.g., diaphoresis, palpitations, tremors, anxiety), and (3) improvement in symptoms with resolution of hypoglycemia [1, 24]. Hypoglycemia due to insulinomas is often related to exercise or periods of fasting [24]; a subset of patients experience postprandial hypoglycemia [25].

Laboratory Evaluation

Before pursuing imaging or invasive procedures, it is important to exclude other more common causes of hypoglycemia, including factitious hypoglycemia or that which is secondary to other medical conditions such as severe liver or renal impairment or sepsis. Insulinomas can be diagnosed based on biochemical evaluation during medically supervised fasting periods, which traditionally can last up to 72 h. A positive fasting test that is consistent with excess endogenous insulin includes a confirmatory negative oral hypoglycemic agent screen, plasma concentrations of glucose less than 55 mg/dl (3.0 mmol/L), insulin of at least 3.0 µU/mL (18 pmol/L), C-peptide of at least 0.6 ng/mL (0.2 nmol/L), and proinsulin of at least 5.0 pmol/L [26, 27].

Gastrinoma

Etiology/Pathophysiology

Gastrinomas are PETs that secrete excessive amounts of gastrin. This peptide hormone stimulates gastric parietal cells directly and indirectly by way of histamine-secreting enterochromaffin-like (ECL) cells with the ultimate response of overproduction of gastric acid. High volumes of gastric acid overwhelm the pancreas's ability to neutralize intestinal contents. Drastically increased acidity of intestinal contents weakens pancreatic digestive enzymes and damages intestinal epithelial cells and villi, hindering digestion and reabsorption of intestinal contents, leading to diarrhea [28, 29].

Epidemiology

The incidence of gastrinomas is 1–3 per million per year, with 75% localized to the duodenum and 25% arising in the pancreas [1, 18, 30]. Studies have shown a slightly higher incidence of gastrinomas in men compared to women [28]. The majority of gastrinomas are sporadic; however, it is the most common functional PET in MEN1 syndrome [31]. Forty percent of patients with MEN1 have either the Zollinger-Ellison syndrome or asymptomatic elevation in serum gastrin concentrations. Gastrinomas in MEN1 are often multiple, and most are malignant, with 50% of patients having metastatic disease at the time of diagnosis. Primary pancreatic gastrinomas have a poor prognosis. Relative to duodenal gastrinomas, they are more aggressive, larger in size, and more frequently metastasize (usually to the liver) [32].

Clinical Evaluation

The clinical manifestations of gastrinomas are related to increased gastric acid secretion and its effects on the lining of the esophagus, stomach, and intestines. The common presenting symptoms include abdominal pain, recurrent peptic ulcer disease, severe gastroesophageal reflux that may lead to dysphagia, diarrhea, and weight loss. These constellations of symptoms are often referred to as Zollinger-Ellison syndrome [1, 27].

Laboratory Evaluation

Gastrinomas are diagnosed by biochemical evaluation showing gastrin levels elevated during fasting and hypersecretion of gastric acid. In patients not on anti-acid treatment, fasting gastrin levels >500 pg/mL or greater than 5 times the upper limit of normal are suggestive of gastrinoma, and levels >1000 pg/mL are highly suggestive [24, 33].

Prior to biochemical evaluation, patients must stop protein pump inhibitor (PPI) therapies as they may alter testing sensitivity and specificity [6]. If initial gastrin levels are equivocal, provocative testing such as secretin stimulation testing can be performed. Secretin provocative testing requires a period of fasting and intravenous administration of secretin followed by serial measurements of gastrin levels. Results showing a gastrin level rising above 200 pg/mL or a doubling of baseline fasting gastrin is strongly suggestive of a gastrinoma [24]. Additionally, basal gastric acid output greater than 115 mEq/h in the general population, without history of bariatric surgery, is characteristic of gastrinomas [27]. Intravenous calcium administration has also been shown to increase gastrin levels [34]. Provocative testing may help distinguish gastrinomas from other medical conditions associated with higher levels of gastrin, including *Helicobacter pylori* infections, G cell hyperplasia, chronic atrophic gastritis, or pernicious anemia [27].

Glucagonomas

Etiology/Pathophysiology

Glucagonomas are PETs that secrete excessive amounts of glucagon, a peptide that causes upregulation of gluconeogenesis and lipolysis pathways [35].

Epidemiology

Glucagonomas are much less common than insulinomas and gastrinomas, with an annual incidence of less than 0.1 per million [18, 36]. The majority of glucagonomas are sporadic, with approximately 10–20% occurring in association with MEN1; however, glucagonomas occur in only 3% of patients with MEN1 [31].

Sporadic glucagonomas most commonly occur in the 5th decade of life, while those associated with MEN1 occur earlier [37]. Glucagonomas are usually solitary tumors and are larger than other PETs. Approximately 50–80% are metastatic at the time of diagnosis [31].

Clinical Evaluation

Clinical manifestations of glucagonomas include new-onset diabetes mellitus or worsening of glycemic control in patients with diabetes. The catabolic effects of high levels of glucagon often result in significant weight loss. Patients with glucagonomas are also at higher risk for acute deep vein thrombosis and pulmonary embolism [1, 27]. The most distinct feature of glucagonomas and often the initial presenting symptom is necrolytic migratory erythema, a painful pruritic erythematous rash that varies from vesicles and bullae to plaques [2, 37].

Laboratory Evaluation

The diagnosis of a glucagonoma requires the demonstration of increased plasma glucagon levels (>500 pg/mL), or 10 to 20-fold elevation above normal reference ranges (normal <50 pg/mL). Concentrations above 1000 pg/mL are virtually diagnostic of glucagonoma. Before undergoing extensive biochemical testing and imaging, it is important to rule out other causes of elevations in serum glucagon, including hypoglycemia, fasting, trauma, sepsis, acute pancreatitis, abdominal surgery, Cushing's syndrome, renal failure, and liver failure [37].

Somatostatinomas

Etiology/Pathophysiology

Somatostatinomas are PETs that secrete excessive amounts of somatostatin, a tetradecapeptide involved in inhibiting secretions of several hormones, including gastrin, glucagon, growth hormone, and insulin, in addition to other gastrointestinal hormones such as cholecystokinin and pancreatic enzymes.

Epidemiology

Somatostatinomas are estimated to have an annual incidence of less than 0.1 per million [18]. The mean age of diagnosis is in the 5th decade [38]. The majority of somatostatinomas are sporadic, but slightly over one third of somatostatinomas occur in association with MEN1 syndrome or other familial syndromes such as neurofibromatosis type 1, von Hippel-Lindau, and tuberous sclerosis [38, 39].

Like glucagonomas, somatostatinomas tend to have larger primary tumors, with the median size of a pancreatic tumor being 4.25 cm [39]. It has previously been documented that over 70% of somatostatinomas are malignant, with the majority having metastasized at the time of diagnosis [40].

Clinical Evaluation

Somatostatin-secreting tumors are associated with several gastrointestinal symptoms. However, due to the intermittent secreting pattern of this tumor, initially, symptoms may be nonspecific. The most common presentation is abdominal pain. Less often, patients present with somatostatin syndrome, which is characterized by the triad of glucose intolerance/diabetes mellitus, cholelithiasis, and steatorrhea. Steatorrhea is due to compromised lipid absorption. Increased risk of cholelithiasis is due to reduced gallbladder contraction secondary to inhibition of cholecystokinin release [27, 39].

Laboratory Evaluation

Somatostatinomas are diagnosed by detecting elevated fasting plasma levels of somatostatin (usually exceeding 30 pg/mL); however, they are more commonly identified on imaging for workup of nonspecific complaints such as abdominal pain or weight loss [38].

VIPoma

Etiology/Pathophysiology

VIPomas are PETs that secrete excessive amounts of vasoactive intestinal peptide (VIP), a polypeptide known to bind to receptors widely in the human body, including in the gastrointestinal system, resulting in increased fluid and electrolyte secretion into the gastrointestinal lumen leading to diarrhea. VIP is also involved in other pathways that result in vasodilation, increased glycogenolysis, and bone resorption. Somatostatinomas are diagnosed by detecting elevated fasting plasma levels of somatostatin (usually exceeding 30 pg/mL). However, they are more commonly found on initial imaging for work up of nonspecific complaints such as abdominal pain or weight loss [41].

Epidemiology

The annual incidence of VIP-secreting tumors is 0.1 per million [18]. The majority of VIPomas are sporadic, with only 5% being associated with MEN1 syndrome. VIPomas are usually diagnosed between the third and fifth decades of life. The majority of VIPomas have metastasized at the time of diagnosis [42].

Clinical Evaluation

Patients with VIPomas often present with recurrent episodes of facial flushing, severe watery diarrhea that persists during fasting periods, and volume depletion. This collection of symptoms is often referred to as pancreatic cholera syndrome or watery diarrhea, hypokalemia, and hypochlorhydria or achlorhydria (WDHA) syndrome [41]. Patients often present with symptoms of dehydration and manifestations of hypokalemia such as weakness, fatigue, and muscle cramps.

Laboratory Evaluation

VIP-secreting PETs can be diagnosed by eliciting a detailed history of symptoms in the setting of VIP levels higher than 500 pg/mL. These patients have severe secretory diarrhea, which may reach a volume of several liters a day and with a low fecal osmotic gap (<50 mOsm/kg). VIPomas may secrete hormones intermittently, so it may be necessary to repeat testing when patients are symptomatic to confirm the diagnosis [41].

Imaging Evaluation

Imaging plays a pivotal role in the diagnosis and workup of PETs. The typical imaging features of a PET include a well-defined, homogeneously hyperenhancing mass without pancreatic ductal obstruction. Peak enhancement of these tumors typically occurs in the early arterial phase. Larger tumors can show internal cystic or necrotic change but usually retain a hypervascular rim. Unlike pancreatic adenocarcinoma, PETs do not commonly invade or obstruct adjacent structures.

Computerized tomography (CT) scans are the initial imaging modality of choice at many medical centers. CT can be performed quickly, is readily available, and is a highly sensitive examination to detect both primary pancreatic lesions and metastatic disease [18, 43, 44]. CT protocols are typically multiphasic with unenhanced imaging to detect intratumoral calcification or hemorrhage and arterial and portovenous phase imaging to detect enhancement characteristics (Fig. 5.1). Given the high vascularity of these tumors, most lesions are detected on arterial phase imaging when they reach peak enhancement, but the use of portovenous phase imaging has shown to increase overall detection rates. Like other morphological imaging modalities, sensitivity depends on tumor size, with higher rates of success with larger tumors. Sensitivity of CT for the detection of PETs ranges from 64% to 100% [45].

Although not as readily available and more costly, magnetic resonance imaging (MRI) offers a few advantages to multiphasic CT, including better soft tissue differentiation, improved detection of hepatic metastases, and lack of ionizing radiation (Fig. 5.2). As with CT, the success of PETs detection with MRI depends on tumor size, with higher rates of success for larger tumors. Sensitivity is high at 93% with a specificity of 88% [4]. Of note, long scan times and narrow bores may prohibit the use of this imaging technique in patients with claustrophobia, especially as MRI is degraded by motion artifact.

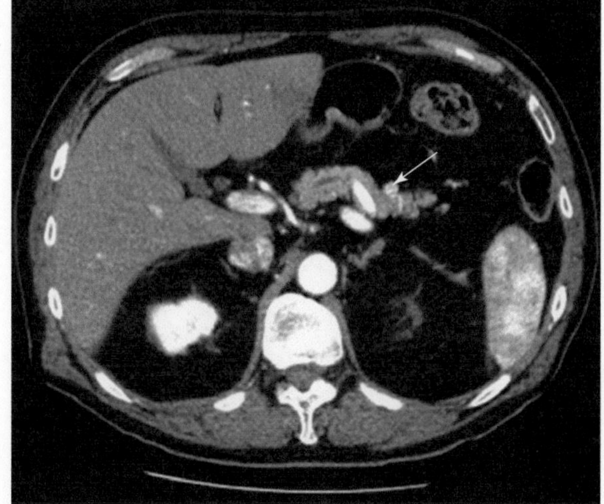

Fig. 5.1 Single axial contrast-enhanced CT image of the upper abdomen in arterial phase demonstrating a 1 cm hyperenhancing mass along the anterior aspect of the pancreatic tail (arrow). Pathologic evaluation confirmed an islet cell tumor

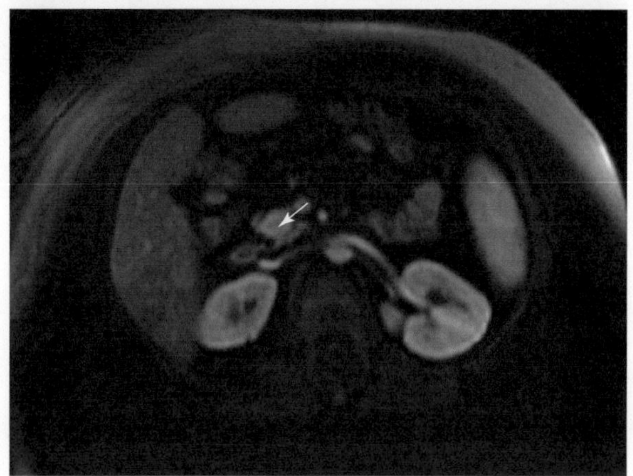

Fig. 5.2 Single axial post-contrast T1-weighted volumetric interpolated breath-hold examination (VIBE) image of the upper abdomen demonstrating a 1.6 cm hyperenhancing mass within the pancreatic head on arterial phase imaging. Pathologic confirmation at endoscopic US was consistent with an insulinoma

The majority of well-differentiated PETs overexpress somatostatin receptors allowing for functional imaging to play a role in detection. Functional imaging techniques use ^{111}In-pentetreotide or [68]Gallium to localize NETs. Octreoscan using ^{111}In demonstrates a sensitivity ranging between 60% and 80% and a specificity of 92–100% [18, 44].

More recently, 68Ga-DOTA positron emission tomography has become the functional imaging modality of choice due to high sensitivity and specificity of 93% and 91%, respectively [46] (Fig. 5.3). One advantage of this technique is the detection of whole-body distant metastases, which may not be included in the field of view on cross-sectional imaging alone. Of note, functional imaging requires the tumors to overexpress somatostatin receptors, so in cases of poorly differentiated PETs and

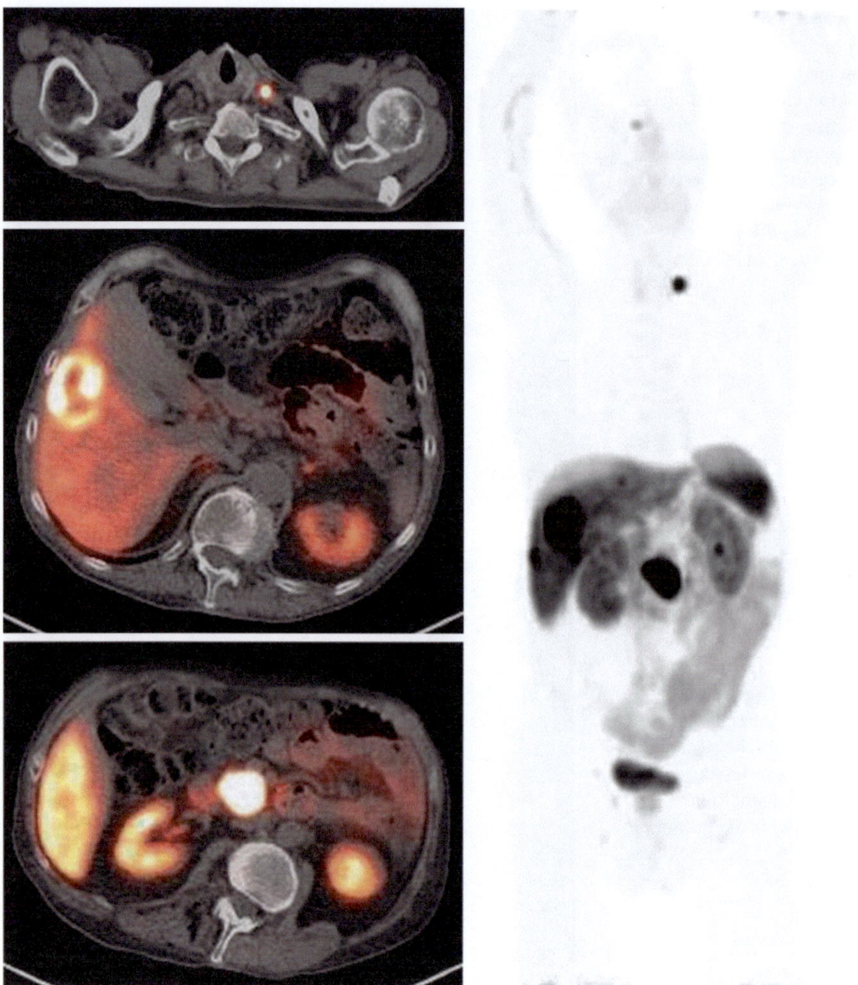

Fig. 5.3 Selected images from an Octreoscan positron emission tomography/CT with ^{111}In-pentetreotide demonstrating foci of uptake within the primary pancreatic neuroendocrine tumor in the uncinate process of the pancreas, an inferior right hepatic lobe metastasis, and a distant left supraclavicular metastatic lymph node. (Images c/o Dr. Amir Khandani)

benign insulinomas, these imaging techniques may be falsely negative. Conversely, there are nonneoplastic processes that may lead to false positive findings including infection and other inflammatory processes, granulomatous disease, and thyroid disease [44, 47].

Finally, in cases of high suspicion but negative imaging, endoscopic ultrasound has a role in the detection of small tumors. Although invasive, this technique can both detect tumors and allow for simultaneous biopsy of PETs. The drawbacks of endoscopic ultrasound are that it is a user-dependent skill with results depending on the experience of the physician and requires sedation [4].

Conclusion

Neuroendocrine cells arise from lineage of sensory and secretory cells and are present all over the body. The incidence of functional and non-functional PETs has slowly increased over the past decades. The process of diagnosing PETs requires a thorough history and physical examination. Biochemical evaluations for PETs include baseline hormone levels and may require provocative testing. It is important for clinicians to do thorough medication reviews as some drugs may hinder biochemical evaluation. Imaging also plays a pivotal role in the diagnosis and workup of PETs, with CT often being the initial modality of choice. Due to the unique changes in protein expressions, functional imaging has become a helpful adjunct for the detection of distant metastases.

References

1. Hofland J, Kaltsas G, de Herder WW. Advances in the diagnosis and management of well-differentiated neuroendocrine neoplasms. Endocr Rev. 2020;41(2):371–403.
2. Asa SL. Pancreatic endocrine tumors. Mod Pathol. 2011;24(Suppl 2):S66–77.
3. Ramage JK, Ahmed A, Ardill J, Bax N, Breen DJ, Caplin ME, et al. Guidelines for the management of gastroenteropancreatic neuroendocrine (including carcinoid) tumours (NETs). Gut. 2012;61(1):6–32.
4. Lee L, Ito T, Jensen RT. Imaging of pancreatic neuroendocrine tumors: recent advances, current status, and controversies. Expert Rev Anticancer Ther. 2018;18(9):837–60.
5. Ito T, Lee L, Jensen RT. Treatment of symptomatic neuroendocrine tumor syndromes: recent advances and controversies. Expert Opin Pharmacother. 2016;17(16):2191–205.
6. Ito T, Cadiot G, Jensen RT. Diagnosis of Zollinger-Ellison syndrome: increasingly difficult. World J Gastroenterol. 2012;18(39):5495–503.
7. Ito T, Igarashi H, Jensen RT. Zollinger-Ellison syndrome: recent advances and controversies. Curr Opin Gastroenterol. 2013;29(6):650–61.
8. Williams ED, Sandler M. The classification of carcinoid tumours. Lancet. 1963;1(7275):238–9.
9. Utiger R. Pancreas. Britannica: Encyclopædia Britannica; 2020.
10. Hauso O, Gustafsson BI, Kidd M, Waldum HL, Drozdov I, Chan AK, et al. Neuroendocrine tumor epidemiology: contrasting Norway and North America. Cancer. 2008;113(10):2655–64.
11. Kim JY, Hong SM. Recent updates on neuroendocrine tumors from the gastrointestinal and pancreatobiliary tracts. Arch Pathol Lab Med. 2016;140(5):437–48.
12. Schmitt AM, Riniker F, Anlauf M, Schmid S, Soltermann A, Moch H, et al. Islet 1 (Isl1) expression is a reliable marker for pancreatic endocrine tumors and their metastases. Am J Surg Pathol. 2008;32(3):420–5.
13. Bergsland EK, Woltering EA, Rindo G. Neuroendocrine tumors of the pancreas. In: AJCC cancer staging manual. 8th ed. Chicago: Springer International; 2017.

14. Dasari A, Shen C, Halperin D, Zhao B, Zhou S, Xu Y, et al. Trends in the incidence, prevalence, and survival outcomes in patients with neuroendocrine tumors in the United States. JAMA Oncol. 2017;3(10):1335–42.

15. Leoncini E, Boffetta P, Shafir M, Aleksovska K, Boccia S, Rindi G. Increased incidence trend of low-grade and high-grade neuroendocrine neoplasms. Endocrine. 2017;58(2):368–79.

16. Lee MR, Harris C, Baeg KJ, Aronson A, Wisnivesky JP, Kim MK. Incidence trends of gastroenteropancreatic neuroendocrine tumors in the United States. Clin Gastroenterol Hepatol. 2019;17(11):2212–7 e1.

17. Yao JC, Hassan M, Phan A, Dagohoy C, Leary C, Mares JE, et al. One hundred years after "carcinoid": epidemiology of and prognostic factors for neuroendocrine tumors in 35,825 cases in the United States. J Clin Oncol. 2008;26(18):3063–72.

18. Young K, Iyer R, Morganstein D, Chau I, Cunningham D, Starling N. Pancreatic neuroendocrine tumors: a review. Future Oncol. 2015;11(5):853–64.

19. Mulvey CK, Van Loon K, Bergsland EK, Masharani U, Nakakura EK. Complicated case presentation: Management of Pancreatic Neuroendocrine Tumors in multiple endocrine Neoplasia type 1. Pancreas. 2017;46(3):416–26.

20. Fraenkel M, Kim M, Faggiano A, de Herder WW, Valk GD, Knowledge N. Incidence of gastroenteropancreatic neuroendocrine tumours: a systematic review of the literature. Endocr Relat Cancer. 2014;21(3):R153–63.

21. Kuo JH, Lee JA, Chabot JA. Nonfunctional pancreatic neuroendocrine tumors. Surg Clin North Am. 2014;94(3):689–708.

22. Petersen MC, Shulman GI. Mechanisms of insulin action and insulin resistance. Physiol Rev. 2018;98(4):2133–223.

23. Vortmeyer AO, Huang S, Lubensky I, Zhuang Z. Non-islet origin of pancreatic islet cell tumors. J Clin Endocrinol Metab. 2004;89(4):1934–8.

24. Melmed S, Auchus RJ, Goldfine AB, Koenig RJ, Rosen CJ. Williams textbook of endocrinology. 14th ed. Philadelphia: Elsevier, Inc.; 2019.

25. Placzkowski KA, Vella A, Thompson GB, Grant CS, Reading CC, Charboneau JW, et al. Secular trends in the presentation and management of functioning insulinoma at the Mayo Clinic, 1987-2007. J Clin Endocrinol Metab. 2009;94(4):1069–73.

26. Cryer PE, Axelrod L, Grossman AB, Heller SR, Montori VM, Seaquist ER, et al. Evaluation and management of adult hypoglycemic disorders: an Endocrine Society clinical practice guideline. J Clin Endocrinol Metab. 2009;94(3):709–28.

27. Lairmore TC, Moley JF. Endocrine pancreatic tumors. Scand J Surg. 2004;93(4):311–5.

28. Berna MJ, Hoffmann KM, Serrano J, Gibril F, Jensen RT. Serum gastrin in Zollinger-Ellison syndrome: I. Prospective study of fasting serum gastrin in 309 patients from the National Institutes of Health and comparison with 2229 cases from the literature. Medicine (Baltimore). 2006;85(6):295–330.

29. Norton JA, Foster DS, Ito T, Jensen RT. Gastrinomas: medical or surgical treatment. Endocrinol Metab Clin N Am. 2018;47(3):577–601.

30. Rehfeld JF, Bardram L, Hilsted L, Goetze JP. An evaluation of chromogranin A versus gastrin and progastrin in gastrinoma diagnosis and control. Biomark Med. 2014;8(4):571–80.

31. Levy-Bohbot N, Merle C, Goudet P, Delemer B, Calender A, Jolly D, et al. Prevalence, characteristics and prognosis of MEN 1-associated glucagonomas, VIPomas, and somatostatinomas: study from the GTE (Groupe des Tumeurs Endocrines) registry. Gastroenterol Clin Biol. 2004;28(11):1075–81.

32. Brandi ML, Gagel RF, Angeli A, Bilezikian JP, Beck-Peccoz P, Bordi C, et al. Guidelines for diagnosis and therapy of MEN type 1 and type 2. J Clin Endocrinol Metab. 2001;86(12):5658–71.

33. Run Y. Neuroendocrine tumor syndromes. In: Endocrinology: adult and pediatric [internet]; 2016. Seventh. [2606-14].

34. Berna MJ, Hoffmann KM, Long SH, Serrano J, Gibril F, Jensen RT. Serum gastrin in Zollinger-Ellison syndrome: II. Prospective study of gastrin provocative testing in 293 patients from the National Institutes of Health and comparison with 537 cases from the literature. Evaluation

of diagnostic criteria, proposal of new criteria, and correlations with clinical and tumoral features. Medicine (Baltimore). 2006;85(6):331–64.

35. John AM, Schwartz RA. Glucagonoma syndrome: a review and update on treatment. J Eur Acad Dermatol Venereol. 2016;30(12):2016–22.

36. Jensen RT, Cadiot G, Brandi ML, de Herder WW, Kaltsas G, Komminoth P, et al. ENETS consensus guidelines for the management of patients with digestive neuroendocrine neoplasms: functional pancreatic endocrine tumor syndromes. Neuroendocrinology. 2012;95(2):98–119.

37. Wermers RA, Fatourechi V, Wynne AG, Kvols LK, Lloyd RV. The glucagonoma syndrome. Clinical and pathologic features in 21 patients. Medicine (Baltimore). 1996;75(2):53–63.

38. Vinik A, Pacak K, Feliberti E, Perry RR. Somatostatinoma. In: Feingold KR, Anawalt B, Boyce A, Chrousos G, de Herder WW, Dungan K, et al., editors. Endotext. South Dartmouth: MDText.com, Inc; 2000.

39. Garbrecht N, Anlauf M, Schmitt A, Henopp T, Sipos B, Raffel A, et al. Somatostatin-producing neuroendocrine tumors of the duodenum and pancreas: incidence, types, biological behavior, association with inherited syndromes, and functional activity. Endocr Relat Cancer. 2008;15(1):229–41.

40. Doherty GM. Rare endocrine tumours of the GI tract. Best Pract Res Clin Gastroenterol. 2005;19(5):807–17.

41. Vinik A. Vasoactive intestinal peptide tumor (VIPoma). In: Feingold KR, Anawalt B, Boyce A, Chrousos G, de Herder WW, Dungan K, et al., editors. Endotext. South Dartmouth: MDText.com, Inc; 2000.

42. Perry RR, Vinik AI. Clinical review 72: diagnosis and management of functioning islet cell tumors. J Clin Endocrinol Metab. 1995;80(8):2273–8.

43. Falconi M, Eriksson B, Kaltsas G, Bartsch DK, Capdevila J, Caplin M, et al. ENETS consensus guidelines update for the management of patients with functional pancreatic neuroendocrine tumors and non-functional pancreatic neuroendocrine tumors. Neuroendocrinology. 2016;103(2):153–71.

44. Sundin A, Arnold R, Baudin E, Cwikla JB, Eriksson B, Fanti S, et al. ENETS consensus guidelines for the standards of care in neuroendocrine tumors: radiological, nuclear medicine & hybrid imaging. Neuroendocrinology. 2017;105(3):212–44.

45. Rockall AG, Reznek RH. Imaging of neuroendocrine tumours (CT/MR/US). Best Pract Res Clin Endocrinol Metab. 2007;21(1):43–68.

46. Maxwell JE, Howe JR. Imaging in neuroendocrine tumors: an update for the clinician. Int J Endocr Oncol. 2015;2(2):159–68.

47. Hofman MS, Lau WF, Hicks RJ. Somatostatin receptor imaging with 68Ga DOTATATE PET/CT: clinical utility, normal patterns, pearls, and pitfalls in interpretation. Radiographics. 2015;35(2):500–16.

Part II
Selective Venous Sampling

Chapter 6
Adrenal Vein Sampling

Hyeon Yu and Clayton W. Commander

Introduction

Primary Aldosteronism

Dr. Jerome W. Conn first described primary aldosteronism (PA) in 1954 in a patient with an adrenocortical tumor [1–4]. PA is an endocrine disorder widely recognized as the most common form of secondary hypertension [5–7]. It is caused by excess secretion of aldosterone from one or both adrenal glands [8]. Initially, PA was believed to be quite rare, with reported prevalence rates of 1–2%, mostly from retrospective cohort studies [9, 10]. However, in a prospective study, Rossi et al. showed that PA is far more common than previously believed, with a prevalence rate of 11.2% in patients with newly diagnosed hypertension [7]. In this report, unilateral aldosterone-producing adenoma (APA) was found in 4.8% of patients, demonstrating PA as the most common cause of a curable endocrine form of hypertension [7]. Despite this, it remains underdiagnosed and undertreated with significant morbidity and mortality associated with renal and cardiovascular injury [5, 11].

Diagnosis of Primary Aldosteronism

According to the Endocrine Society guidelines, PA is diagnosed by a three-step approach, consisting of screening, confirmation testing, and subtyping [5, 8]. For initial screening, a positive plasma aldosterone-to-renin ratio (ARR) is used to

H. Yu (✉) · C. W. Commander
Division of Vascular and Interventional Radiology, Department of Radiology, University of North Carolina at Chapel Hill School of Medicine, Chapel Hill, NC, USA
e-mail: hyeon_yu@med.unc.edu; clayton_commander@med.unc.edu

© The Author(s), under exclusive license to Springer Nature Switzerland AG 2022
H. Yu et al. (eds.), *Diagnosis and Management of Endocrine Disorders in Interventional Radiology*, https://doi.org/10.1007/978-3-030-87189-5_6

differentiate PA from essential hypertension [8, 12]. Next, the adrenal gland's unsuppressed production of aldosterone should be demonstrated by confirmatory tests, such as fludrocortisone suppression test, oral sodium loading test, saline infusion test, and captopril challenge test [8]. Once PA is confirmed, identifying a curable subtype of PA is crucial because only patients with PA caused by unilateral adrenal abnormality benefit from surgery. Subtypes of PA include unilateral APA, unilateral adrenal hyperplasia, unilateral multiple adrenocortical nodular hyperplasias, bilateral APA, and bilateral adrenal hyperplasia [13–19]. Unilateral APAs and bilateral adrenal hyperplasia are the most common types with prevalence rates of 55–65% and 35–45%, respectively [20].

Imaging of Primary Aldosteronism

Computed tomography (CT) is considered the primary imaging technique to identify adrenal nodules/hyperplasia and exclude adrenocortical carcinoma [13, 21]. High-resolution adrenal CT with contrast is preferred over magnetic resonance imaging (MRI) because of the limited spatial resolution of MRI. However, differentiating PA subtypes with CT is still challenging due to low sensitivity for the detection of micro APAs (<10 mm in diameter) and low specificity for the distinction of APAs from incidental nonsecretory nodules [8]. In a systematic review evaluating 950 patients from 38 studies, Kempers et al. showed that CT and MRI misdiagnosed the subtype of PA in 37.8% of patients [22]. More recently, a retrospective study evaluating a total of 342 patients reported high discordance rates of 22–28% between CT/MRI and adrenal vein sampling (AVS) [23]. A study of 367 patients with PA demonstrated that AVS changed the management in 43% of cases [24]. In this study, patients with discordant cross-sectional imaging and AVS would have undergone wrong-side adrenalectomy and unnecessary surgery and would have been incorrectly excluded from surgery in 3%, 25%, and 16% of cases, respectively [24]. Several other similar studies also conclude that cross-sectional imaging is not optimal in identifying surgically curable PA subtypes due to the lack of sensitivity and specificity [23, 25, 26]. Dekkers et al. later challenged this finding in a prospective randomized study evaluating the outcomes of 184 patients who underwent treatments based on either CT or AVS [27]. The results of their study showed that there was no significant difference in the intensity of hypertensive medication required to control blood pressure between patients with CT-based and those with AVS-based treatments. However, this study has been criticized for its substantial referral bias, suboptimal primary endpoint (improvement in blood pressure control instead of biochemical cure), and insufficient statistical power, such that the results should be interpreted with caution [28–30]. There has been an attempt to lateralize the source of PA with PET-CT using various tracers, including ^{11}C-metomidate, ^{68}Ga-pentixafor, and ^{18}F-CDP2230 [31–33]. The efficacy of ^{131}I-6β-iodomethyl-19-norcholesterol adrenal scintigraphy has also been suggested for PA workup [34]. However, their accuracies are still inferior to AVS and are not suitable for routine clinical use.

Adrenal Vein Sampling

Since AVS was first introduced in 1967, it has been the only reliable technique for differentiating PA subtypes [35]. The Endocrine Society recommends AVS as the gold standard to distinguish unilateral from bilateral forms of PA before considering surgery [8, 28]. However, the frequency of AVS performed in patients with PA varied widely among institutions due to various levels of expertise and practice. Also, AVS is technically demanding and is regarded as an invasive procedure. In the Adrenal Vein Sampling International Study (AVIS), including 2064 AVS procedures in 24 centers from Asia, Australia, North America, and Europe, Rossi et al. found that AVS is not systematically performed even at major referral centers worldwide [36]. The mean rate of the systemic use of AVS was only 77% (19–100%) in patients with PA [36]. Factors associated with the low frequency of AVS included the reliance on cross-sectional imaging, high costs of AVS, lack of experience in AVS or surgery, and the use of medical treatment only [36]. The technical success of AVS depends on the interventional radiologists' experience and skills. A safe and successful procedure requires familiarity with normal and variant anatomy of the adrenal veins, patient selection and preparation, stimulation and sampling techniques, well-organized specimen handling, and consistent criteria for results interpretation. Also, collaboration among interventional radiology, surgery, and endocrinology is essential for developing an efficient clinical practice [37].

Anatomy

Embryology

The development of the venous system begins during the fourth week of gestation, with the two anterior and two posterior cardinal veins [38, 39]. The posterior cardinal veins drain the venous flow from the caudal portion of the embryonic body and the mesonephroi (Wolffian bodies), which later develop the adrenal glands, kidneys, and gonads [38, 40]. In the fifth week, subcardinal veins arise from the mesonephroi, and venous flow gradually changes from the posterior cardinal veins to the subcardinal veins [41, 42]. During this transition, the posterior cardinal veins begin to regress distally. Simultaneously, the mesonephroi enlarge and migrate medially with the subcardinal vein, connecting to the contralateral subcardinal vein through the intersubcardinal anastomoses [38, 40]. The intersubcardinal anastomoses then grow into the subcardinal sinuses, forming the renal veins [38].

In the seventh week, the supracardinal veins replace the regressing posterior cardinal veins and start draining venous flow from the caudal embryonic body [41]. The supracardinal vein subsequently enlarges on the right side, forming the infrarenal segment of the inferior vena cava (IVC) [39]. The cranial part of the right subcardinal vein becomes the suprarenal segment of the IVC. In the embryonic liver area, hepatic sinusoids drain into the right subcardinal vein forming the hepatic segment of the IVC [43]. During the IVC formation, bilateral mesonephroi and subcardinal veins gradually regress, leaving the short segments of the subcardinal veins on both sides of the IVC [38–40]. The left adrenal vein develops from the remnant of the left subcardinal vein, which is associated with the left adrenal gland and subsequently drains into the subcardinal sinus [42]. The remnant of the right subcardinal vein, between the subcardinal sinus and the hepatic segment of the IVC, becomes the right adrenal vein, draining directly into the suprarenal segment of the IVC [42]. In each adrenal gland center, a prominent central adrenomedullary vein is formed from the tributaries draining both cortex and medulla [44].

Right Adrenal Vein

Most commonly, the single right adrenal vein (RAV) drains directly into the IVC (Fig. 6.1a). The orifice of the RAV locates most commonly in the IVC's right posterior quadrant at a level between the T11 and L1 vertebral bodies. The RAV takes

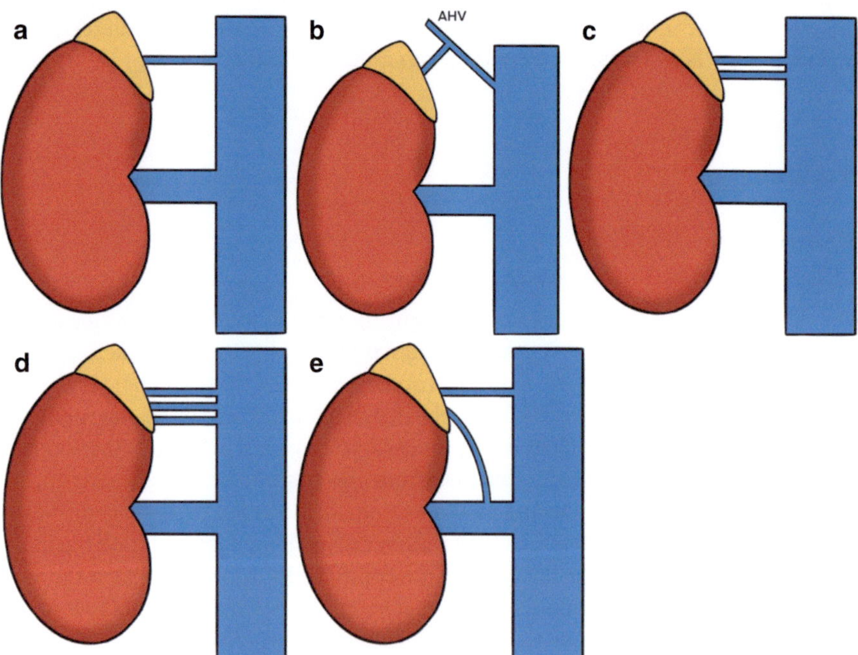

Fig. 6.1 Anatomical variations of the right adrenal vein (RAV). (**a**) The single RAV drains directly into the IVC. (**b**) The RAV drains into the accessory hepatic vein, which drains into the IVC. (**c**) Two RAVs drain into the IVC independently. (**d**) The RAV is tripled and draining into the IVC. (**e**) Two RAVs with one vein drain directly into the IVC, and the other vein drains into the right renal vein

a cranial, anterior, and medial course from the right adrenal gland to join the IVC approximately 4–5 cm above the right renal vein. The RAV's reported mean length and diameter are 3.8 ± 1.7 mm and 1.7 ± 0.6 mm, respectively [45]. The RAV communicates with multiple small superficial veins from the glandular surface, surrounding fat, and retroperitoneal veins [40, 46–48]. Most of the superficial veins of the right adrenal gland join the right inferior phrenic vein (IPV) at the gland's superior border [48]. These communicating veins drain into the accessory hepatic vein (AHV) or azygos vein, providing a collateral venous channel when the RAV is occluded [49]. The RAV also communicates with the portal venous network, playing an essential role as a portosystemic shunt when the portal venous pressure increases [50, 51].

Contrast-enhanced CT is frequently used to identify the RAV before AVS to determine appropriate catheter shape. The RAV is best visualized in the late arterial phase of CT, with the detection rate of 76–95% [45, 52]. In a retrospective study evaluating the RAV's radiologic anatomy, Matsuura et al. demonstrated that the RAV joined the IVC at a level between the middle third of the T12 and the superior third of the L1 vertebral body in 69% of the cases [45]. The reported mean distance between the RAV orifice and the vertebral body's right margin was 9.3 ± 4.5 mm. Later, the same group evaluated the RAV's anatomic variations in a total of 440 consecutive patients using MDCT and catheter venography [52]. They found that the RAV formed a common trunk with the AHV on MDCT in 20% of the patients (Fig. 6.1b). The common trunk's most frequent angle was a posterior, rightward, and nearly horizontal from the IVC. The AHV was absent, located within 3 mm of the RAV orifice, located >3 mm from the RAV orifice in 32%, 13%, and 35% of the patients, respectively [52]. When the RAV and AHV form a trunk, or their orifices locate near within 3 mm, the AHV may be misinterpreted as the RAV on the venous sampling if the anatomy and relationship are not thoroughly evaluated on CT before the procedure. Other variations of the RAV include (1) two RAVs draining separately into the IVC (Fig. 6.1c), (2) three RAVs (Fig. 6.1d), and (3) two RAV with one draining into the IVC and the other into the right renal vein (Fig. 6.1e) [53]. It was reported that the variants occurred more often on the RAV (17%) compared to the left side (9%) [51].

Left Arenal Vein

The left adrenal vein (LAV) receives the left IPV to form a common trunk before entering the left renal vein (Fig. 6.2a). The LAV courses inferomedially and posterior to the pancreas body to join the left renal vein's superior border approximately 2.5–5 cm from the IVC [53, 54]. The mean lengths of the LAV from the adrenal gland to the junction with the IPV and from the junction to the left renal vein are 1.4 cm (0.2–3.2 cm) and 1.6 cm (0.9–2.8 cm), respectively [48, 54]. The diameter of the LAV changes from ~3 mm between the adrenal gland and the junction with the IPV to 4–5 mm between the junction and the left renal vein [54]. Similar to the

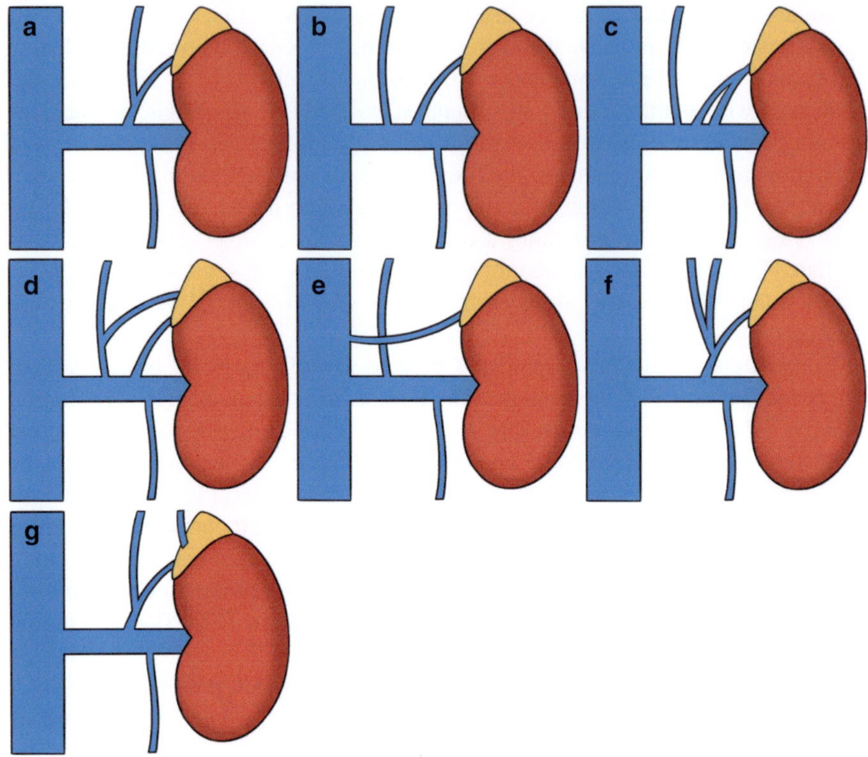

Fig. 6.2 Anatomical variations of the left adrenal vein (LAV). (**a**) The LAV receives the left IPV to form a common trunk before entering into the left renal vein. (**b**) The left IPV and LAV drain independently into the left renal vein. (**c**) Two LAVs join the left renal vein separately. (**d**) The LAV is doubled, with only one joining the left IPV before entering into the left renal vein. (**e**) The LAV drains directly into the IVC. (**f**) Two left IPVs merge with the LAV, forming the common trunk, and drain into the left renal vein. (**g**) The left IPV is doubled, with one joining the LAV and the other entering the adrenal gland, draining into the left renal vein

right side, the LAV communicates with multiple small veins from the glandular surface and the retroperitoneal veins [48]. These small communications drain into the azygos or hemiazygos vein [53]. At the posterior surface of the gland, the small superficial veins join the perirenal veins and occasionally drain into the left renal vein [48]. The portal venous network also communicates with the LAV through the left inferior phrenic vein (IPV) and create a portosystemic shunt in patients with portal hypertension [51].

In a small cadaver study for the LAV's anatomical variations, the left IPV joined the LAV before entering into the left renal vein in 100% of the cases (Fig. 6.2a) [55]. However, they could not find any case with anastomoses between the LAV and the lumbar-azygos system. In a similar but more extensive study of 300 cadavers evaluating the IPV's anatomy, Loukas et al. reported that the left IPV joined the LAV and entered into the left renal vein as a common trunk in only 34% of the cases (Fig. 6.2a) [56].

The left IPV was also drained directly into the IVC (Fig. 6.2e), the left renal vein, the left hepatic vein in 37%, 15%, and 14% of the cases. Other rare variations of the LAV include (1) two LAVs joining the left renal vein independently (Fig. 6.2c), (2) two LAVs with only one joining the left IPV before entering into the left renal vein (Fig. 6.2d), (3) the LAV draining directly into the IVC (Fig. 6.2e), (4) two left IPVs merging with the LAV forming the common trunk (Fig. 6.2f), and (5) two IPVs with one joining the LAV and the other entering into the adrenal gland, draining into the left renal vein (Fig. 6.2g) [53]. Rarely, the LAV drains into the left renal capsular vein, leading to unsuccessful AVS [57].

AVS Procedure

Preparation of Patients

Any medications that could potentially stimulate renin secretion should be discontinued or replaced by the medications that have no or minimal effects on renin secretion before AVS. The preferred drugs that do not interfere with the renin-angiotensin system include long-acting calcium channel blockers (verapamil or diltiazem) and α1-adrenergic receptor blockers [58–60]. Similarly, β-blockers, angiotensin-converting enzyme inhibitors, and angiotensin II receptor blockers can also be used in most cases [58]. However, loop and thiazide diuretics, amiloride, and mineralocorticoid receptor antagonists should be discontinued at least 4 weeks before sampling [28]. If plasma renin activity is suppressed, AVS can be safely performed regardless of the duration of the withdrawal of the medication. A 2-week withdrawal protocol has been reported to be feasible in patients who cannot tolerate the withdrawal of the medications for 4–6 weeks [61]. AVS should be performed early in the morning when the highest value of cortisol and aldosterone is observed. If the patient is allergic to contrast media, proper prophylactic premedication with corticosteroid and diphenhydramine is needed.

ACTH Stimulation

Cosyntropin is a synthetic adrenocorticotropic hormone (ACTH 1–24) used to stimulate adrenal hormone secretion and minimize the confounding effects of stress resulting in fluctuation of the hormone during AVS [62, 63]. It has been reported that ACTH stimulation improves the successful catheterization in AVS [64, 65]. Wolley et al. tested whether ACTH stimulation improved AVS's diagnostic performance for subtyping PA [66]. They found a significant increase in adrenal/peripheral cortisol concentration gradients in both sides between before and after an intravenous bolus of 250 µg of ACTH, resulting in a reduction of nondiagnostic studies. Later, in a systematic review and meta-analysis, Laurent et al. confirmed that AVS with ACTH stimulation significantly reduced the number of unsuccessful catheterization of both adrenal veins more than AVS without ACTH stimulation ($p < 0.001$) [67]. ACTH stimulation is also recommended: (1) for patients with ongoing glucocorticoid therapy, (2) for patients with concomitant subclinical hypercortisolism, (3) when AVS is performed after 10 AM, and (4) to avoid bilaterally lower adrenal vein aldosterone levels than in IVC due to temporary quiescent aldosterone secretion [28]. ACTH stimulation is achieved via either continuous infusion of ACTH at 50 μg/h, starting 30 min before AVS, or a bolus of 250 μg of ACTH, 15 min before AVS.

Technique

Our institution uses a continuous infusion of cosyntropin (50 μg/h), initiated approximately 30 min before the AVS procedure. Under ultrasound guidance, the common femoral vein is accessed with a 21-gauge needle, and a 5- or 6-Fr vascular sheath is placed. The right internal jugular vein can be accessed when both femoral veins are not patent or AVS is not successful via a transfemoral approach. Using a 5-Fr Mikaelsson (Beacon Tip, Cook, Bloomington, IN) or Cobra-2 (Imager, Boston Scientific, Natick, MA) catheter, the RAV is selected under fluoroscopy. Digital subtraction venography (DSV) is performed to verify the correct catheter position. When performing DSV, a gentle manual injection of a small volume of contrast media (~3 mL) is essential to avoid adrenal hemorrhage or vein injury [68]. If the target vein is identified, further injection of contrast media for opacifying the entire gland is not necessary. A 2.8- or 2.4-Fr microcatheter is subsequently advanced through the 5-Fr catheter into the central vein, from which two blood samples are collected by slow aspiration. We do not create a side hole at the tip or distal portion of the catheter to minimize the sample's potential dilution by IVC blood. Instead, we use a microcatheter for the collection of blood samples in most cases. A Simmons-1, Cobra-1, or other reverse-curve catheters, such as RDC, MK Adrenal-R shape, MK-X, and MK-1B, can also be used [68, 69].

The selection of the LAV is relatively easy compared to the RAV. A 5-Fr Simmons-2 catheter (Cordis, Miami Lakes, FL) is commonly used for the LAV. The Simmons-2 catheter is first advanced into the left renal vein over a guidewire, and DSV is performed to identify the common trunk of the left IPV and LAV. The catheter is then slowly pulled back until the tip is engaged in the common trunk at the left renal vein's superior border. A gentle DSV is repeated from the common trunk to confirm the LAV. The selection of the LAV and collecting blood samples are performed similarly using a microcatheter. Lastly, the catheter is pulled down to the lower IVC at the confluence of the bilateral common iliac veins and collect the final set of blood samples. Each blood sample is collected in a properly labeled test tube containing a serum separator, and all samples are transferred immediately to the endocrinology lab for rapid cortisol assay.

Venography of RAV

Successful RAV sampling requires comprehensive knowledge of the various venographic findings of the RAV. Daunt et al. described the RAV's five unique patterns on DSV, including (1) classic gland-like pattern with a central vein and numerous small feathery branches and glandular blush (Fig. 6.3a); (2) delta pattern with two or three prominent branches, but no filling of glandular structure (Fig. 6.3b); (3) triangular pattern with crowded branches showing a "blush-like" appearance (Fig. 6.3c); (4) spiderweb-like branches without a glandular blush (Fig. 6.3d); and (5) irregular branches with no discernible pattern (Fig. 6.3e) [68]. In addition to the RAV's different patterns, recognizing the communicating vessels between the RAV and surrounding capsular branches is also essential to avoid inadequate blood sampling. The capsular veins of the right adrenal gland commonly course inferolaterally and drain into the right renal vein, IPV, intercostal vein, or IVC [68]. If the AHV is accidentally catheterized and injected with contrast media, the venogram shows the intrahepatic branches with an upward and medial course (Fig. 6.4a), joining the right hepatic vein with large irregular hepatic parenchymal blushes (Fig. 6.4b). The AHV has been reported to be the most common cause of inadequate RAV sampling [70]. However, if the AHV is used as an anatomic landmark, the catheterization of the RAV can be greatly improved [71].

Rapid Cortisol Assay

AVS is a technically challenging procedure, mainly due to difficulties in catheterization of the RAV. The technical success depends on the interventional radiologist's experience [72, 73]. Besides identifying the RAV on venography, no other confirming methods were available before completing the procedure [74]. However, studies have shown that rapid cortisol assay allowed immediate resampling of the RAV, resulting in markedly improved AVS success rates [74–77]. Rapid cortisol assay is performed during AVS while the patient and the interventional radiologist are waiting in the angiography suite for immediate feedback from the endocrinology lab [77]. At our institution, while the cortisol assay is being performed, the patient is transferred to the recovery room with the vascular sheath in place until the preliminary results are available [74]. If the results show successful catheterization of the bilateral adrenal veins, the vascular sheath is removed, and hemostasis is achieved with manual compression. If not successful, the patient is transferred back to the angiography suite for repeat AVS. In two similar retrospective studies, the reported success rates significantly improved from 55–73% to 85–97% after introducing rapid cortisol assay [76]. Another new method, an on-site quick cortisol assay, was recently introduced by Yoneda et al. [78]. They showed a semiquantitative and quantitative cortisol assay using immunochromatography and gold nanoparticles, which was completed within 6 min in

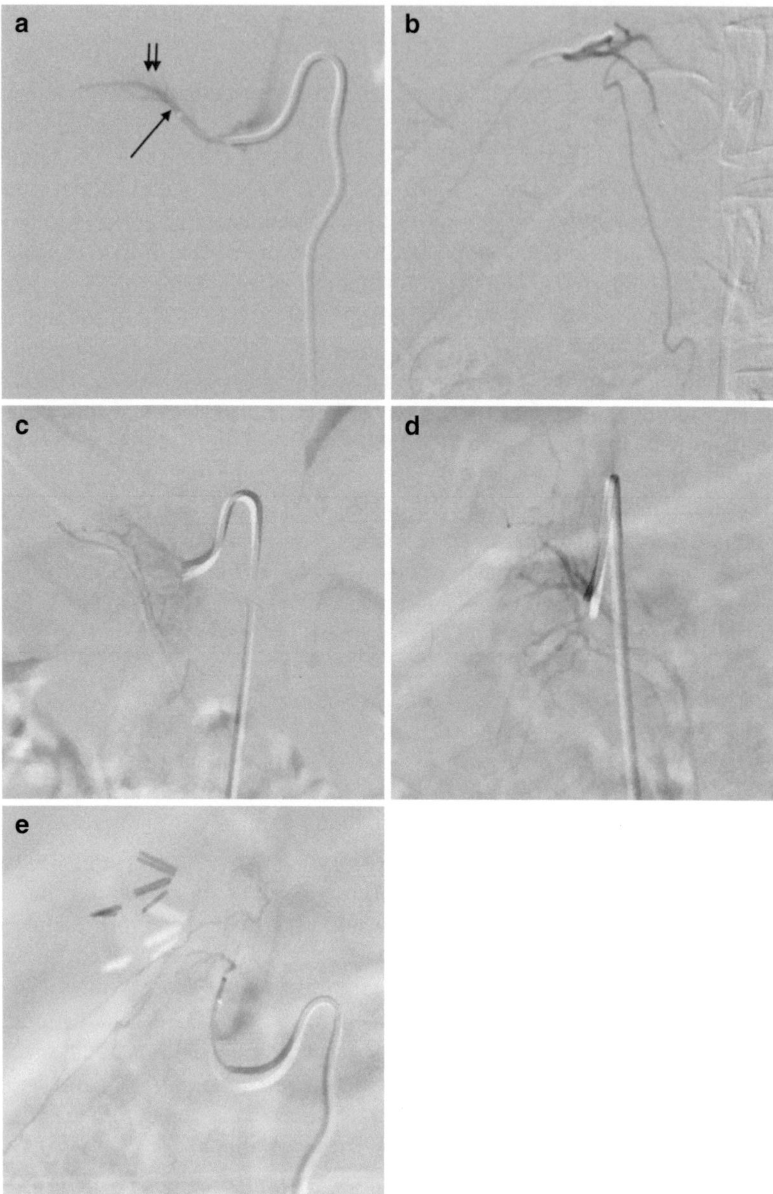

Fig. 6.3 Digital subtraction venographic (DSV) findings of the right adrenal vein (RAV). (**a**) DSV shows a typical gland-like pattern of the RAV with the central vein (long arrow), small branches (small arrows), and a faint gland-like blush. (**b**) DSV demonstrates a delta pattern of the RAV with multiple prominent veins without small branches or glandular structures. (**c**) DSV demonstrates a triangular pattern of the RAV with multiple crowded branches, showing a triangular "blush-like" appearance. (**d**) DSV demonstrates a spiderweb pattern of the RAV. (**e**) DSV demonstrates the RAV with no discernible pattern. There are multiple irregular branches without a pattern or gland-like blush

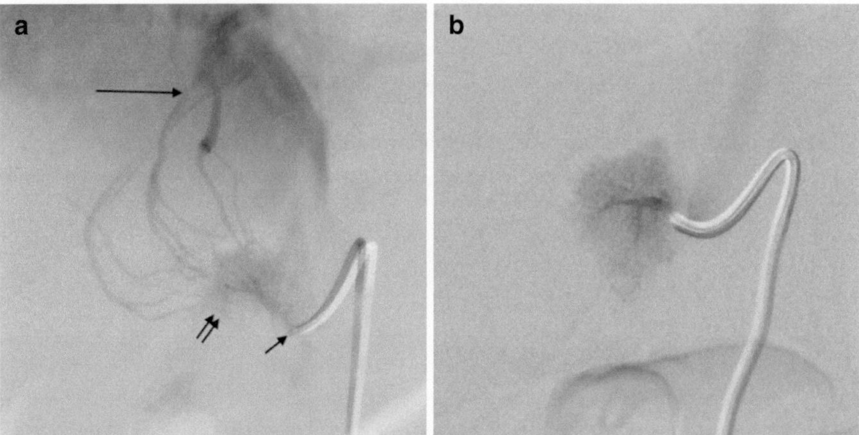

Fig. 6.4 Digital subtraction venographic (DSV) findings of the accessory hepatic vein (AHV). (**a**) DSV of the AHV (short arrow) shows a hepatic parenchymal blush (double arrow) and multiple intraparenchymal collateral veins draining into the right hepatic vein (long arrow) with a supero-medial course. (**b**) DSV of the AHV shows a hepatic parenchymal blush with irregular outer margins

the angiography suite. As a result, the success rates were significantly improved (93–94%) compared to AVS without quick cortisol assay (60–63%).

Sequential vs. Simultaneous AVS

Sequential AVS involves a single puncture of the femoral vein with sequential catheterization of the adrenal veins and samplings. The AVS usually starts from the RAV, followed by LAV, and completed with infrarenal IVC. This technique requires a continuous infusion of cosyntropin (50 µg/h) during the procedure to minimize the stress-induced fluctuation in hormone secretion [79, 80]. Simultaneous AVS, on the other hand, involves two separate accesses in the femoral vein, two different types of catheters for bilateral adrenal veins, and a collection of all three sets of blood samples at the same time for eliminating bias from stress-induced hormone fluctuation [36, 80–83]. Therefore, simultaneous AVS can potentially obviate the need for cosyntropin stimulation. Also, it allows multiple samplings for comparing values between before and after a bolus of cosyntropin (250 µg) without reentering the veins. However, simultaneous AVS is relatively more invasive, technically demanding, and time-consuming and has an increased risk of adrenal vein thrombosis due to prolonged catheterization [58, 80]. According to the 2012 AVIS, sequential AVS has been the primary technique adopted by most centers, with simultaneous AVS performed only in 35% of the centers worldwide [36]. Several studies have advocated using simultaneous AVS over sequential AVS, without comparing two methods [81, 84, 85]. To date, only two studies compared two methods and concluded that the results from both techniques were concordant without compromising the reliability of time-sensitive AVS [80, 86]. In a most recent study evaluating simultaneous and simulated sequential AVS, Rossitto et al. recommended primarily simultaneous AVS if the time delay between the RAV and LAV is longer than 15 min [84]. We use sequential AVS at our institution approximately 30 min after initiating continuous infusion of cosyntropin, with an average time delay between two adrenal veins of less than 10 min.

C-Arm Cone-Beam CT

Cone-beam CT (CBCT) generates a volumetric data set in a single gantry rotation using a two-dimensional, digital flat-panel detector system [87, 88]. The CBCT mounted on a C-arm (C-arm CBCT) produces projection radiography, fluoroscopy, digital subtraction angiography, and three-dimensional CT images in a single patient setup in the angiography suite. C-arm CBCT has been used to improve AVS's diagnostic outcomes by confirming an appropriate catheter position before collecting blood samples, especially in the RAV [89–91]. In a retrospective study of 156 patients with PA, the rate of adequate bilateral AVS increased from 40.6% to 88.7% when C-arm CBCT was used [90]. Also, the rate of catheterization failure from the RAV decreased significantly. In a similar study of 91 AVS, Meyrignac et al. demonstrated an improved overall success rate of AVS from 44% to 80% with C-arm CBCT [91]. However, the patient's radiation dose can be significant in C-arm CBCT due to the automatic exposure control system [88]. When it is performed repeatedly to confirm the catheter position, the patient's radiation exposure further increases. Therefore, C-arm CBCT is usually recommended when the institutional overall AVS success rate is below 50% or for an inexperienced interventional radiologist [92].

Interpretation of AVS

Successful AVS is defined by the correct catheterization of the adrenal vein measured by the selectivity index (SI). The SI is the ratio of plasma cortisol concentration (PCC) in the adrenal vein and IVC (right SI = PCC_{RAV}/PCC_{IVC}, left SI = PCC_{LAV}/PCC_{IVC}) [65]. Although different SI values are used during AVS in most centers, studies have shown that higher SI is more reliable, and the obtained results are more accurate and reproducible [93, 94]. The Endocrine Society Guidelines recommend $SI \geq 2$ without ACTH stimulation and $SI \geq 5$ with ACTH stimulation as benchmarks for correct adrenal vein catheterization [28, 67].

The lateralization index (LI) is used to identify the source of excess secretion of aldosterone. It is calculated by dividing the aldosterone-to-cortisol (A/C) ratio from the adrenal vein by the A/C ratio from the IVC (right LI = $[A_{RAV}/C_{RAV}]/[A_{IVC}/C_{IVC}]$, left LI = $[A_{LAV}/C_{LAV}]/[A_{IVC}/C_{IVC}]$) [95, 96]. To date, there is no consensus on the ideal cutoff values of the LI to select the patients for surgery [28]. Based on the retrospective studies and the Endocrine Society Guidelines, LI of 4 is recommended to lateralize the source of aldosterone, regardless of the ACTH stimulation [28, 58, 83]. Although ACTH stimulation could potentially reduce the LI by increasing aldosterone secretion from the suppressed adrenal gland, the systematic review showed that the number of incorrect lateralization was similar between the groups with and without ACTH stimulation [28, 67].

Complications

Complications associated with AVS include adrenal hemorrhage resulted from adrenal vein rupture or dissection, infarction of the adrenal gland, and adrenal vein thrombosis. The reported overall complication rate was 0.61% in the AVIS [36]. When an extreme outlier was excluded, the corrected complication rate was only 0.51%. In this international study, the number of AVS performed by each interventional radiologist and the number of AVS performed per center were the major predictors for adrenal vein rupture. Also, the higher number of attempts necessary to select the adrenal vein contributes to the higher rate of adrenal hemorrhage, especially in the RAV due to anatomical complexity [97]. Abdominal pain is the most common symptom associated with adrenal hemorrhage, requiring conservative management with opioids in most cases. If the symptom persists, follow-up CT is recommended to rule out major retroperitoneal hemorrhage. Major complications, such as adrenal insufficiency or hypertensive crisis, requiring long-term treatment, are extremely rare [97].

Conclusion

Despite the advanced imaging technologies, AVS is still the only reliable method for differentiating unilateral versus bilateral subtypes of PA before surgery. AVS is a safe procedure with a low complication rate, but technically challenging. Therefore, successful AVS requires experience, skills, and knowledge of adrenal venous anatomy, variations, and venographic findings. A combination of cosyntropin stimulation and rapid or on-site quick cortisol assay should be considered to improve the success rate. C-arm CBCT can also be considered for interventional radiologists with limited experience or a center with a small number of AVS procedures.

References

1. Conn JW, Cohen EL, Rovner DR, Nesbit RM. Normokalemic primary aldosteronism. A detectable cause of curable "essential" hypertension. JAMA. 1965;193:200–6.
2. Conn JW, Cohen EL, Rovner DR. Suppression of plasma renin activity in primary aldosteronism. JAMA. 1964;190:213–21.
3. Conn JW, Louis LH. Primary aldosteronism, a new clinical entity. Ann Intern Med. 1956;44(1):1–15.
4. Conn JW, Louis LH. Primary aldosteronism: a new clinical entity. Trans Assoc Am Phys. 1955;68:215–31. discussion 31–3
5. Mulatero P, Monticone S, Deinum J, et al. Genetics, prevalence, screening and confirmation of primary aldosteronism: a position statement and consensus of the Working Group on Endocrine Hypertension of The European Society of Hypertension. J Hypertens. 2020;38(10):1919–28.
6. Monticone S, Burrello J, Tizzani D, et al. Prevalence and clinical manifestations of primary aldosteronism encountered in primary care practice. J Am Coll Cardiol. 2017;69(14):1811–20.
7. Rossi GP, Bernini G, Caliumi C, et al. A prospective study of the prevalence of primary aldosteronism in 1,125 hypertensive patients. J Am Coll Cardiol. 2006;48(11):2293–300.
8. Funder JW, Carey RM, Mantero F, et al. The management of primary aldosteronism: case detection, diagnosis, and treatment: an Endocrine Society clinical practice guideline. J Clin Endocrinol Metab. 2016;101(5):1889–916.
9. Rossi GP, Seccia TM, Pessina AC. Primary aldosteronism – part I: prevalence, screening, and selection of cases for adrenal vein sampling. J Nephrol. 2008;21(4):447–54.
10. Streeten DH, Tomycz N, Anderson GH. Reliability of screening methods for the diagnosis of primary aldosteronism. Am J Med. 1979;67(3):403–13.
11. Mulatero P, Monticone S, Burrello J, Veglio F, Williams TA, Funder J. Guidelines for primary aldosteronism: uptake by primary care physicians in Europe. J Hypertens. 2016;34(11):2253–7.
12. Denimal D, Duvillard L. 2016 Endocrine Society guidelines update for the diagnosis of primary aldosteronism: are the proposed aldosterone-to-renin ratio cut-off values relevant in the era of fully automated immunoassays? Ann Clin Biochem. 2016;53(6):714–5.
13. Rossi GP, Seccia TM, Pessina AC. Primary aldosteronism: part II: subtype differentiation and treatment. J Nephrol. 2008;21(4):455–62.
14. Morioka M, Kobayashi T, Sone A, Furukawa Y, Tanaka H. Primary aldosteronism due to unilateral adrenal hyperplasia: report of two cases and review of the literature. Endocr J. 2000;47(4):443–9.
15. Katayama Y, Takata N, Tamura T, et al. A case of primary aldosteronism due to unilateral adrenal hyperplasia. Hypertens Res. 2005;28(4):379–84.
16. Ito A, Yamazaki Y, Sasano H, et al. A case of primary aldosteronism caused by unilateral multiple adrenocortical micronodules presenting as muscle cramps at rest: the importance of functional histopathology for identifying a culprit lesion. Pathol Int. 2017;67(4):214–21.
17. Hirono Y, Doi M, Yoshimoto T, et al. A case with primary aldosteronism due to unilateral multiple adrenocortical micronodules. Endocr J. 2005;52(4):435–9.
18. Omura M, Sasano H, Fujiwara T, Yamaguchi K, Nishikawa T. Unique cases of unilateral hyperaldosteronemia due to multiple adrenocortical micronodules, which can only be detected by selective adrenal venous sampling. Metabolism. 2002;51(3):350–5.
19. Haenel LC, Hermayer KL. A case of unilateral adrenal hyperplasia: the diagnostic dilemma of hyperaldosteronism. Endocr Pract. 2000;6(2):153–8.
20. Doppman JL, Gill JR Jr, Miller DL, et al. Distinction between hyperaldosteronism due to bilateral hyperplasia and unilateral aldosteronoma: reliability of CT. Radiology. 1992;184(3):677–82.
21. Gordon RD. Primary aldosteronism. J Endocrinol Investig. 1995;18(7):495–511.
22. Kempers MJ, Lenders JW, van Outheusden L, et al. Systematic review: diagnostic procedures to differentiate unilateral from bilateral adrenal abnormality in primary aldosteronism. Ann Intern Med. 2009;151(5):329–37.

23. Sam D, Kline GA, So B, Leung AA. Discordance between imaging and adrenal vein sampling in primary aldosteronism irrespective of interpretation criteria. J Clin Endocrinol Metab. 2019;104(6):1900–6.
24. Wachtel H, Zaheer S, Shah PK, et al. Role of adrenal vein sampling in primary aldosteronism: impact of imaging, localization, and age. J Surg Oncol. 2016;113(5):532–7.
25. Magill SB, Raff H, Shaker JL, et al. Comparison of adrenal vein sampling and computed tomography in the differentiation of primary aldosteronism. J Clin Endocrinol Metab. 2001;86(3):1066–71.
26. Espiner EA, Ross DG, Yandle TG, Richards AM, Hunt PJ. Predicting surgically remedial primary aldosteronism: role of adrenal scanning, posture testing, and adrenal vein sampling. J Clin Endocrinol Metab. 2003;88(8):3637–44.
27. Dekkers T, Prejbisz A, Kool LJS, et al. Adrenal vein sampling versus CT scan to determine treatment in primary aldosteronism: an outcome-based randomised diagnostic trial. Lancet Diabetes Endocrinol. 2016;4(9):739–46.
28. Mulatero P, Sechi LA, Williams TA, et al. Subtype diagnosis, treatment, complications and outcomes of primary aldosteronism and future direction of research: a position statement and consensus of the Working Group on Endocrine Hypertension of the European Society of Hypertension. J Hypertens. 2020;38(10):1929–36.
29. Young WF Jr. Diagnosis and treatment of primary aldosteronism: practical clinical perspectives. J Intern Med. 2019;285(2):126–48.
30. Beuschlein F, Mulatero P, Asbach E, et al. The SPARTACUS trial: controversies and unresolved issues. Horm Metab Res. 2017;49(12):936–42.
31. Burton TJ, Mackenzie IS, Balan K, et al. Evaluation of the sensitivity and specificity of (11) C-metomidate positron emission tomography (PET)-CT for lateralizing aldosterone secretion by Conn's adenomas. J Clin Endocrinol Metab. 2012;97(1):100–9.
32. Heinze B, Fuss CT, Mulatero P, et al. Targeting CXCR4 (CXC Chemokine Receptor Type 4) for molecular imaging of aldosterone-producing adenoma. Hypertension. 2018;71(2):317–25.
33. Abe T, Naruse M, Young WF Jr, et al. A novel CYP11B2-specific imaging agent for detection of unilateral subtypes of primary aldosteronism. J Clin Endocrinol Metab. 2016;101(3):1008–15.
34. Yen RF, Wu VC, Liu KL, et al. 131I-6beta-iodomethyl-19-norcholesterol SPECT/CT for primary aldosteronism patients with inconclusive adrenal venous sampling and CT results. J Nucl Med. 2009;50(10):1631–7.
35. Melby JC, Spark RF, Dale SL, Egdahl RH, Kahn PC. Diagnosis and localization of aldosterone-producing adenomas by percutaneous bilateral adrenal vein catheterization. Prog Clin Cancer. 1970;4:175–84.
36. Rossi GP, Barisa M, Allolio B, et al. The Adrenal Vein Sampling International Study (AVIS) for identifying the major subtypes of primary aldosteronism. J Clin Endocrinol Metab. 2012;97(5):1606–14.
37. Monroe EJ, Carney BW, Ingraham CR, Johnson GE, Valji K. An interventionist's guide to endocrine consultations. Radiographics. 2017;37(4):1246–67.
38. Clemente CD. Gray's anatomy of the human body. 30th ed. Philadelphia: Lea & Febiger; 1985. p. 788–836.
39. Moore KL, Persaud TVN. The developing human. 7th ed. Philadelphia: Saunders; 2003. p. 331–5.
40. Anson MJ. Morris' human anatomy. 12th ed. New York: McGraw-Hill; 1966. p. 834–9.
41. Spentzouris G, Zandian A, Cesmebasi A, et al. The clinical anatomy of the inferior vena cava: a review of common congenital anomalies and considerations for clinicians. Clin Anat. 2014;27(8):1234–43.
42. McClure CFW, Butler EG. The development of the vena cava inferior in man. Am J Anat. 1925;35:331–83.
43. Fernandez-Cuadrado J, Alonso-Torres A, Baudraxler F, Sanchez-Almaraz C. Three-dimensional contrast-enhanced magnetic resonance angiography of congenital inferior vena cava anomalies. Semin Pediatr Surg. 2005;14(4):226–32.

44. Ross MH, Pawlina W. Histology; a text and atlas. 6th ed. Philadelphia: Lippincott Williams & Wilkins; 2011. p. 762–71.
45. Matsuura T, Takase K, Ota H, et al. Radiologic anatomy of the right adrenal vein: preliminary experience with MDCT. AJR Am J Roentgenol. 2008;191(2):402–8.
46. Pearl M. Image-guided interventions: abdominal aorta and the inferior vena cava. Philadelphia: Saunders; 2008. p. 415–27.
47. Hollinshead WH. In: Hollinshead WH, editor. Anatomy for surgeons. New York: Hoeber-Harper; 1956. p. 573–9.
48. Monkhouse WS, Khalique A. The adrenal and renal veins of man and their connections with azygos and lumbar veins. J Anat. 1986;146:105–15.
49. Kahn SL, Angle JF. Adrenal vein sampling. Tech Vasc Interv Radiol. 2010;13(2):110–25.
50. Avisse C, Marcus C, Patey M, Ladam-Marcus V, Delattre JF, Flament JB. Surgical anatomy and embryology of the adrenal glands. Surg Clin North Am. 2000;80(1):403–15.
51. Scholten A, Cisco RM, Vriens MR, Shen WT, Duh Q-Y. Variant adrenal venous anatomy in 546 laparoscopic adrenalectomies. JAMA Surg. 2013;148(4):378.
52. Omura K, Ota H, Takahashi Y, et al. Anatomical variations of the right adrenal vein: concordance between multidetector computed tomography and catheter venography. Hypertension. 2017;69(3):428–34.
53. Cesmebasi A, Du Plessis M, Iannatuono M, Shah S, Tubbs RS, Loukas M. A review of the anatomy and clinical significance of adrenal veins. Clin Anat. 2014;27(8):1253–63.
54. Johnstone FRC. The suprarenal veins. Am J Surg. 1957;94(4):615–20.
55. Siebert M, Robert Y, Didier R, et al. Anatomical variations of the venous drainage from the left adrenal gland: an anatomical study. World J Surg. 2017;41(4):991–6.
56. Loukas M, Louis RG Jr, Hullett J, Loiacano M, Skidd P, Wagner T. An anatomical classification of the variations of the inferior phrenic vein. Surg Radiol Anat. 2005;27(6):566–74.
57. Araki T, Imaizumi A, Okada H, Onishi H. Unusual anatomical variants of the left adrenal vein via the renal capsular vein preventing successful adrenal vein sampling. Cardiovasc Intervent Radiol. 2017;40(8):1296–8.
58. Monticone S, Viola A, Rossato D, et al. Adrenal vein sampling in primary aldosteronism: towards a standardised protocol. Lancet Diabetes Endocrinol. 2015;3(4):296–303.
59. Funder J, Carey R, Fardella C, et al. Withdrawn: case detection, diagnosis, and treatment of patients with primary aldosteronism: an Endocrine Society clinical practice guideline. Eur J Endocrinol. 2009; https://doi.org/10.1530/EJE-09-0870.
60. Mulatero P, Rabbia F, Milan A, et al. Drug effects on aldosterone/plasma renin activity ratio in primary aldosteronism. Hypertension. 2002;40(6):897–902.
61. Ching KC, Cohen DL, Fraker DL, Trerotola SO. Adrenal vein sampling for primary aldosteronism: a 2-week protocol for withdrawal of renin-stimulating antihypertensives. Cardiovasc Intervent Radiol. 2017;40(9):1367–71.
62. Weinberger MH, Grim CE, Higgins JT Jr. Diagnosis, localization, and treatment of primary aldosteronism. Compr Ther. 1977;3(5):12–7.
63. Seccia TM, Miotto D, De Toni R, et al. Adrenocorticotropic hormone stimulation during adrenal vein sampling for identifying surgically curable subtypes of primary aldosteronism: comparison of 3 different protocols. Hypertension. 2009;53(5):761–6.
64. El Ghorayeb N, Mazzuco TL, Bourdeau I, et al. Basal and post-ACTH aldosterone and its ratios are useful during adrenal vein sampling in primary aldosteronism. J Clin Endocrinol Metabol. 2016;101(4):1826–35.
65. Rossi GP, Pitter G, Bernante P, Motta R, Feltrin G, Miotto D. Adrenal vein sampling for primary aldosteronism: the assessment of selectivity and lateralization of aldosterone excess baseline and after adrenocorticotropic hormone (ACTH) stimulation. J Hypertens. 2008;26(5):989–97.
66. Wolley MJ, Ahmed AH, Gordon RD, Stowasser M. Does ACTH improve the diagnostic performance of adrenal vein sampling for subtyping primary aldosteronism? Clin Endocrinol. 2016;85(5):703–9.

67. Laurent I, Astère M, Zheng F, et al. Adrenal venous sampling with or without adrenocorticotropic hormone stimulation: a meta-analysis. J Clin Endocrinol Metabol. 2019;104(4):1060–8.
68. Daunt N. Adrenal vein sampling: how to make it quick, easy, and successful. Radiographics. 2005;25(suppl_1):S143–S58.
69. Makita K, Nishimoto K, Kiriyama-Kitamoto K, et al. A novel method: super-selective adrenal venous sampling. J Vis Exp. 2017;(127):55716.
70. Miotto D, De Toni R, Pitter G, et al. Impact of accessory hepatic veins on adrenal vein sampling for identification of surgically curable primary aldosteronism. Hypertension. 2009;54(4):885–9.
71. Trerotola SO, Smoger DL, Cohen DL, Fraker DL. The inferior accessory hepatic vein: an anatomic landmark in adrenal vein sampling. J Vasc Interv Radiol. 2011;22(9):1306–11.
72. Young WF. Primary aldosteronism: renaissance of a syndrome. Clin Endocrinol. 2007;66(5):607–18.
73. Young WF Jr. Minireview: primary aldosteronism--changing concepts in diagnosis and treatment. Endocrinology. 2003;144(6):2208–13.
74. Auchus RJ, Michaelis C, Wians FH Jr, et al. Rapid cortisol assays improve the success rate of adrenal vein sampling for primary aldosteronism. Ann Surg. 2009;249(2):318–21.
75. Mengozzi G, Rossato D, Bertello C, et al. Rapid cortisol assay during adrenal vein sampling in patients with primary aldosteronism. Clin Chem. 2007;53(11):1968–71.
76. Betz MJ, Degenhart C, Fischer E, et al. Adrenal vein sampling using rapid cortisol assays in primary aldosteronism is useful in centers with low success rates. Eur J Endocrinol. 2011;165(2):301–6.
77. Monticone S, Mulatero P. Rapid cortisol assay increases the success of adrenal vein sampling. Am J Hypertens. 2011;24(12):1265.
78. Yoneda T, Karashima S, Kometani M, et al. Impact of new quick gold nanoparticle-based cortisol assay during adrenal vein sampling for primary aldosteronism. J Clin Endocrinol Metab. 2016;101(6):2554–61.
79. Young WF Jr, Stanson AW, Grant CS, Thompson GB, van Heerden JA. Primary aldosteronism: adrenal venous sampling. Surgery. 1996;120(6):913–9; discussion 9–20
80. Carr CE, Cope C, Cohen DL, Fraker DL, Trerotola SO. Comparison of sequential versus simultaneous methods of adrenal venous sampling. J Vasc Interv Radiol. 2004;15(11):1245–50.
81. Doppman JL, Gill JR Jr. Hyperaldosteronism: sampling the adrenal veins. Radiology. 1996;198(2):309–12.
82. Seccia TM, Miotto D, Battistel M, et al. A stress reaction affects assessment of selectivity of adrenal venous sampling and of lateralization of aldosterone excess in primary aldosteronism. Eur J Endocrinol. 2012;166(5):869–75.
83. Rossi GP, Auchus RJ, Brown M, et al. An expert consensus statement on use of adrenal vein sampling for the subtyping of primary aldosteronism. Hypertension. 2014;63(1):151–60.
84. Rossitto G, Battistel M, Barbiero G, et al. The subtyping of primary aldosteronism by adrenal vein sampling: sequential blood sampling causes factitious lateralization. J Hypertens. 2018;36(2):335–43.
85. Lupi A, Battistel M, Barbiero G, Miotto D, Rossi GP, Quaia E. Simultaneous bilateral adrenal vein sampling for primary aldosteronism: useful tips to make it simple and safe. Eur Radiol. 2019;29(11):6330–5.
86. Almarzooqi MK, Chagnon M, Soulez G, et al. Adrenal vein sampling in primary aldosteronism: concordance of simultaneous vs sequential sampling. Eur J Endocrinol. 2017;176(2):159–67.
87. Jaffray DA, Siewerdsen JH. Cone-beam computed tomography with a flat-panel imager: initial performance characterization. Med Phys. 2000;27(6):1311–23.
88. Orth RC, Wallace MJ, Kuo MD. C-arm cone-beam CT: general principles and technical considerations for use in interventional radiology. J Vasc Interv Radiol. 2008;19(6):814–20.
89. Georgiades CS, Hong K, Geschwind JF, et al. Adjunctive use of C-arm CT may eliminate technical failure in adrenal vein sampling. J Vasc Interv Radiol. 2007;18(9):1102–5.

90. Park CH, Hong N, Han K, et al. C-arm computed tomography-assisted adrenal venous sampling improved right adrenal vein cannulation and sampling quality in primary aldosteronism. Endocrinol Metab (Seoul). 2018;33(2):236–44.
91. Meyrignac O, Arcis E, Delchier MC, et al. Impact of cone beam – CT on adrenal vein sampling in primary aldosteronism. Eur J Radiol. 2020;124:108792.
92. Bai HX, Trerotola SO. Adrenal Vein Sampling. In: Advances in treatment and management in surgical endocrinology. Elsevier; 2020. p. 187–98.
93. Mulatero P, Bertello C, Sukor N, et al. Impact of different diagnostic criteria during adrenal vein sampling on reproducibility of subtype diagnosis in patients with primary aldosteronism. Hypertension. 2010;55(3):667–73.
94. Lethielleux G, Amar L, Raynaud A, Plouin PF, Steichen O. Influence of diagnostic criteria on the interpretation of adrenal vein sampling. Hypertension. 2015;65(4):849–54.
95. Tagawa M, Ghosn M, Wachtel H, et al. Lateralization index but not contralateral suppression at adrenal vein sampling predicts improvement in blood pressure after adrenalectomy for primary aldosteronism. J Hum Hypertens. 2017;31(7):444–9.
96. Shibayama Y, Wada N, Naruse M, et al. The occurrence of apparent bilateral aldosterone suppression in adrenal vein sampling for primary aldosteronism. J Endocr Soc. 2018;2(5):398–407.
97. Monticone S, Satoh F, Dietz AS, et al. Clinical management and outcomes of adrenal hemorrhage following adrenal vein sampling in primary aldosteronism. Hypertension. 2016;67(1):146–52.

Chapter 7
Selective Venous Sampling for Hyperparathyroidism

Takayuki Yamada and Akiyuki Kotoku

Introduction

Surgical dissection of the responsible parathyroid gland is the curative treatment for primary hyperparathyroidism (pHPT). The conventional approach requires bilateral neck exploration (BNE), but recently minimally invasive parathyroidectomy (MIP) has become the preferred option. Both BNE and MIP are effective in terms of cure rate; however, the safety profile of MIP is superior to BNE with lower rates of hypocalcemia and recurrent laryngeal nerve injury [1]. MIP does require precise preoperative localization of the abnormal parathyroid gland [2]. This preoperative localization can be performed with a variety of noninvasive and invasive imaging studies. The noninvasive studies include ultrasound, computed tomography (CT), magnetic resonance imaging (MRI), and ^{99m}Tc-sestamibi (MIBI). When noninvasive studies are inadequate, venous sampling is a minimally invasive study that can be used.

Selective venous sampling (SVS) was initially reported in 1970 [3]. Taking advantage of the fact that venous drainage of the four parathyroid glands is into the adjacent thyroid veins [4], SVS identifies the area of venous drainage of a hyperactive gland rather than its exact anatomical location [5]. Despite potential anatomic variations, both radiology and surgical studies confirm the utility of SVS. Nevertheless, improvements in noninvasive imaging techniques have reduced the utilization of SVS over time. Yet, there continue to be situations in which SVS continues to have a role in the localization of abnormal glands for pHPT. For these situations, a thorough understanding of the complex anatomy and potential variants, as well as the ability to selectively catheterize small veins draining the thyroid gland, is paramount to accurately localize the abnormal parathyroid gland.

T. Yamada (✉) · A. Kotoku
Department of Radiology, St. Marianna University School of Medicine, Yokohama City Seibu Hospital, Yokohama, Kanagawa, Japan
e-mail: yamataka@marianna-u.ac.jp

© The Author(s), under exclusive license to Springer Nature Switzerland AG 2022

H. Yu et al. (eds.), *Diagnosis and Management of Endocrine Disorders in Interventional Radiology*, https://doi.org/10.1007/978-3-030-87189-5_7

Indications

A noninvasive imaging study is the first step for localizing the responsible parathyroid gland containing the adenoma. Ultrasound and 99mTc-MIBI are the standard first-line noninvasive imaging studies, while CT and MRI are reserved for patients requiring further workup. 99mTc-MIBI single-photon emission computed tomography (SPECT) remains a valuable tool in identifying parathyroid adenomas. In a recent meta-analysis, SPECT was found to have a pooled sensitivity of 78.9% (CI: 64–90.6%) and PPV of 90.7% [6]. Recently, four-dimensional (4D) CT, a dynamic contrast-enhanced CT, has been used to detect parathyroid adenomas [7–11]. Parathyroid adenomas are identified by their early contrast enhancement with washout on the delayed phase. 4D-CT has also been shown to be effective in multiglandular disease [11]. For this reason, many radiologists have adopted 4D-CT as the first- or second-line study for pHPT [12]. With advances such as this in noninvasive imaging technique, SVS has taken on a reduced role for localizing the adenoma [13].

Despite the advances in noninvasive imaging, SVS continues to have an essential role in evaluating postoperative patients with persistent or recurrent HPT [5, 14–24]. For these patients, 99mTc-MIBI scans have limited utility due to low sensitivities, reported to be as low as 50% [25, 26].

For those patients presenting with de novo hyperparathyroidism, there are studies supporting the use of SVS in localizing the adenoma. The noninvasive imaging studies mentioned above provide good detectability; however, there remain patients with nonlocalizing or discordant results. In a systematic review, studies of 99mTc-MIBI showed a wide range of sensitivities with values as low as 39% to over 90% [27], whereas SVS has generally been shown to have high sensitivity with values reported at 94.7% and 87% [28–30]. Therefore, at present, SVS is indicated for patients with recurrent or persistent HPT after resection as well as for patients with negative or discordant results on noninvasive imaging studies.

Techniques

Anatomy

The venous drainage of the parathyroid glands is via the thyroid plexus and then centrally via the inferior thyroid veins [3]. The thyroid plexus forms under the capsule on the anterior surface of the thyroid gland [31, 32]. The thyroid plexus gives rise to three pairs of thyroid veins: superior, middle, and inferior veins. Knowledge of three thyroid veins is imperative for conducting successful SVS procedures.

The anatomy of the superior thyroid veins is similar bilaterally based on studies using either cadavers or multi-detector row helical CT (MDCT) [33, 34]. In most people, there is a single superior thyroid vein bilaterally (83.3%), while a minority of people have duplicated superior thyroid veins (16.7%) [34]. The superior thyroid veins typically drain the upper pole of the thyroid gland and drain directly into the IJV (97.2%), either as a single vein or after joining other veins, most commonly the lingual vein.

The middle thyroid veins run parallel to the inferior thyroid arteries and drain the mid-thyroid gland into the ipsilateral IJV. This vein was identified in 43.3% of people in a cadaver study [34] and was identified in 36% of people on the left side and 49% on the right side by MDCT [33]. Similarly, a surgical study also showed the middle thyroid vein in only 36.7% of people on the left side and in 40.7% on the right [35].

The inferior thyroid veins are typically the largest of the thyroid veins, coursing from the lower thyroid gland in 34.1% and the upper and medial thyroid gland in 58.7%. The inferior thyroid vein is consistently present though variable in number, ranging from one (common trunk) to five [33, 34, 36]. The left inferior thyroid veins and common trunk drain into the left BCV (Fig. 7.1a, b). The right inferior thyroid vein less commonly flows into the right BCV. The supernumerary vein often accompanies the inferior thyroid veins or common trunks on either side [33] (Fig. 7.2a–d). The previously mentioned study using MDCT showed the distance between the junction of both BCVs and orifice of inferior thyroid veins ranged from 0.63 to

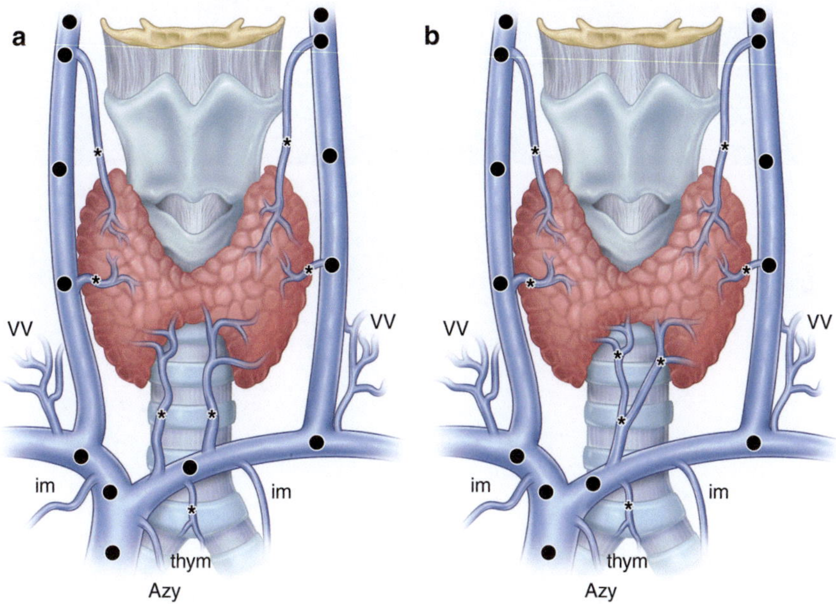

Fig. 7.1 Illustration of venous anatomy. *thym* thymic vein, *vv* vertebral vein, *im* intermammary vein, *Azy* azygos vein. (**a**) The pattern with two inferior thyroid veins. (**b**) The pattern with the common trunk of the inferior thyroid vein. The asterisks represent the sampling points in the small neck veins, while the black dots represent the sampling points in the large central neck veins. The site of black dots needs to be adjusted to aim at detecting the step-up of iPTH value draining from the certain small neck vein

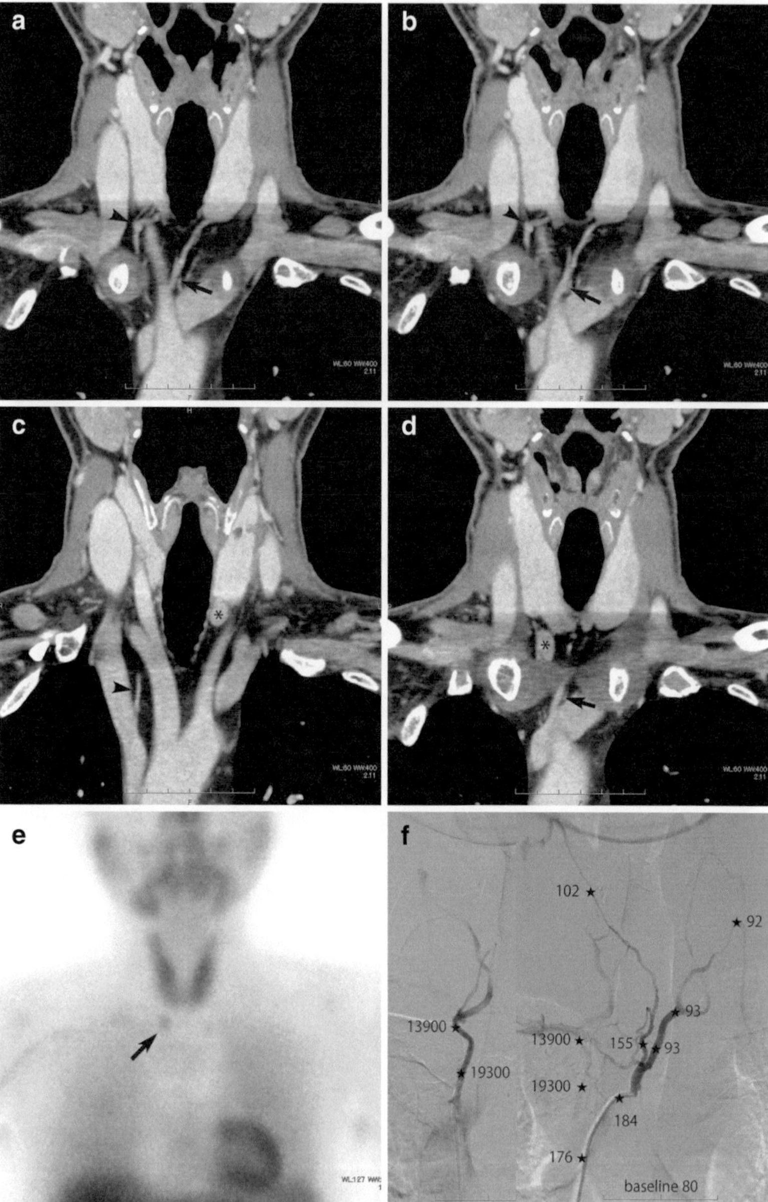

Fig. 7.2 A 40-year-old male with primary hyperparathyroidism. (**a–d**) Coronal CT images. The common trunk of the inferior thyroid veins is noted (arrows). The right inferior thyroid vein is also noted (arrowheads). The two nodules are identified near the lower pole of both thyroid glands (asterisks). An ultrasound image shows the two nodules adjacent to the lower pole of the thyroid gland (not shown). (**e**) 99mTc-MIBI scintigraphy. A scintigraphic image shows an uptake in the lower right lobe of the thyroid gland (arrow). There is no uptake in the nodule on the left side. (**f**) Retrograde venography. Venograms from the right inferior thyroid vein (left image) and the left inferior thyroid vein (right image). Both thyroid veins are similar to those on the coronal CT images (**a–d**)

2.94 cm (mean 1.65 cm) for the right vein, from 0.5 to 6.19 cm (mean 3.01 cm) for the left vein, and from 0.5 to 4.4 cm (mean 2.04 cm) for the common trunk [33].

The anatomy and anastomotic connections of the venous drainage in the mediastinum are variable. Mediastinal glands drain into the thymic veins. The left thymic vein drains into the anteroinferior aspect of the left BCV in the midline, while the right thymic vein drains directly into the superior vena cava and cannot be catheterized [32]. However, these mediastinal glands occasionally will drain into the internal mammary vein or the common trunk of the inferior thyroid vein [37]. This pattern leads to the elevation of iPTH in the inferior thyroid vein even with mediastinal adenoma, making it impossible to discriminate the mediastinal adenoma from an adenoma in the neck by venous sampling alone [37] (Fig. 7.3).

In the postsurgical neck, venous anatomy is altered. In patients who have undergone surgical exploration, the middle and, often, the inferior thyroid veins generally are ligated. Therefore, the venous drainage from the thyroid bed may be via the vertebral veins [32].

Approaches

Three SVS techniques have been reported: a conventional SVS (cSVS) with samples obtained only from the large central neck veins (jugular, subclavian, and innominate veins) [14, 23, 38], super-selective venous sampling (sSVS) with sampling of smaller neck veins (superior, middle, and inferior thyroid veins and thymic veins) [15, 17, 21, 22, 24], and direct percutaneous bilateral IJV sampling (BIJVS) [39, 40].

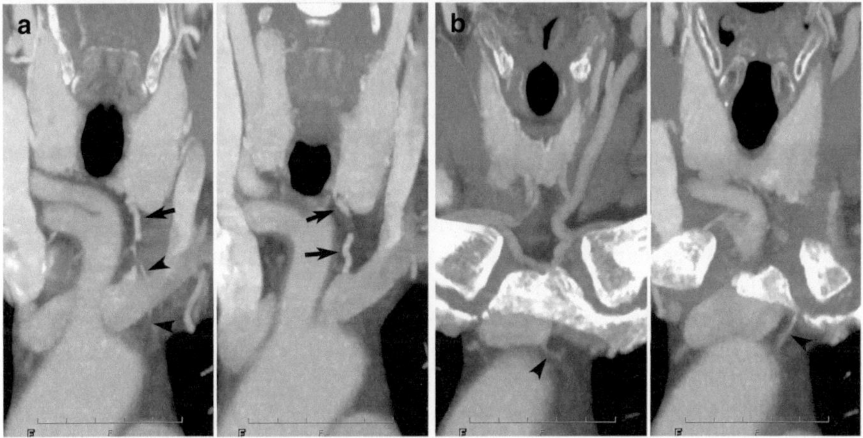

Fig. 7.3 Anastomoses between the left inferior thyroid and thymic veins. Partial maximum intensity projections of coronally reformatted CT images. (**a**) At the middle of the left thyroid vein (arrows), a small vein (arrowhead) joins. (**b**) The opposite end of the small vein continues to the thymic vein, which drains into the left brachiocephalic vein

Figure 7.1 illustrates the sampling points in the large central neck veins and small neck veins (Fig. 7.1a, b). More precise localization can be achieved with sSVS but cSVS can capture the drainage from the unsuccessful or unknown missed veins. The sampling points in the large central neck veins are modified based on the venous anatomy to detect elevated hormones from suspected small draining veins. While the thyroid veins are imperative for sSVS, the thymic vein is also important. This fact justifies the extensive efforts at catheterizing this small vein, even though it may be difficult [32]. Knowledge of the venous anatomy is essential before SVS to determine the proper sampling points in the IJV and BCV where the thyroid veins join and show the step-up values of iPTH. This information helps identify the thyroid vein for further interrogation using super-selective catheterization. The middle thyroid vein is not constantly present. Therefore, one can avoid an attempt to catheterize the middle thyroid vein if the anatomy is reviewed on available imaging studies before the procedure. Also, one study employed a quickPTH assay and added sSVS to the small veins in the relevant area with an increase in PTH to save time [20].

Given the anatomic variability, pre-procedure MDCT can help identify the location of the thyroid veins as well as suggest possible locations of the abnormal parathyroid gland. At present, vascular mapping by MDCT is routinely recommended before performing an SVS procedure. Both axial and coronal CT images help locate the thyroid veins and map the confluence with the IJV or BCV (Fig. 7.2). Sagittal images can also help identify the venous confluence level relative to the nearby vertebral bodies [41], thus providing a guide when probing the IJV, since the level of connection between the IJV and thyroid vein can be variable. On the other hand, MDCT is insufficient to define the anatomy of the thyroid venous plexus and typically requires retrograde thyroidal venography. The appearance of the thyroid venous plexus is variable, affected by different connections and flow patterns of the thyroid veins (Fig. 7.4). This flow pattern can be helpful, though, since potentially significant thyroid veins may be opacified through this plexus.

Technical Considerations

The approach of SVS is usually via the right femoral vein. Conventional 4-Fr. catheters such as Berenstein, Multipurpose, or Headhunter catheter (100-cm long) are used to catheterize the BCV and IJV and the larger thyroid veins. Microcatheters are typically also needed for sSVS in order to access the distal portion of thyroid veins and sample from other smaller veins in the neck. Any microcatheter with a thin tip allowing high flow is convenient for collecting the blood sample in sSVS.

The tip of conventional catheters tends to angle upward, which may not be conducive to selecting the superior and middle thyroid veins. Superior thyroid veins sometimes require a catheter with a downward angle. The left middle thyroid vein arising from the lower part of the left IJV often requires a catheter with a more winding shape. Various other catheter configurations, like Hilal Spinal 2 or Cobra,

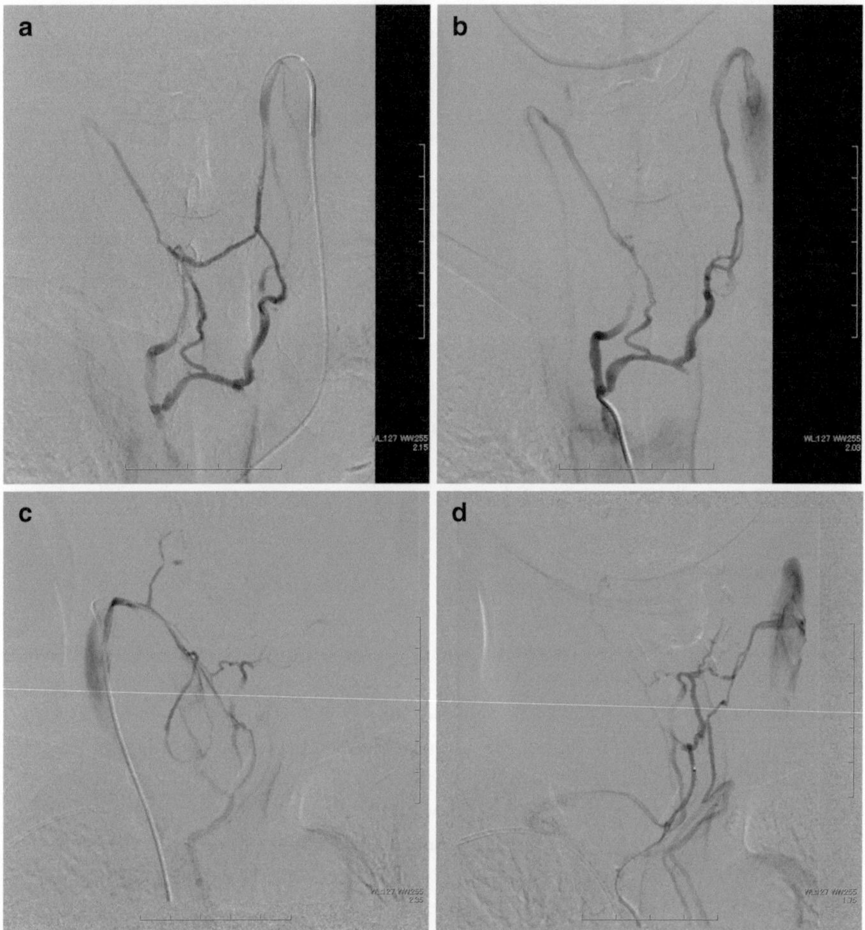

Fig. 7.4 Thyroid venous plexus on retrograde venography. (**a, b**) Retrograde venograms obtained from the left superior thyroid and right lower thyroid veins, respectively. The opacification of the thyroid plexus is different between (**a**) and (**b**), affected by the venous flow in the plexus. Contralateral flow is demonstrated to the thyroid veins on the right side. (**c, d**) Retrograde venograms from the right superior thyroid and right inferior thyroid veins, respectively. The opacification of the thyroid plexus is quite different between c and d, affected by the venous flow in the plexus. Contralateral flow is demonstrated to the thyroid veins on the left side

that have a large curve and downward tip can be helpful in accessing the superior and middle thyroid veins. We sometimes modify the curve or angle of the frequently used catheters by heating; however, this adjustment of the shape can make withdrawing the blood in the central neck veins difficult due to the catheter's wedging to the venous wall. If the catheter's angle or curve does not fit the veins despite these modifications, performing the venous sampling through a microcatheter should be considered.

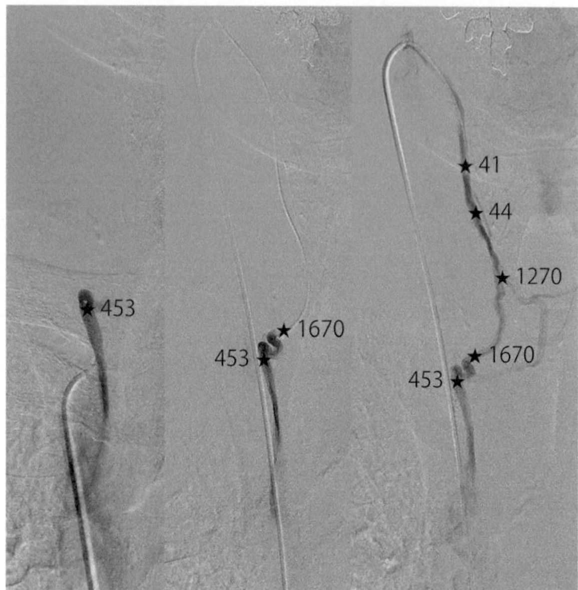

Fig. 7.5 A 72-year-old male with primary hyperparathyroidism. The middle and right images are the venograms obtained from the right superior thyroid vein. The microcatheter was advanced through the right superior thyroid vein to the tortuous point (middle). Four blood samples were collected in the right superior thyroid vein. Below the tortuosity, another sample was collected from the right inferior thyroid vein (left image). A steep gradient of iPTH was detected along the right inferior thyroid veins (453 vs. 1670)

The blood samples from the distal portion of the thyroid vein may be added when it is possible, improving the ability to precisely localize the offending adenoma. The steep gradient of iPTH in the same thyroid vein is occasionally observed (Figs. 7.5 and 7.6) [41]. In addition, the contralateral thyroid vein can be sampled by advancing a microcatheter through the venous plexus across the midline (Figs. 7.5 and 7.6), which can obviate the need to selectively catheterize the contralateral side. However, we occasionally encounter a situation in that the microguidewire advances but the microcatheter will not follow. In this case, the rotation of microcatheter rather than pushing may enable it to proceed.

Interpretation

A 1.5–2-fold increase in iPTH level compared to baseline (periphery, IVC or SVC) is considered an abnormal elevation. 1.4- or 1.5-fold was employed for cSVS [5, 18, 21, 38]; however, most studies that included sSVS have adopted a twofold gradient of iPTH to baseline as significant [15, 17, 19, 22–24, 28, 30].

SVS does not identify the culprit gland itself; rather, it allows "regionalization" by defining a territory drained by a specific vein or veins from the abnormal gland [32]. There has been no established way to determine the responsible gland in the previous reports. Some reports divided the thyroid gland into regions, such as right (upper and lower) side, left (upper and lower) side, bilateral or thymic-mediastinum, and report the area in which the positive gradient is recognized [5, 15, 17, 18, 30]. Others conducting sSVS regard the area containing the gland with the highest

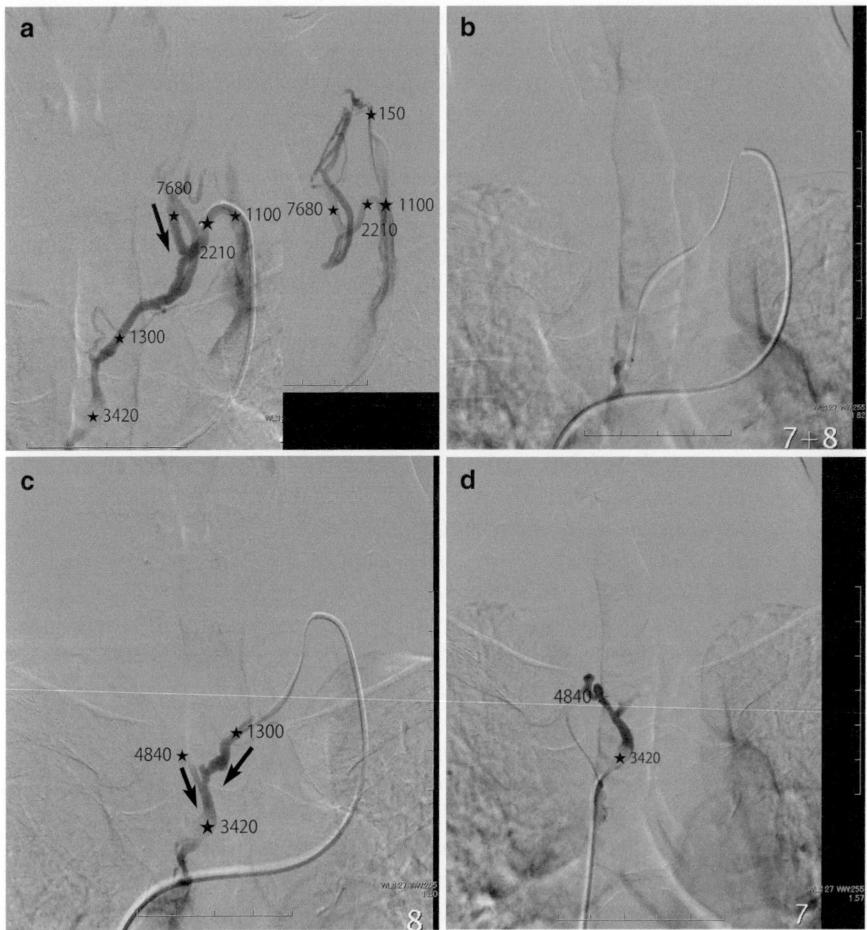

Fig. 7.6 A 77-year-old male with primary hyperparathyroidism. (**a**) Venogram from the proximal region of the left superior and middle thyroid veins. The flow from the middle thyroid vein to the common trunk of the inferior thyroid vein is demonstrated. (**b, c**) The microcatheter was proceeded to the common trunk and the part of the superior thyroid vein. Blood samples were obtained along the vein from the common trunk the superior thyroid vein and the middle thyroid vein. (**d**) The right thyroid vein could not be catheterized from the left side. Therefore, it was selected from the common trunk

gradient as the abnormal lesion [16, 20, 24]. This would be effective method if multiple samples are obtained along the small neck veins (Figs. 7.2, 7.5, and 7.6). One study performing cSVS just determined laterality of the lesion [38], which is the least useful result.

Attention should be paid to the flow direction of the thyroid venous plexus and thyroid veins when the gradient map is analyzed. Occasionally, the primary route of venous drainage during venography will be to the contralateral side [22]. In this situation, the solitary parathyroid adenoma result in bilateral gradients. This cross-flow occurs through the thyroid plexus, as well as through the vertebral venous plexus posteriorly and the jugular veins anteriorly [4]. The venous flow toward the opposite side could cause the false-positive gradient of thyroid and/or large central neck veins.

Another challenge is the occasional draining of thymic veins into the internal mammary vein or the common trunk of the inferior thyroid vein [37]. This leads to the elevation of iPTH in the inferior thyroid vein even with mediastinal adenoma, making it impossible to discriminate the mediastinal adenoma from the neck adenoma by venous sampling [37].

Complications

SVS is a minimally invasive procedure, and the risk of complication is quite low. Possible complications include contrast reactions and post-contrast acute kidney injury. One should monitor the amount of contrast used during sSVS, since the challenging nature of the procedure can easily result in one using large volumes of contrast. It is no surprise that the amount of contrast needed for sSVS is greater than with cSVS. Morris et al. reported using 204 mL of contrast in sSVS procedures, compared to 63 mL for non-super-selective sampling [21]. Other potential complications include groin hematoma, pain, deep vein thrombosis, infection, and cardiac arrythmia.

There are a few procedure-specific complications that can occur. A catheter or guidewire-induced venous injury is one of them. It is rare to see contrast extravasation with retrograde contrast venography. When it does occur, it is usually caused by either a catheter position wedged against the wall of the vein or an overly enthusiastic injection of contrast. This complication can often be avoided or minimized with careful attention to technique and gentle contrast injections when in the smaller neck veins.

An area of concern, which is not exactly a complication, is radiation exposure. These can be technically challenging procedures and the protracted effort to catheterize these smaller neck veins can result in high radiation exposures. Thus, it is important to practice safe radiation techniques, such as minimizing fluoroscopic frame rates and proper shielding.

Outcomes

A meta-analysis of 12 studies showed the sensitivity of SVS to be 74% (range 32–100%) and the specificity to be 41% (range 0–100%) [42]. SVS could be considered a reliable test for determining disease location; however, as indicted by the

Table 7.1 Previous studies on selective venous sampling for hyperparathyroidism

Author	Year	Cases	Sensitivity (%)	Technique
Jones [15]	2002	64	75	sSVS
Udelsman [16]	2003	13	88.8	sSVS
Estella [17]	2003	7	83	sSVS
Seehofer [18]	2004	21	90	cSVS
				Optional sSVS
Liew [43]	2004	9	78	N/A
Chaffanjon [28]	2004	23	94.7	sSVS
Eloy [29]	2006	8	87.5	N/A
Reidel [19]	2006	51	83.3	sSVS
Witteveen [5]	2010	18 (20; procedure)	75	cSVS
Gimm [20]	2012	5	80	sSVS with quickPTH assay
Morris [21]	2012	19	80	sSVS with arteriography
Lebastchi [22]	2015	31	89	sSVS with rapid PTH assay
Sun [23]	2016	18	93	sSVS
Habibollahi [24]	2018	32	96	sSVS
			28	Simulated cSVS
Lee [38]	2020	59	61.8	cSVS

cSVS conventional selective venous sampling, *sSVS* super-selective venous sampling, *N/A* no available

low specificity value, it also has a high rate of false positives [42]. Table 7.1 summarizes the studies included in the meta-analysis showing their results and techniques (Table 7.1).

Moreover, the results of SVS differed depending on the techniques employed. sSVS showed higher pooled sensitivity (89%) than cSVS (44%) or BISVS (69%). Habibollahi et al. published a study in which the simulated cSVS showed a positive gradient in only 28% of patients, but that number increased to 96% when using the sSVS technique [24]. This is a much different result than a study published by Morris et al. In their study, non-super-selective sampling resulted in a positive gradient in 95% of patients. However, sSVS still provided superior correlation with operative finding and guidance for the surgery [21]. When compared with noninvasive imaging studies, the pooled sensitivity (89%) of sSVS is higher than that of 99mTc-MIBI (71%) and comparable with US (87%) and MRI (89%) [42]. However, the actual sensitivity of localizing studies varied among each report, and it is difficult to say which modality is superior. Rather, the important thing is that sSVS can yield positive results in discordant and non-detectable results on noninvasive imaging studies. Ikuno et al. studied 14 patients with pHPT. In this group, there were four patients with discordant results on noninvasive imaging and one patient in which the noninvasive tests were negative. For these patients, sSVS was able to localize the adenoma to the correct quadrant of thyroid at parathyroidectomy [30].

Conclusion

Selective venous sampling is an effective technique to localize parathyroid adenomas in patients with primary hyperparathyroidism. This procedure can be challenging due to the variability in the venous anatomy encountered when performing the procedure and the small veins that must be catheterized if performing super-selective venous sampling. Understanding this variable anatomy, along with pre-procedure mapping with MDCT, will save time and increase the likelihood of locating the adenoma. Thorough mapping becomes even more critical in patients with ectopic parathyroid glands or a history of prior surgical resections. However, once the anatomy is well-defined, the procedure can be straightforward and poses minimal risk of complications.

References

1. Singh Ospina NM, Rodriguez-Gutierrez R, Maraka S, Espinosa de Ycaza AE, Jasim S, Castaneda-Guarderas A, et al. Outcomes of parathyroidectomy in patients with primary hyperparathyroidism: a systematic review and meta-analysis. World J Surg. 2016;40(10):2359–77.
2. Noureldine SI, Gooi Z, Tufano RP. Minimally invasive parathyroid surgery. Gland Surg. 2015;4(5):410–9.
3. Doppman JL, Hammond WG. The anatomic basis of parathyroid venous sampling. Radiology. 1970;95(3):603–10.
4. Dunlop DA, Papapoulos SE, Lodge RW, Fulton AJ, Kendall BE, O'Riordan JL. Parathyroid venous sampling: anatomic considerations and results in 95 patients with primary hyperparathyroidism. Br J Radiol. 1980;53(627):183–91.
5. Witteveen JE, Kievit J, van Erkel AR, Morreau H, Romijn JA, Hamdy NA. The role of selective venous sampling in the management of persistent hyperparathyroidism revisited. Eur J Endocrinol. 2010;163(6):945–52.
6. Cheung K, Wang TS, Farrokhyar F, Roman SA, Sosa JA. A meta-analysis of preoperative localization techniques for patients with primary hyperparathyroidism. Ann Surg Oncol. 2012;19(2):577–83.
7. Chazen JL, Gupta A, Dunning A, Phillips CD. Diagnostic accuracy of 4D-CT for parathyroid adenomas and hyperplasia. AJNR Am J Neuroradiol. 2012;33(3):429–33.
8. Hunter GJ, Schellingerhout D, Vu TH, Perrier ND, Hamberg LM. Accuracy of four-dimensional CT for the localization of abnormal parathyroid glands in patients with primary hyperparathyroidism. Radiology. 2012;264(3):789–95.
9. Kelly HR, Hamberg LM, Hunter GJ. 4D-CT for preoperative localization of abnormal parathyroid glands in patients with hyperparathyroidism: accuracy and ability to stratify patients by unilateral versus bilateral disease in surgery-naive and re-exploration patients. AJNR Am J Neuroradiol. 2014;35(1):176–81.
10. Sepahdari AR, Yeh MW, Rodrigues D, Khan SN, Harari A. Three-phase parathyroid 4-dimensional computed tomography initial experience: inexperienced readers have high accuracy and high interobserver agreement. J Comput Assist Tomogr. 2013;37(4):511–7.
11. Sho S, Yilma M, Yeh MW, Livhits M, Wu JX, Hoang JK, et al. Prospective validation of two 4D-CT-based scoring systems for prediction of multigland disease in primary hyperparathyroidism. AJNR Am J Neuroradiol. 2016;37(12):2323–7.
12. Hoang JK, Williams K, Gaillard F, Dixon A, Sosa JA. Parathyroid 4D-CT: multi-institutional international survey of use and trends. Otolaryngol Head Neck Surg. 2016;155(6):956–60.

13. Uruno T, Kebebew E. How to localize parathyroid tumors in primary hyperparathyroidism? J Endocrinol Investig. 2006;29(9):840–7.
14. Sugg SL, Fraker DL, Alexander R, Doppman JL, Miller DL, Chang R, et al. Prospective evaluation of selective venous sampling for parathyroid hormone concentration in patients undergoing reoperations for primary hyperparathyroidism. Surgery. 1993;114(6):1004–9; discussion 9–10
15. Jones JJ, Brunaud L, Dowd CF, Duh QY, Morita E, Clark OH. Accuracy of selective venous sampling for intact parathyroid hormone in difficult patients with recurrent or persistent hyperparathyroidism. Surgery. 2002;132(6):944–50; discussion 50–1
16. Udelsman R, Aruny JE, Donovan PI, Sokoll LJ, Santos F, Donabedian R, et al. Rapid parathyroid hormone analysis during venous localization. Ann Surg. 2003;237(5):714–9; discussion 9–21
17. Estella E, Leong MS, Bennett I, Hartley L, Wetzig N, Archibald CA, et al. Parathyroid hormone venous sampling prior to reoperation for primary hyperparathyroidism. ANZ J Surg. 2003;73(10):800–5.
18. Seehofer D, Steinmuller T, Rayes N, Podrabsky P, Riethmuller J, Klupp J, et al. Parathyroid hormone venous sampling before reoperative surgery in renal hyperparathyroidism: comparison with noninvasive localization procedures and review of the literature. Arch Surg. 2004;139(12):1331–8.
19. Reidel MA, Schilling T, Graf S, Hinz U, Nawroth P, Buchler MW, et al. Localization of hyperfunctioning parathyroid glands by selective venous sampling in reoperation for primary or secondary hyperparathyroidism. Surgery. 2006;140(6):907–13; discussion 13
20. Gimm O, Arnesson LG, Olofsson P, Morales O, Juhlin C. Super-selective venous sampling in conjunction with quickPTH for patients with persistent primary hyperparathyroidism: report of five cases. Surg Today. 2012;42(6):570–6.
21. Morris LF, Loh C, Ro K, Wiseman JE, Gomes AS, Asandra A, et al. Non-super-selective venous sampling for persistent hyperparathyroidism using a systemic hypocalcemic challenge. J Vasc Interv Radiol: JVIR. 2012;23(9):1191–9.
22. Lebastchi AH, Aruny JE, Donovan PI, Quinn CE, Callender GG, Carling T, et al. Real-time super selective venous sampling in remedial parathyroid surgery. J Am Coll Surg. 2015;220(6):994–1000.
23. Sun PY, Thompson SM, Andrews JC, Wermers RA, McKenzie TJ, Richards ML, et al. Selective parathyroid hormone venous sampling in patients with persistent or recurrent primary hyperparathyroidism and negative, equivocal or discordant noninvasive imaging. World J Surg. 2016;40(12):2956–63.
24. Habibollahi P, Shin B, Shamchi SP, Wachtel H, Fraker DL, Trerotola SO. Eleven-year retrospective report of super-selective venous sampling for the evaluation of recurrent or persistent hyperparathyroidism in 32 patients. Cardiovasc Intervent Radiol. 2018;41(1):63–72.
25. Chen CC, Skarulis MC, Fraker DL, Alexander R, Marx SJ, Spiegel AM. Technetium-99m-sestamibi imaging before reoperation for primary hyperparathyroidism. J Nucl Med. 1995;36(12):2186–91.
26. Rotstein L, Irish J, Gullane P, Keller MA, Sniderman K. Reoperative parathyroidectomy in the era of localization technology. Head Neck. 1998;20(6):535–9.
27. Gotthardt M, Lohmann B, Behr TM, Bauhofer A, Franzius C, Schipper ML, et al. Clinical value of parathyroid scintigraphy with technetium-99m methoxyisobutylisonitrile: discrepancies in clinical data and a systematic meta-analysis of the literature. World J Surg. 2004;28(1):100–7.
28. Chaffanjon PC, Voirin D, Vasdev A, Chabre O, Kenyon NM, Brichon PY. Selective venous sampling in recurrent and persistent hyperparathyroidism: indication, technique, and results. World J Surg. 2004;28(10):958–61.
29. Eloy JA, Mitty H, Genden EM. Preoperative selective venous sampling for nonlocalizing parathyroid adenomas. Thyroid. 2006;16(8):787–90.

30. Ikuno M, Yamada T, Shinjo Y, Morimoto T, Kumano R, Yagihashi K, et al. Selective venous sampling supports localization of adenoma in primary hyperparathyroidism. Acta Radiol Open. 2018;7(2):2058460118760361.
31. Mohebati A, Shaha AR. Anatomy of thyroid and parathyroid glands and neurovascular relations. Clin Anat (New York, NY). 2012;25(1):19–31.
32. Taslakian B, Trerotola SO, Sacks B, Oklu R, Deipolyi A. The essentials of parathyroid hormone venous sampling. Cardiovasc Intervent Radiol. 2017;40(1):9–21.
33. Tomita H, Yamada T, Murakami K, Hashimoto K, Tazawa Y, Kumano R, et al. Anatomical variation of thyroid veins on contrast-enhanced multi-detector row computed tomography. Eur J Radiol. 2015;84(5):872–6.
34. Wafae N, Hirose K, Franco C, Wafae GC, Ruiz CR, Daher L, et al. The anatomy of the human thyroid veins and its surgical application. Folia Morphol (Warsz). 2008;67(4):221–5.
35. Dionigi G, Congiu T, Rovera F, Boni L. The middle thyroid vein: anatomical and surgical aspects. World J Surg. 2010;34(3):514–20.
36. Belli AM, Ingram CE, Heron CW, Husband JE. The appearance of the inferior thyroid veins on computed tomography. Br J Radiol. 1988;61(722):125–7.
37. Doppman JL, Mallette LE, Marx SJ, Monchik JM, Broadus A, Spiegel AM, et al. The localization of abnormal mediastinal parathyroid glands. Radiology. 1975;115(1):31–6.
38. Lee J, Hong N, Kim BM, Kim DJ, Yun M, Jeong JJ, et al. Evaluation of an optimal cutoff of parathyroid venous sampling gradient for localizing primary hyperparathyroidism. J Bone Miner Metab. 2020;38(4):570–80.
39. Alvarado R, Meyer-Rochow G, Sywak M, Delbridge L, Sidhu S. Bilateral internal jugular venous sampling for parathyroid hormone determination in patients with nonlocalizing primary hyperparathyroidism. World J Surg. 2010;34(6):1299–303.
40. Bergenfelz A, Algotsson L, Roth B, Isaksson A, Tibblin S. Side localization of parathyroid adenomas by simplified intraoperative venous sampling for parathyroid hormone. World J Surg. 1996;20(3):358–60.
41. Yamada T, Ikuno M, Shinjo Y, Hiroishi A, Matsushita S, Morimoto T, et al. Selective venous sampling for primary hyperparathyroidism: how to perform an examination and interpret the results with reference to thyroid vein anatomy. Jpn J Radiol. 2017;35(8):409–16.
42. Ibraheem K, Toraih EA, Haddad AB, Farag M, Randolph GW, Kandil E. Selective parathyroid venous sampling in primary hyperparathyroidism: a systematic review and meta-analysis. Laryngoscope. 2018;128(11):2662–7.
43. Liew V, Gough IR, Nolan G, Fryar B. Re-operation for hyperparathyroidism. ANZ J Surg. 2004;74(9):732–40.

Chapter 8
Ovarian Venous Sampling for Hyperandrogenism

Clayton W. Commander

Introduction

Hyperandrogenism is the most common endocrine disorder in females [1]. Polycystic ovarian syndrome (PCOS) is by far the most common etiology occurring in 2–20% of all women ages 18–44 [2]. Androgen-secreting ovarian tumors account for a minuscule percentage of overall cases of hyperandrogenism. Among all ovarian tumors, virilizing Sertoli-Leydig cell tumors account for less than 0.5% of all cases [3], with Leydig cell tumors accounting for <0.1% of all ovarian tumors [4].

Ovarian venous sampling is a minimally invasive technique used to localize and confirm the presence of unilateral androgen-secreting ovarian tumors. When combined with adrenal vein sampling, it is possible to detect both androgen-secreting ovarian and adrenal masses.

Diagnosis of Hyperandrogenism

Clinical signs of hyperandrogenism include secondary amenorrhea, infertility, impaired glucose tolerance, alopecia, hirsutism, acne, deepening of the voice, increased libido, and clitoromegaly [5].

Women with suspected hyperandrogenism should have a physical examination and laboratory tests to confirm the diagnosis. Typical diagnostic workup includes, at a minimum, obtaining basal peripheral serum androgen levels, including testosterone (T), androstenedione (A4), dehydroepiandrosterone sulfate (DHEA-S),

C. W. Commander (✉)
Division of Vascular and Interventional Radiology, Department of Radiology, University of North Carolina at Chapel Hill School of Medicine, Chapel Hill, NC, USA
e-mail: clayton_commander@med.unc.edu

© The Author(s), under exclusive license to Springer Nature Switzerland AG 2022

H. Yu et al. (eds.), *Diagnosis and Management of Endocrine Disorders in Interventional Radiology*, https://doi.org/10.1007/978-3-030-87189-5_8

cortisol, and 17-hydroxyprogesterone. These values alone are often not enough to diagnose a hypersecretory tumor as some tumors secrete androgens at a low rate with symptoms that can mimic nontumoral hyperandrogenism. Kaltsas et al. [6] report that a single serum T level over 3 nmol/L (87 ng/dL) can predict tumoral hyperandrogenism with a sensitivity of 100% but a specificity of only 53%. Therefore, patients with elevated androgens require further workup to investigate whether a tumor is the source of their androgen excess. This is done by interrogating the hypothalamic-pituitary-gonadal axis (Fig. 8.1).

Such evaluation is usually performed by a 48-h low-dose dexamethasone suppression test (LDDST). Under physiologic circumstances, testosterone production provides negative feedback to the hypothalamus and pituitary gland to inhibit further secretion of gonadotropin-releasing hormone (GnRH) from the former and luteinizing hormone (LH) and follicle-stimulating hormone (FSH) from the latter. In general, androgen-producing adrenal or ovarian tumors secrete hormone and do

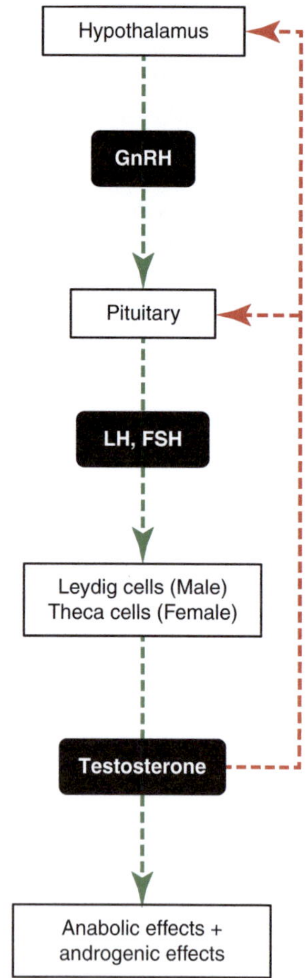

Fig. 8.1 The hypothalamic-pituitary-gonadal axis is depicted. Green arrows depict positive feedback with downstream production of hormones dependent upon secretion of upstream hormones. Red arrows depict negative feedback, whereby upstream hormone secretion is inhibited by downstream release

not have feedback from the hypothalamic-pituitary-gonadal axis (Fig. 8.1). As such, hormones secreted from a tumoral source will not diminish with suppressed LH secretion caused by exogenous steroids (such as dexamethasone), in the same way that adrenocorticotropic hormone secretion is suppressed when evaluating a patient with hypercortisolism. After the LDDST, persistently elevated peripheral serum T levels (e.g., exceeding 80 ng/dL) are suggestive of hyperandrogenism. Furthermore, post-LDDST T levels exceeding 4.51 nmol/L (130 ng/dL) are suggestive of a neo-plastic source with a sensitivity of 94% and specificity of 78% [7]. Another com-monly used diagnostic criteria for the LDDST is the failure of androgens to suppress to normal levels or reduce by at least 40% from baseline [6]. Using these criteria, the LDDST has a sensitivity of 100% and specificity of 88% for identifying patients with androgen-secreting tumors [6].

Imaging Evaluation

In patients in whom an androgen-secreting tumor is felt likely, cross-sectional imag-ing should include contrast-enhanced CT or MRI of the adrenal glands and pelvis. The most common adrenal cause of hyperandrogenism is congenital adrenal hyper-plasia, which results in marked bilateral adrenal enlargement and is easily detect-able on CT and MRI. Androgen-secreting adrenal tumors are rare entities and likely to be carcinomas rather than benign adenomas, the most common adrenal tumor seen in hyperaldosteronism [8]. Androgen-producing adrenal tumors are cortically based and usually larger than 2 cm in diameter, making them easily detected on CT and MRI. The sensitivity and specificity of CT are reported to be >95% [9] and between 89% and 100% for MRI, depending on the density of the lesion on CT [10].

While unilateral in 97% of cases [3], virilizing ovarian tumors are difficult to localize as they are usually less than 2 cm in diameter and often lie within the ovar-ian parenchyma [11]. This often renders CT and MRI nondiagnostic of these small lesions. Color Doppler ultrasound, however, can offer some diagnostic utility. One study of 38 hyperandrogenemic women, five of whom had androgen-secreting ovar-ian tumors, found that pelvic ultrasound had a sensitivity of 80% and specificity of 93% by detecting the mass or marked asymmetry in ovarian size [12]. However, despite advances in imaging technology, small lesions may remain occult on cross-sectional imaging and even diagnostic laparoscopy [13, 14].

Indications

Most agree that ovarian vein sampling should not be routinely performed for women with hyperandrogenism. Rather, the procedure should be reserved for patients in whom both laboratory and imaging evaluations fail to identify the source of andro-gen excess as small ovarian tumors cannot be excluded based on laboratory and imaging tests alone [12]. If pursued, concomitant adrenal vein sampling should also be performed. The details (and associated challenges) of adrenal vein sampling are discussed in a separate chapter.

Contraindications

As selective venous sampling is safe and minimally invasive, there are few contra-indications. Patients with known ovarian vein thrombus should not undergo attempted venous sampling. However, given that the procedure is elective, it should be avoided in patients with uncorrectable coagulopathy. Patients with allergies to iodinated contrast media should also be identified, and alternative contrast agents (e.g., CO2, gadolinium) should be used.

Technique

Anatomy

Two gonadal (ovarian) veins originate from a venous (pampiniform) plexus within the broad ligament of the uterus and ascend with the ovarian arteries on the left and right sides of the pelvis along the anterior surface of the psoas muscles, converging to a single vein on both sides before terminating [15]. The right ovarian vein, arising from the right pampiniform plexus, lies lateral to the right ureter. It parallels the right ureter as it ascends into the abdomen crossing the ureter anteromedially, approximately halfway between its confluence with the inferior vena cava (IVC) and the IVC bifurcation. The right ovarian vein drains directly into the anterior IVC, forming an acute angle just caudal to the right renal vein [16]. The left ovarian vein drains into the left renal vein at a 90-degree angle before the left renal vein crosses the aorta [15]. Normal ovarian vein anatomy is depicted in Fig. 8.2.

There are few published studies examining variant gonadal vein anatomy in women, with most studies investigating variants in men (see references [17, 18] for examples). That said, Lechter et al. [18] did submit that this was not by design. They claim that the 100 cadavers dissected were obtained from a medical institute that predominantly receives bodies of individuals who suffered violent deaths, a cohort that is heavily skewed toward males.

In a study of 60 cadavers (40 men, 20 women), Ghosh et al. [19] found variations in testicular vein anatomy in 45% of cases but no variant ovarian venous anatomy. Another cadaveric study also demonstrated rare variant ovarian venous anatomy, occurring in less than 0.5% of cases [19]. Reported variants include the right ovarian vein emptying into the right renal vein and the left ovarian vein draining directly into the inferior vena cava. The ovarian veins may also be duplicated or partially duplicated [20]. In the cases of duplicated IVC, the left ovarian vein will drain into the left IVC.

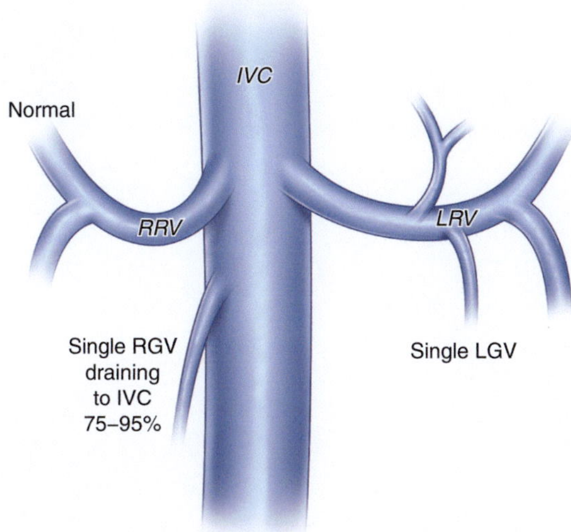

Fig. 8.2 Normal anatomy of the juxtarenal inferior vena cava (IVC). The single left ovarian vein arises orthogonally from the left renal vein. The right ovarian vein arises acutely from the IVC just inferior to the right renal vein

Identification of the ovarian veins on CT and MRI is important for identifying the ovaries, localizing adnexal masses, and looking for thrombus in patients with pulmonary embolism without a clear thrombotic source [21]. When attempting to identify the ovarian veins on contrast-enhanced CT, they are best visualized at the level of the origin of the inferior mesenteric artery [22]. The veins are both surrounded by retroperitoneal fat at this level and can be identified in 98% of cases. Normal ovarian vein diameter on CT and MRI is 3–4 mm [23, 24]. These measurements have also been corroborated in a recent cadaveric study [19].

Procedure Technique

Both jugular and femoral access can be utilized for ovarian vein sampling; however, since concomitant adrenal vein sampling is performed, a femoral approach is more commonly utilized. Access is obtained using a 21-gauge needle under direct ultrasound guidance and using the Seldinger technique, after which either a 5- or 6-French sheath is placed.

A forward-looking catheter, such as a Cobra, is used to access the left ovarian vein (Fig. 8.3a). The catheter is advanced into the left renal vein and then retracted until the tip engages the ostium of the ovarian vein (Fig. 8.3b). The right ovarian vein can be cannulated using a reverse-curve catheter (e.g., Simmons-1, Simmons-2, Sos-1, Michaelson) or a Cobra-style catheter (Fig. 8.4a). Gentle injection of dilute

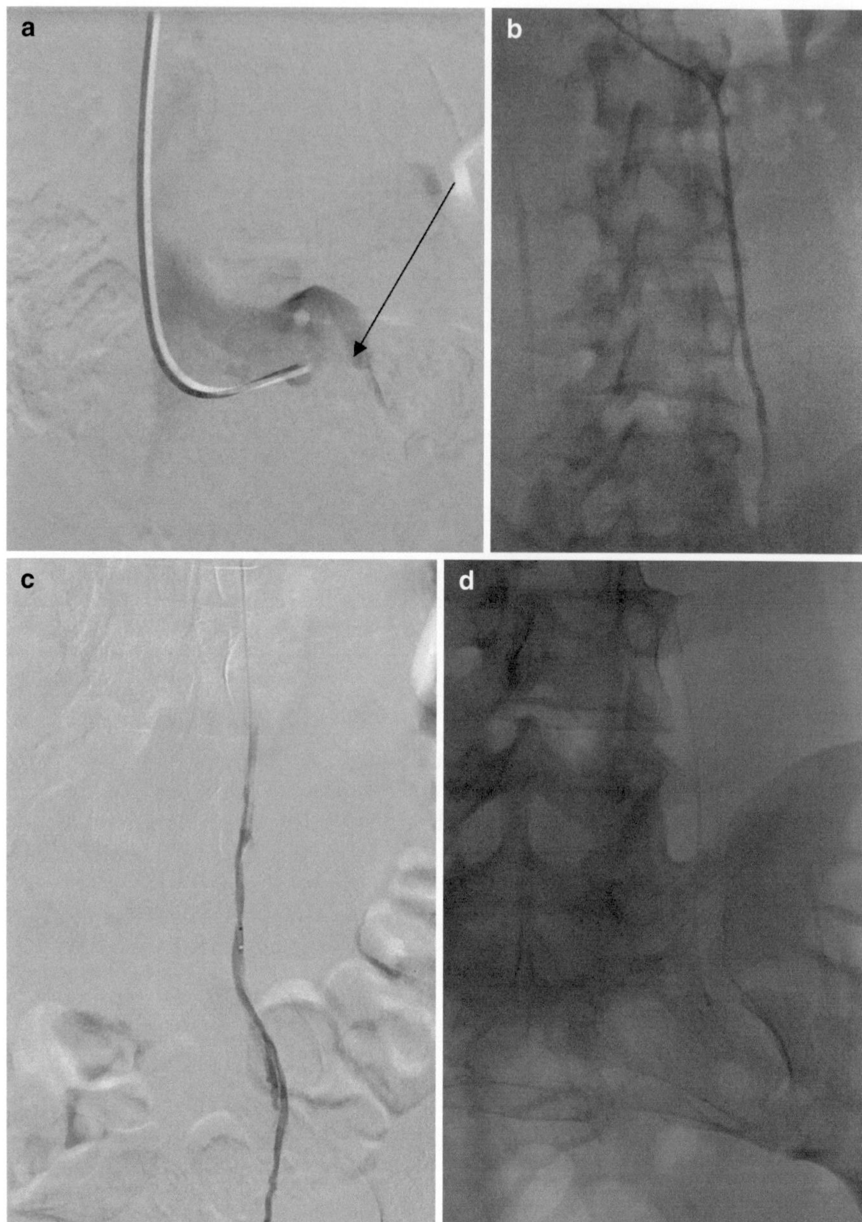

Fig. 8.3 Left ovarian vein sampling. (**a**) The left renal vein is catheterized and a digital subtraction venogram performed. Note the dilution of contrast secondary to inflow from the ovarian vein (arrow). (**b**) The catheter has been advanced into the proximal ovarian vein, and venography performed confirming position. (**c**) A microcatheter has been advanced into the ovarian vein, and repeat venography confirms appropriate position for sampling. (**d**) Sampling is performed with the microcatheter in the distal ovarian vein

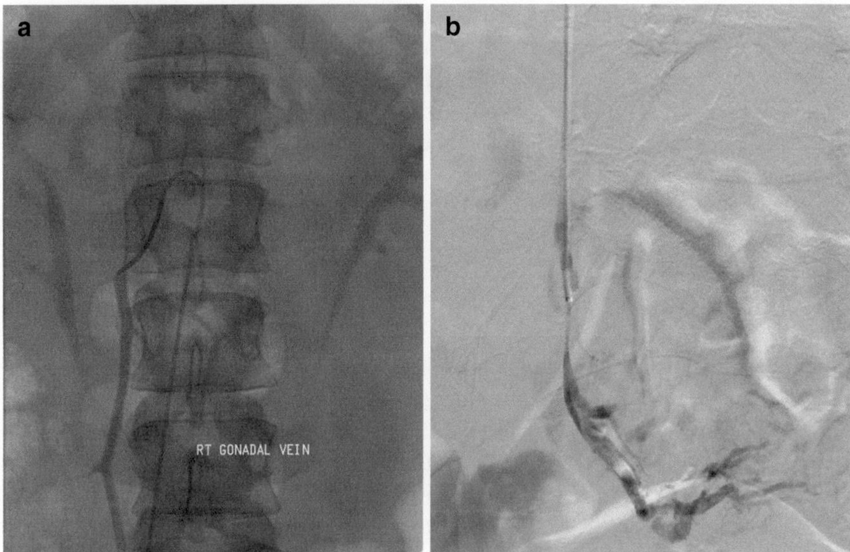

Fig. 8.4 Right ovarian vein sampling. (**a**) The right ovarian vein is catheterized and venography performed to confirm. (**b**) A microcatheter is advanced into the distal ovarian vein. Venography confirms appropriate positioning for sampling

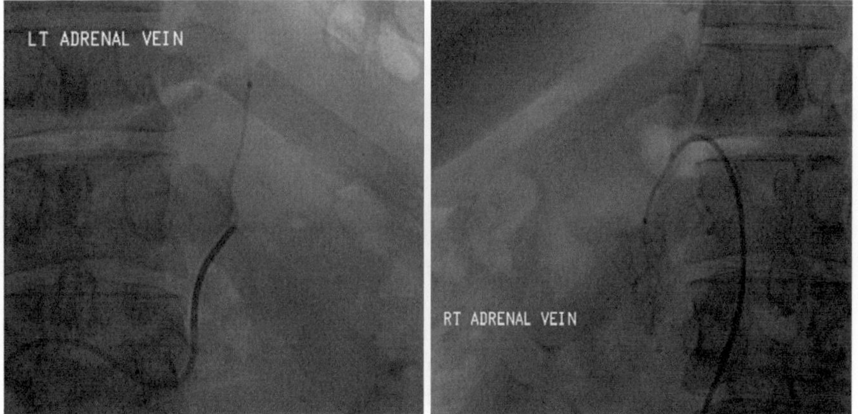

Fig. 8.5 Representative images from adrenal vein sampling

contrast is performed to confirm location within the desired vessel. If a spasm is encountered, injection of nitroglycerin in 100 μg aliquots can be helpful. Samples are usually aspirated from the ostia of the veins, though a microcatheter can be advanced deeper into the vessel if desired (Figs. 8.3c, d, and 8.4b). There are no data to suggest that technical success rates are improved when a microcatheter is used. Representative venography of adrenal vein sampling is shown in Fig. 8.5, though the specifics of this challenging procedure are discussed in Chap. 6.

In addition to the adrenal and ovarian venous effluents, peripheral blood samples taken from the sheath are also sent for analysis. Some authors also take samples from the right renal vein and the proximal and distal left renal vein [12]. To confirm proper cannulation of the adrenal and ovarian veins, samples are sent for cortisol and estradiol (E2), respectively. Samples from each vein are also sent for T, DHEA-S, and A4.

Challenges

Like other selective venous sampling procedures, ovarian vein sampling is technically challenging. To complete a full diagnostic evaluation, successful sampling of the bilateral ovarian veins as well as the bilateral adrenal veins is required [16]. Technical success rates vary with cannulation and sampling of all four vessels, ranging from 27% to 45% in two reported series [1, 12]. In [12], the authors report successful cannulation rates of 42% for the right ovarian vein and 73% for the left ovarian vein. The success rates of catheterization of the adrenal veins were similar, with reported values of 50% on the right and 87% on the left. Interpretation of the results of the combined adrenal and ovarian vein sampling is also challenging as there are no validated guidelines for localizing androgen-secreting tumors, as described below.

Results Interpretation

Consistent and reliable interpretation of the results of ovarian venous sampling remains a challenging task and a major barrier to a more widespread implementation of the procedure in the diagnostic workup of suspected neoplastic hyperandrogenism. Presently, there is no consensus or guideline from any professional society specifying diagnostic criteria for localizing unilateral androgen-producing ovarian tumors. One reason for this is that reported values distinguishing this pathology from nonneoplastic hyperandrogenism have a large variance.

In a small case series, Moltz et al. report on seven patients with androgen-secreting ovarian masses [11]. They found that peripheral T levels were greater than 5.2 nmol/L (150 ng/dL) for all patients with a unilateral ovarian vein-to-peripheral T gradient of greater than 9.4 nmol/L (270 ng/dL) for six of the seven cases. For the seventh patient, sampling ruled out an adrenal tumor, but suboptimal ovarian vein sampling prevented lateralization. All tumors in this series ranged from 0.6 to 2.2 cm in diameter.

Surrey et al. presented a series of ten patients with androgen-secreting neoplasms who underwent selective venous sampling [25]. Of these, nine patients had ovarian tumors, and one patient had an adrenal tumor. In this series, only 50% of patients had peripheral T > 6.9 nmol/L (200 ng/dL). Instead, more credence was given to abnormal ovarian venous effluent-to-peripheral androgen gradients to predict the presence of a neoplasm. Based on their results, the authors suggest an ovarian-to-peripheral T gradient of greater than 9.5 nmol/L (274 ng/dL) for detecting a unilateral hormone source. However, this threshold was unable to be validated in further studies, as detailed below.

Moltz et al. [26] also reported the results of 60 women with hyperandrogenism and no clear evidence of a hypersecretory tumor who underwent selective ovarian and adrenal vein sampling. Excess androgen secretion was assumed when at least one of the ovarian (adrenal)-to-peripheral vein gradients exceed the upper 95% confidence limit of normal based on an earlier study from the same group [27]. The most common finding was combined ovarian and adrenal hypersecretion (42%), with purely ovarian causes (27%) and purely adrenal causes (12%) being less likely. Normal glandular steroid production was found in 20% of patients. In this cohort, an ovarian-to-peripheral vein gradient of 9.5 nmol/L (274 ng/dL) was found in four out of ten women with histologically proven hyperthecosis. Similarly, Kaltas et al. [12] demonstrated an ovarian-to-peripheral vein gradient of >9.5 nmol/L (274 ng/dL) in five out of eight patients with the histologically proven polycystic ovarian syndrome.

In [7], Levens et al. report on four cases of selective venous sampling performed on hyperandrogenemic women performed at the United States National Institutes of Health. Additionally, they analyzed laboratory values from 132 published cases and established sensitive and specific values for lateralizing androgen-producing tumors. In this series, basal peripheral T $\geq$ 4.51 nmol/L (130 ng/dL) discriminated ovarian tumors from other pathology with a sensitivity of 93.8% and specificity of 77.8%. For all 18 women with right ovarian tumors, a peripheral T $\geq$ 4.51 nmol/L (130 ng/dL) and a right-to-left ovarian vein T ratio $\geq$ 1.44 correctly lateralized all lesions. Using this cutoff, two women with bilateral tumors were misclassified. When applying the converse, i.e., using a right-to-left ovarian vein effluent ratio of <1.44, 12 of 14 women with left-sided or bilateral tumors were correctly classified. For women with strictly left ovarian tumors, a left-to-right ovarian vein effluent ratio of >15 correctly lateralized three of seven cases. The left and right ovarian vein T levels were similar in the remaining four cases of left ovarian tumors.

From these data, using a peripheral T $\geq$ 4.51 nmol/L (130 ng/dL), a right-to-left ovarian vein effluent ratio greater than 1.44, and a left-to-right ovarian vein effluent ratio greater than 15, 66% of all cases could be correctly lateralized. It is important to remember that when using these cutoffs, patients with left-sided tumors, PCOS, and hyperthecosis may be misdiagnosed [7].

Complications

Complications of ovarian vein sampling are rare. Access site hematoma and thrombosis should be monitored. Given that adrenal vein sampling is also performed, the risk of injury to the adrenal glands, while rare, should also be considered.

Conclusions

Ovarian vein sampling is a minimally invasive procedure, which, when performed on a highly selective patient population, can aid in the diagnosis and localization of androgen-secreting ovarian tumors. It should be considered for patients in whom an androgen-secreting tumor is suspected only if cross-sectional imaging fails to provide a diagnosis. Due to the technical difficulty of the procedure, it is recommended that it be performed at centers with high volume to ensure successful sampling. However, as ovarian vein sampling is a rare procedure, such centers are scarce. On the other hand, given that adrenal vein sampling is performed at the same time as ovarian vein sampling and is a more commonly performed procedure, it can be argued that centers performing large volumes of adrenal vein sampling should also be referral centers for ovarian vein sampling.

References

1. Sorensen R, Moltz L, Schwartz U. Technical difficulties of selective venous blood sampling in the differential diagnosis of female hyperandrogenism. Cardiovasc Intervent Radiol. 1986;9(2):75–82.
2. Teede H, Deeks A, Moran L. Polycystic ovary syndrome: a complex condition with psychological, reproductive and metabolic manifestations that impacts on health across the lifespan. BMC Med. 2010;8:41.
3. Penick E, Hamilton CA, Maxwell GL, Marcus CS, Cell G. Stromal, and other ovarian tumors. In: Philip WTC, DiSaia J, Mannell RS, McMeekin S, Mutch DG, editors. Clinical gynecologic oncology. Philadelphia: Elsevier; 2018. p. 290–313.
4. Nardo LG, et al. Ovarian Leydig cell tumor in a peri-menopausal woman with severe hyperandrogenism and virilization. Gynecol Endocrinol. 2005;21(4):238–41.
5. Yildiz BO. Diagnosis of hyperandrogenism: clinical criteria. Best Pract Res Clin Endocrinol Metab. 2006;20(2):167–76.
6. Kaltsas GA, et al. The value of the low-dose dexamethasone suppression test in the differential diagnosis of hyperandrogenism in women. J Clin Endocrinol Metab. 2003;88(6):2634–43.
7. Levens ED, et al. Selective venous sampling for androgen-producing ovarian pathology. Clin Endocrinol. 2009;70(4):606–14.
8. Reznek RH, Armstrong P. The adrenal gland. Clin Endocrinol. 1994;40(5):561–76.
9. Sangwaiya MJ, et al. Incidental adrenal lesions: accuracy of characterization with contrast-enhanced washout multidetector CT--10-minute delayed imaging protocol revisited in a large patient cohort. Radiology. 2010;256(2):504–10.
10. Nandra G, et al. Technical and interpretive pitfalls in adrenal imaging. Radiographics. 2020;40(4):1041–60.
11. Moltz L, et al. Ovarian and adrenal vein steroids in seven patients with androgen-secreting ovarian neoplasms: selective catheterization findings. Fertil Steril. 1984;42(4):585–93.
12. Kaltsas GA, et al. Is ovarian and adrenal venous catheterization and sampling helpful in the investigation of hyperandrogenic women? Clin Endocrinol. 2003;59(1):34–43.
13. Northrop G, et al. Adrenal and ovarian vein androgen levels and laparoscopic findings in hirsute women. Am J Obstet Gynecol. 1975;122(2):192–8.
14. Dickerson RD, et al. Selective ovarian vein sampling to localize a Leydig cell tumor. Fertil Steril. 2005;84(1):218.

15. De Boo D, Koukounaras J. Vascular anatomy of the abdominal aorta and inferior vena cava. In: Mauro M, Morgan R, Murphy K, Thomson K, Venbrux T, editors. Image-guided interventions. Philadelphia: Elsevier; 2021. p. 163–70.
16. Lau JH, Drake W, Matson M. The current role of venous sampling in the localization of endocrine disease. Cardiovasc Intervent Radiol. 2007;30(4):555–70.
17. Wishahi MM. Detailed anatomy of the internal spermatic vein and the ovarian vein. Human cadaver study and operative spermatic venography: clinical aspects. J Urol. 1991;145(4):780–4.
18. Lechter A, et al. Anatomy of the gonadal veins: a reappraisal. Surgery. 1991;109(6):735–9.
19. Ghosh A, Chaudhury S. A cadaveric study of ovarian veins: variations, measurements and clinical significance. Anat Cell Biol. 2019;52(4):385–9.
20. Monroe EJ, et al. An interventionist's guide to endocrine consultations. Radiographics. 2017;37(4):1246–67.
21. Karaosmanoglu D, et al. MDCT of the ovarian vein: normal anatomy and pathology. AJR Am J Roentgenol. 2009;192(1):295–9.
22. Govil S, Justus A. Using the ovarian vein to find the ovary. Abdom Imaging. 2006;31(6):747–50.
23. Coakley FV, Varghese SL, Hricak H. CT and MRI of pelvic varices in women. J Comput Assist Tomogr. 1999;23(3):429–34.
24. Nascimento AB, Mitchell DG, Holland G. Ovarian veins: magnetic resonance imaging findings in an asymptomatic population. J Magn Reson Imaging. 2002;15(5):551–6.
25. Surrey ES, et al. Preoperative localization of androgen-secreting tumors: clinical, endocrinologic, and radiologic evaluation of ten patients. Am J Obstet Gynecol. 1988;158(6 Pt 1):1313–22.
26. Moltz L, et al. Ovarian and adrenal vein steroids in patients with nonneoplastic hyperandrogenism: selective catheterization findings. Fertil Steril. 1984;42(1):69–75.
27. Moltz L, et al. Ovarian and adrenal vein steroids in healthy women with ovulatory cycles-selective catheterization findings. J Steroid Biochem. 1984;20(4A):901–5.

Chapter 9
Selective Venous Sampling for Hypercortisolism

James P. Ho and Sten Y. Solander

Introduction

Cushing's syndrome (CS) is a disorder characterized by prolonged exposure to glucocorticoids. It is associated with several comorbidities, spanning multiple organ systems, including hypertension, glucose intolerance, obesity, cardiovascular disease, infertility, and an increased risk of infections and fractures [1]. These constellations of symptoms are often not pathognomonic for any specific disease process, making diagnosis of the disorder difficult. Furthermore, CS has been shown in population-based studies to be associated with a significant increased risk of morbidity and mortality [2]. A retrospective cohort study by Clayton et al. demonstrated that despite treatment, patients with CS are at an increased risk of overall mortality for at least 10 years relative to the normal population, with the main driver of this risk being from cardiovascular disease [3]. This underscores the importance of prompt diagnosis and treatment in these patients.

Cushing's syndrome can be broadly divided into exogenous and endogenous hypercortisolism. Exogenous hypercortisolism is typically secondary to iatrogenic administration of corticosteroids, while endogenous hypercortisolism can be further separated into ACTH-dependent and ACTH-independent disease. Cushing's disease (CD) is the most common cause of ACTH-dependent CS, being five to six times more common than ectopic ACTH syndrome (EAS). Nevertheless, it is still rare in

J. P. Ho (✉)
Department of Neurology, University of North Carolina at Chapel Hill,
Chapel Hill, NC, USA
e-mail: james_ho@med.unc.edu

S. Y. Solander
Department of Radiology, University of North Carolina at Chapel Hill, Chapel Hill, NC, USA
e-mail: sten_solander@med.unc.edu

© The Author(s), under exclusive license to Springer Nature
Switzerland AG 2022

H. Yu et al. (eds.), *Diagnosis and Management of Endocrine Disorders in Interventional Radiology*, https://doi.org/10.1007/978-3-030-87189-5_9

the United States, with an incidence of approximately 6–7 per million persons per year [4, 5]. CD results in excess ACTH production typically from ACTH-secreting pituitary tumors, whereas EAS is secondary to ACTH-secreting ectopic (i.e., non-pituitary) tumors. The treatment of choice for CD is surgical resection of the pituitary tumor [6]. Therefore, the ability to distinguish Cushing's disease from ectopic causes of ACTH-dependent CS is vital and can spare the patient a potentially unnecessary and invasive neurosurgical procedure.

Laboratory tests and noninvasive cross-sectional imaging have been used to attempt to distinguish between CD and EAS. Assays such as the high-dose dexamethasone suppression test and the corticotropin-releasing hormone (CRH) test are based on differences in biochemical profiles between ACTH-secreting pituitary and ectopic tumors. Overlap in biochemical nature of these tumors leads to reduced sensitivity and specificity of these tests. The high-dose dexamethasone suppression test uses high doses of dexamethasone to suppress pituitary ACTH secretion without suppressing ectopic ACTH secretion; however, it has only approximately a 78–81% sensitivity and a 67–81% specificity [7, 8]. The corticotropin-releasing hormone (CRH) stimulation test involves the administration of CRH to induce ACTH production in pituitary tumors. However, many ectopic ACTH-secreting tumors also respond to CRH, limiting the diagnostic utility of this test [9, 10]. Cross-sectional imaging with contrast-enhanced MRI can allow for imaging of a pituitary tumor; however, some microadenomas may be below the level of resolution of imaging, leading to false-negative exams [11, 12]. Even if a pituitary tumor is identified on imaging, 10–20% are nonfunctioning tumors that do not result in excess ACTH production [13, 14]. Previous studies have demonstrated that pituitary tumor size >6 mm on contrast-enhanced MRI has a 96% specificity for the diagnosis of CD compared to EAS [15, 16]. Therefore, clinical practice guidelines consider pituitary tumors >6 mm in patients with ACTH-dependent hypercortisolism to be diagnostic of CD [6]. In cases where pituitary tumors are ≤6 mm or not detected at all, further diagnostic testing is required.

Inferior petrosal sinus sampling (IPSS) has emerged as the "gold standard" for differentiating between CD and EAS due to its high sensitivity (88–100%) and specificity (67–100%) [17]. IPSS involves selective catheterization and measurement of ACTH levels in the inferior petrosal sinus. Initially performed via individual sampling of each inferior petrosal sinus, the procedure has evolved into a highly coordinated process involving simultaneous sampling of the bilateral inferior petrosal sinuses and peripheral blood [18]. Over time, it was discovered that direct stimulation of the potential tumor through administration of CRH further increased the diagnostic yield of the procedure [19, 20]. In centers where CRH is unavailable, vasopressin is sometimes used instead [21]. Resultant ACTH levels from each inferior petrosal sinus and from peripheral blood are reported as a whole and as an inferior petrosal sinus to peripheral blood ratio (ISP:P). Given the low incidence of Cushing's disease, this procedure is not commonly performed at most hospitals. Regardless, it has tremendous diagnostic utility in a disorder that is associated with significant morbidity and mortality, making it a valuable tool in any neuro-interventionalist's armamentarium.

Indications

Inferior petrosal sinus sampling is indicated in patients with ACTH-dependent hypercortisolism, to differentiate between Cushing's disease and ectopic ACTH syndrome. It is not indicated when the diagnosis of Cushing's disease has been made, such as in cases when contrast-enhanced MRI has demonstrated a pituitary tumor >6 mm. It is important that the diagnosis of ACTH-dependent hypercortisolism be made prior to the procedure as IPSS is unable to reliably differentiate between other causes of hypercortisolism. In fact, pseudo-Cushing's, a variety of conditions including pregnancy, morbid obesity, and chronic alcoholism, can sometimes result in elevated ACTH and cortisol levels, skewing the results of the procedure. Yanovski et al. reported significant crossover in ACTH IPS:P ratios between patients with CD and pseudo-Cushing's, raising the concern for false-positive findings in patients without CD that could potentially lead to unwarranted surgeries [22]. Therefore, it is important to ensure that a diagnosis of ACTH-dependent hypercortisolism has been made prior to proceeding with IPSS.

Contraindications

There are relatively few contraindications to this procedure. Relative contraindications include underlying renal insufficiency, history of severe contrast allergy, or uncorrectable coagulopathy.

Technique

Anatomy

The pituitary gland is an endocrine structure that is located within the sella turcica and is divided into the anterior and posterior lobes. The anterior lobe is responsible for the secretion of trophic hormones, including ACTH, which drain into a venous plexus on the surface of the pituitary gland. This plexus ultimately empties into the cavernous sinus, which in turn drains into the superior petrosal sinus and the inferior petrosal sinus. The inferior petrosal sinus courses posteriorly and inferiorly and empties into the internal jugular vein, usually at the level of the skull base.

Anatomical Variations

Anatomical variants are common with venous anatomy and may alter the diagnostic yield or technical feasibility of inferior petrosal sinus sampling. In most cases, the inferior petrosal sinus drains directly into the internal jugular vein. However, in some cases, condylar emissary veins may drain into the inferior petrosal sinus just before it empties into the internal jugular vein. It is important to recognize this to ensure adequate positioning of the microcatheter to minimize dilution of the sample. Rarely, the inferior petrosal sinus may be hypoplastic, or it may drain into the internal jugular vein via a network of veins, making catheterization of the sinus difficult. Even less common, the inferior petrosal sinus may not drain into the internal jugular vein at all and instead empty into a vertebral venous plexus. In these instances, the inferior petrosal sinus may not be amenable to safe catheterization.

Pathophysiology

The hypothalamic-pituitary-adrenal (HPA) axis is a complex neuroendocrine system that regulates many of the body's processes and reactions to stress. The hypothalamus secretes corticotropin-releasing hormone, which stimulates the anterior lobe of the pituitary gland to produce ACTH. ACTH in turn stimulates adrenal secretion of cortisol. Typically, through a negative feedback loop, cortisol can inhibit the hypothalamus and the pituitary gland from producing CRH and ACTH, respectively. However, patients with a pituitary adenoma are not affected by this negative feedback loop and will continue to produce ACTH despite an excess of cortisol. Administration of CRH can further potentiate the production of ACTH. IPSS is based on this basic understanding of the HPA axis. Measuring the differences in ACTH levels in the bilateral inferior petrosal sinuses as compared to peripheral blood allows for localization of the ACTH-secreting tumor, whether ectopic or pituitary in origin.

Approach

Bilateral inferior petrosal sinus sampling is typically done under conscious or local anesthesia to allow for monitoring of symptoms. Peripheral IV access is obtained in the arm contralateral to the operator. A 5-French, 10-cm sheath is advanced into both right and left femoral veins. Next, 5000 units of heparin are given as an intravenous bolus to reduce the risk of thrombotic complications. A 5-French guide catheter (Envoy, Codman Neuro, Raynham, MA, USA) is advanced through each femoral vein sheath into the ipsilateral internal jugular veins. To avoid confusion during the collection process, it is important to be sure which side the catheter is in, and we find it prudent to keep both guide catheters separate and labeled (R or L). An 0.027″ microcatheter is then advanced through each guide catheter and positioned in the proximal ipsilateral inferior petrosal sinus. Diagnostic venograms are performed via injections through each microcatheter to ensure acceptable position of the microcatheters and to evaluate for aberrant venous anatomy (Fig. 9.1). To ensure simultaneous sampling, we have three separate individuals collecting the samples.

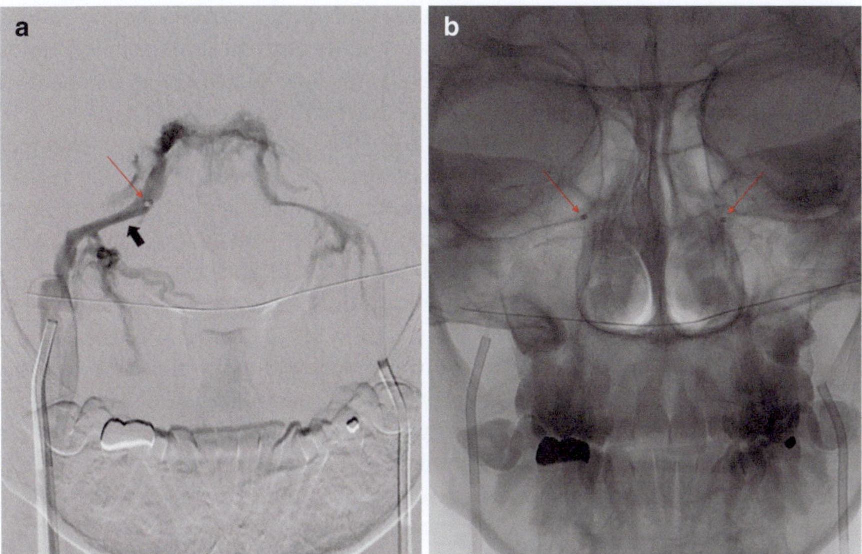

Fig. 9.1 (**a**) Digital subtraction venography from a selective injection of the right inferior petrosal sinus. There is contrast opacification of the cavernous sinus and contralateral inferior petrosal sinus. The microcatheter (red arrow) is positioned in the right inferior petrosal sinus (thick black arrow), distal to the anterior condylar vein. (**b**) Native view demonstrating relative positioning of the right and left microcatheters (red arrows) and guide catheters

Each is assigned to collecting blood either from the microcatheter in the right inferior petrosal sinus (R), the microcatheter in the left interior petrosal sinus (L), or the peripheral IV (P). First, baseline blood samples are taken simultaneously 3 min before and immediately before injection of CRH. CRH (Acthrel, Ben Venue Laboratories, Ohio, USA) is given intravenously at a dose of 1 ug/kg. Next, simultaneous blood samples are obtained at 3, 5, and 10 min after administration of the CRH. Once the sampling is complete, the catheters are removed. The femoral sheaths are removed, and hemostasis is obtained through manual compression. Patients are then rested in the recovery room for 2 h to observe for any delayed complications.

Technical Considerations

- Correct microcatheter positioning is of paramount importance. The goal of IPSS is to obtain venous samples as proximal to the pituitary gland as possible while avoiding potential complications. The microcatheter should be positioned distal to any condylar emissary veins seen on venography, most commonly the anterior condylar vein, to avoid dilution of the sample. Venograms should be obtained prior to sampling to confirm good microcatheter position, and fluoroscopy should be intermittently performed throughout the procedure to double-check positioning. Furthermore, in instances where there is difficulty catheterizing one inferior petrosal sinus but not the contralateral side, roadmap guidance can be obtained from injection of the contralateral inferior petrosal sinus.

- The actual process of venous sampling in IPSS is complex and involves multiple team members. All participants must be diligent about their specific role at each individual step. We find it useful to designate three different individuals to collect the samples, who will then hand the samples to three different assistants to properly label and prepare for the lab. Labels specifying location (R, L, or P) and the time of collection are prepared prior to the procedure. To reduce operator error, the catheter in the right groin is always placed in the right inferior petrosal sinus, and the catheter in the left groin is always placed in the left inferior petrosal sinus. Minus 3 min and 0 min samples are obtained 3 min before and immediately before administration of CRH. Plus 3 min, plus 5 min, and plus 10 min are obtained 3, 5, and 10 min after administration of CRH, respectively. The time and location of each sample is recorded and entered into the electronic medical record. All collected samples are immediately placed into prechilled tubes containing EDTA and kept on ice until processed by the lab.

- Between sampling, there is a risk of microcatheter occlusion due to thrombosis. We attempt to minimize this risk by slowly flushing the microcatheters by hand with heparinized saline in between sampling times. Immediately prior to each sampling time, we then aspirate and waste the volume of the dead space of the microcatheter to ensure true undiluted sampling of the inferior petrosal sinus.

- CRH is typically administered at a dose of 1 ug/kg with a maximum dose of 100 ug. Desmopressin (DDAVP), at a dose of 10 ug, is sometimes used as an alternative to CRH. DDAVP acts on the V2R receptor subtype, promoting secretion of ACTH in a similar fashion as CRH. Several small studies have demonstrated similar clinical experiences between CRH and DDAVP, with a similar increased diagnostic yield following the administration of DDAVP [21, 23]. A single center study by Machado et al. reported good sensitivity and specificity (92.1% and 100%, respectively), following the administration of DDAVP for bilateral IPSS in the differential diagnosis of ACTH-dependent Cushing's syndrome [24]. In centers where CRH is unavailable, DDAVP may be considered as an alternative.

- The results of IPSS are difficult to interpret in the absence of sustained hypercortisolism. Some patients with Cushing's disease may have cyclical secretion of ACTH. This results in "trough" periods of decreased ACTH secretion by the pituitary tumor and decreased ACTH secretion by normal pituitary glandular tissue due to recent hypercortisolism. Cortisol levels are also decreased during these trough periods. This may lead to an absent IPS:P ratio, a false-negative finding in this case [25, 26]. Therefore, it is important for the neurointerventionalist to work with their endocrinology counterpart to ensure that the IPSS is performed during a period of sustained hypercortisolism. Potential strategies include testing of serum cortisol on the morning of the scheduled procedure or testing of midnight salivary cortisol the night prior to the procedure [27, 28]. If hypercortisolism is not detected, the procedure should be canceled and rescheduled.

- There may be situations in which despite apparent proper positioning of the microcatheter(s), inaccurate venous samples are obtained. These situations are typically related to procedural or anatomical abnormalities and include intermittent displacement of the catheter out of the inferior petrosal sinus, dilution of samples from collateral venous drainage, or collecting samples from aberrant collateral veins [26]. If this occurs, elevated ACTH levels may not be captured, resulting in false-negative findings. We believe that the use of microcatheters may improve the accuracy of the samples. Prolactin levels are commonly used to confirm proper microcatheter positioning, with an IPS:P prolactin ratio of $\geq$1.3–1.8 before and after CRH administration, indicative of venous efflux from the pituitary gland [29, 30]. An IPS:P prolactin ratio < 1.3 would then be concerning for improper microcatheter placement or positioning. Therefore, routine sampling of prolactin levels is important, especially when results suggest an ectopic tumor.

Interpretation of Results

Once the venous sampling has been completed, the laboratory will process the samples to report ACTH levels. The ACTH levels are then used to calculate a ratio comparing the ACTH level from each inferior petrosal sinus to peripheral blood (ISP:P ratio). Diagnostic criteria for the diagnosis of CD are a basal IPS:P $\geq$ 2 and/or a post-CRH stimulation IPS:P $\geq$ 3 [20, 23, 31]. IPS:P ratios lower than these thresholds suggest an ectopic source of ACTH.

A note must be made about rare situations in which only one inferior petrosal sinus can be catheterized. Due to variable drainage patterns, pituitary adenomas may not consistently drain into their ipsilateral inferior petrosal sinus. Previously, it had been thought that differences in ACTH levels between the sinuses could assist in predicting tumor lateralization. An inter-sinus ACTH gradient of >1.4 was initially proposed; however, emerging data have reported a poorer predictive value than what was previously thought, only correcting identifying the side of the tumor in 50–70% of cases [32–34]. This suggests that, in many cases, lateralized pituitary microadenomas may drain into the contralateral inferior petrosal sinus. Therefore, when only one inferior petrosal sinus can be catheterized, an absence of an ACTH ISP:P gradient does not necessarily rule out CD. In most cases, both inferior petrosal sinuses will be able to be catheterized successfully; however, in the rare circumstance when only one sinus is catheterized, it is important to note this as the results are interpreted.

Complications

The most common minor complications of IPSS are groin hematomas, occurring in less than 5% of cases [35]. Rarely, more serious complications have been reported, such as a brainstem ischemic stroke, brainstem hemorrhage, and subarachnoid hemorrhage. These are thought to be due to catheterization of anomalous veins or petrosal sinus-to-brainstem bridging veins, leading to rupture of the veins and resultant hemorrhage or venous obstruction and subsequent venous infarcts [17]. One of the largest retrospective studies performed at the NIH evaluated 508 patients and found that major neurologic complications occurred in only 0.2% of procedures [36]. Isolated case reports in the literature have also described thrombotic events, including cavernous sinus thrombosis, deep vein thrombosis, and pulmonary embolism as rare potential complications [37–39].

Conclusion

Inferior petrosal sinus sampling, when performed by an experienced neurointerventionalist, is an especially useful procedure, with a high sensitivity and specificity for the diagnosis of Cushing's disease. It carries a low risk of serious morbidity or mortality. As with most interventional procedures, patient selection is key to avoid unwarranted or unnecessary surgery. During the procedure, great care should be made to ensure appropriate microcatheter position is maintained throughout. Additionally, a preplanned protocol for the correct handling and labeling of the collected venous samples, including the coordination of diligent team members, is key to prevent sampling errors. When performed correctly, IPSS is an important diagnostic test that can be of great diagnostic benefit to patients suffering from Cushing's disease.

References

1. Nieman LK. Recent updates on the diagnosis and management of Cushing's syndrome. Endocrinol Metab. 2018;33:139.
2. Lindholm J, Juul S, Jørgensen JO, et al. Incidence and late prognosis of Cushing's syndrome: a population-based study. J Clin Endocrinol Metab. 2001;86:117–23.
3. Clayton RN, Jones PW, Reulen RC, et al. Mortality in patients with Cushing's disease more than 10 years after remission: a multicentre, multinational, retrospective cohort study. Lancet Diabetes Endocrinol. 2016;4:569–76.
4. Carpenter PC. Diagnostic evaluation of Cushing's syndrome. Endocrinol Metab Clin N Am. 1988;17:445–72.
5. Broder MS, Neary MP, Chang E, Cherepanov D, Ludlam WH. Incidence of Cushing's syndrome and Cushing's disease in commercially-insured patients <65 years old in the United States. Pituitary. 2015;18:283–9.

6. Nieman LK, BMK B, Findling JW, Murad MH, Newell-Price J, Savage MO, Tabarin A, Endocrine Society. Treatment of Cushing's syndrome: an Endocrine Society clinical practice guideline. J Clin Endocrinol Metab. 2015;100:2807–31.

7. Howlett TA, Drury PL, Perry L, Doniach I, Rees LH, Besser GM. Diagnosis and management of ACTH-dependent Cushing's syndrome: comparison of the features in ectopic and pituitary ACTH production. Clin Endocrinol. 1986;24:699–713.

8. Aron DC, Raff H, Findling JW. Effectiveness *versus* efficacy: the limited value in clinical practice of high dose dexamethasone suppression testing in the differential diagnosis of adrenocorticotropin-dependent Cushing's syndrome. J Clin Endocrinol Metabol. 1997;82:1780–5.

9. Barbot M, Trementino L, Zilio M, et al. Second-line tests in the differential diagnosis of ACTH-dependent Cushing's syndrome. Pituitary. 2016;19:488–95.

10. Kaye TB. The Cushing syndrome: an update on diagnostic tests. Ann Intern Med. 1990;112:434.

11. Doppman JL, Frank JA, Dwyer AJ, Oldfield EH, Miller DL, Nieman LK, Chrousos GP, Cutler GB, Loriaux DL. Gadolinium DTPA enhanced MR imaging of ACTH-secreting microadenomas of the pituitary gland. J Comput Assist Tomogr. 1988;12:728–35.

12. Tabarin A, Laurent F, Catargi B, Olivier-Puel F, Lescene R, Berge J, San Galli F, Drouillard J, Roger P, Guerin J. Comparative evaluation of conventional and dynamic magnetic resonance imaging of the pituitary gland for the diagnosis of Cushing's disease: conventional versus dynamic MRI in Cushing's disease. Clin Endocrinol. 1998;49:293–300.

13. Ezzat S, Asa SL, Couldwell WT, Barr CE, Dodge WE, Vance ML, McCutcheon IE. The prevalence of pituitary adenomas: a systematic review. Cancer. 2004;101:613–9.

14. Molitch ME. The pituitary "Incidentaloma.". Ann Intern Med. 1990;112:925.

15. Arnaldi G, Angeli A, Atkinson AB, et al. Diagnosis and complications of Cushing's syndrome: a consensus statement. J Clin Endocrinol Metabol. 2003;88:5593–602.

16. Yogi-Morren D, Habra MA, Faiman C, Bena J, Hatipoglu B, Kennedy L, Weil RJ, Hamrahian AH. Pituitary MRI findings in patients with pituitary and ectopic Acth-dependent Cushing syndrome: does a 6-mm pituitary tumor size cut-off value exclude ectopic Acth syndrome? Endocr Pract. 2015;21:1098–103.

17. Zampetti B, Grossrubatscher E, Dalino Ciaramella P, Boccardi E, Loli P. Bilateral inferior petrosal sinus sampling. Endocr Connect. 2016;5:R12–25.

18. Manni A, Latshaw RF, Page R, Santen RJ. Simultaneous bilateral venous sampling for adrenocorticotropin in pituitary-dependent Cushing's disease: evidence for lateralization of pituitary venous drainage. J Clin Endocrinol Metabol. 1983;57:1070–3.

19. Landolt AM, Valavanis A, Girard J, Eberle AN. Corticotrophin-releasing factor-test used with bilateral, simultaneous inferior PETROSAL sinus blood-sampling for the diagnosis of pituitary-dependent Cushing's disease. Clin Endocrinol. 1986;25:687–96.

20. Oldfield EH, Doppman JL, Nieman LK, Chrousos GP, Miller DL, Katz DA, Cutler GB, Loriaux DL. Petrosal sinus sampling with and without corticotropin-releasing hormone for the differential diagnosis of Cushing's syndrome. N Engl J Med. 1991;325:897–905.

21. Deipolyi AR, Alexander B, Rho J, Hirsch JA, Oklu R. Bilateral inferior petrosal sinus sampling using desmopressin or corticotropic-releasing hormone: a single-center experience. J NeuroIntervent Surg. 2015;7:690–3.

22. Yanovski JA, Cutler GB, Doppman JL, Miller DL, Chrousos GP, Oldfield EH, Nieman LK. The limited ability of inferior petrosal sinus sampling with corticotropin-releasing hormone to distinguish Cushing's disease from pseudo-Cushing states or normal physiology. J Clin Endocrinol Metab. 1993;77:503–9.

23. Javorsky BR, Findling JW. Inferior petrosal sampling for the differential diagnosis of ACTH-dependent Cushing's syndrome. In: Bronstein MD, editor. Cushing's syndrome. Totowa: Humana Press; 2010. p. 105–19.

24. Machado MC, de Sa SV, Domenice S, Fragoso MCBV, Puglia P, Pereira MAA, de Mendonça BB, Salgado LR. The role of desmopressin in bilateral and simultaneous inferior petrosal sinus

sampling for differential diagnosis of ACTH-dependent Cushing's syndrome. Clin Endocrinol. 2006;66(1):136–42.

25. Yamamoto Y, Davis DH, Nippoldt TB, Young WF, Huston J, Parisi JE. False-positive inferior petrosal sinus sampling in the diagnosis of Cushing's disease: report of two cases. J Neurosurg. 1995;83:1087–91.

26. Perlman JE, Johnston PC, Hui F, et al. Pitfalls in performing and interpreting inferior petrosal sinus sampling: personal experience and literature review. J Clin Endocrinol Metabol. 2021; https://doi.org/10.1210/clinem/dgab012.

27. Seltzer J, Lucas J, Commins D, Lerner O, Lerner A, Carmichael JD, Zada G. Ectopic ACTH-secreting pituitary adenoma of the sphenoid sinus: case report of endoscopic endonasal resection and systematic review of the literature. FOC. 2015;38:E10.

28. Atkinson B, Mullan KR. What is the best approach to suspected cyclical Cushing syndrome? Strategies for managing Cushing's syndrome with variable laboratory data: approach to suspected cyclical Cushing syndrome. Clin Endocrinol. 2011;75:27–30.

29. Mulligan GB, Eray E, Faiman C, et al. Reduction of false-negative results in inferior petrosal sinus sampling with simultaneous prolactin and corticotropin measurement. Endocr Pract. 2011;17:33–40.

30. Findling JW, Kehoe ME, Raff H. Identification of patients with Cushing's disease with negative pituitary adrenocorticotropin gradients during inferior petrosal sinus sampling: prolactin as an index of pituitary venous effluent. J Clin Endocrinol Metabol. 2004;89:6005–9.

31. Colao A, Faggiano A, Pivonello R, Giraldi F, Cavagnini F, Lombardi G. Inferior petrosal sinus sampling in the differential diagnosis of Cushing's syndrome: results of an Italian multicenter study. Eur J Endocrinol. 2001;144(5):499–507.

32. Lin L-Y, Teng MM-H, Huang C-I, Ma W-Y, Wang K-L, Lin H-D, Won JGS. Assessment of Bilateral Inferior Petrosal Sinus Sampling (BIPSS) in the diagnosis of Cushing's disease. J Chin Med Assoc. 2007;70:4–10.

33. Bonelli FS, Huston J, Carpenter PC, Erickson D, Young WF, Meyer FB. Adrenocorticotropic hormone-dependent Cushing's syndrome: sensitivity and specificity of inferior petrosal sinus sampling. AJNR Am J Neuroradiol. 2000;21:690–6.

34. Wind JJ, Lonser RR, Nieman LK, DeVroom HL, Chang R, Oldfield EH. The lateralization accuracy of inferior petrosal sinus sampling in 501 patients with Cushing's disease. J Clin Endocrinol Metabol. 2013;98:2285–93.

35. Miller DL, Doppman JL. Petrosal sinus sampling: technique and rationale. Radiology. 1991;178:37–47.

36. Miller DL, Doppman JL, Peterman SB, Nieman LK, Oldfield EH, Chang R. Neurologic complications of petrosal sinus sampling. Radiology. 1992;185:143–7.

37. Obuobie K, Davies JS, Ogunko A, Scanlon MF. Venous thrombo-embolism following inferior petrosal sinus sampling in Cushing's disease. J Endocrinol Investig. 2000;23:542–4.

38. Blevins LS, Clark RV, Owens DS. Thromboembolic complications after inferior petrosal sinus sampling in patients with Cushing's syndrome. Endocr Pract. 1998;4:365–7.

39. Diez JJ, Iglesias P. Pulmonary thromboembolism after inferior petrosal sinus sampling in Cushing's syndrome. Clin Endocrinol. 1997;46:777.

Chapter 10
Arterial Stimulation Venous Sampling for Pancreatic Endocrine Tumors

Charles T. Burke

Introduction

Arterial stimulation venous sampling (ASVS) is a technique to identify and locate functional pancreatic endocrine tumors. Imamura and colleagues first described this approach in 1987 as a means of localizing gastrinomas in patients with Zollinger-Ellison syndrome [1]. In their paper, the researchers describe injecting secretin in three patients in whom cross-sectional imaging had failed to identify the lesion. Through this test, they were able to locate the functioning gastrinoma in all three patients. Over time, this approach became a useful adjunct in the evaluation of patients with elevated gastrin levels [2, 3].

In 1991, Doppman et al. published the first report of using ASVS to localize insulinomas [4]. At that time, angiography alone or angiography combined with portal venous sampling was the best option for identifying small insulinomas. However, these methods had shortcomings: angiography alone was positive only in 50–60% of patients and required the insulinomas to be of sufficient size to be detected. Portal vein sampling did increase the positive rate to 75–80% of patients but at the cost of increased procedural complexity and complications [5, 6].

Doppman et al. theorized that the same technique that worked for gastrinomas could also work for insulinomas if an effective stimulating agent was used [4]. This agent is calcium. In 1975, Gaeke et al. reported that calcium injections could promote the release of insulin, making this an attractive stimulating agent for the ASVS procedure [7]. Replicating Imamura's technique, using calcium rather than secretin,

C. T. Burke (⌧)
Division of Vascular and Interventional Radiology, Department of Radiology, University of North Carolina at Chapel Hill School of Medicine, Chapel Hill, NC, USA
e-mail: charles_burke@med.unc.edu

© The Author(s), under exclusive license to Springer Nature Switzerland AG 2022

H. Yu et al. (eds.), *Diagnosis and Management of Endocrine Disorders in Interventional Radiology*, https://doi.org/10.1007/978-3-030-87189-5_10

Doppman showed that the injection of calcium into the arteries supplying specific regions of the pancreas caused the release of high concentrations of insulin that could be collected via the hepatic veins, enabling both the diagnosis and localization of symptomatic insulinomas.

In the early 1990s, the diagnosis of small neuroendocrine tumors of the pancreas was limited by the quality of the imaging available. Since then, there have been significant technical advancements in both the imaging equipment and protocols that have led to the improvement in the detection of even small lesions using CT and MRI [8–14]. Also, endoscopic ultrasound has become a valuable tool in not only localizing these lesions but providing an approach for image-guided biopsy [15–17]. Nevertheless, the arterial stimulation venous sampling procedure continues to have a role in the evaluation of patients with symptomatic pancreatic endocrine tumors.

Indications

Insulinomas

ASVS is typically used to identify and localize symptomatic pancreatic endocrine tumors, most commonly insulinomas.

Consensus guidelines recommend that patients with suspected pancreatic endocrine tumors have cross-sectional imaging as the initial imaging study [18]. The consensus guidelines also recommend endoscopic ultrasound for patients in whom the initial imaging studies fail to identify the culprit lesion. However, since many insulinomas are small and can occur anywhere within the pancreas, some lesions may not be seen with these modalities. For these patients, in whom the biochemical markers may suggest insulinoma, and the imaging modalities do not show a discreet mass, ASVS can provide a reliable method for confirming the diagnosis and localizing the tumor.

There are also some indications for which ASVS is appropriate even when the tumor is visible on imaging. First, in settings where multiple tumors are present, cross-sectional imaging typically does not identify which tumors are functional. ASVS can help differentiate those functional tumors from nonfunctional tumors [19]. Also, in patients who have had prior attempted resection with continued symptoms, ASVS may help localize a previously unidentified lesion.

Also, in some cases, ASVS is used to assist in determining the surgical approach. Lesion localization to the right or left of the SMA can be the difference between surgical options, such as enucleation, distal pancreatectomy, or pancreatoduodenectomy [20].

Finally, some authors recommend that all patients with insulinomas who are planning to undergo resection have ASVS performed before surgery to confirm functionality. In a retrospective review, Morganstein et al. concluded that ASVS altered the management of several patients [19]. By identifying lesions that were not visible on other forms of imaging, ASVS prompted some patients to undergo surgery who otherwise would not have had a surgical option. Also, by using ASVS to localize small lesions, surgeons were able to avoid more extensive surgical resections.

Gastrinomas

Gastrinomas are typically larger than insulinomas at the time of diagnosis, making them more likely to be identified on imaging [21]. Also, gastrinomas commonly have somatostatin receptors. Thus, somatostatin scintigraphy is a useful tool for identifying and localizing these tumors. However, there remain patients with strong clinical suspicion for gastrinoma and negative imaging evaluation who should undergo ASVS to localize the lesion. Also, in patients with multiple lesions on imaging, ASVS may be used to identify which mass is a functional gastrinoma and, therefore, a candidate for resection.

Nesidioblastosis

Nesidioblastosis is a condition first described in 1938, though it wasn't until 1981 that this condition was reported as causing hyperinsulinemic hypoglycemia in adults [22–24]. It is characterized by islet cell hypertrophy, causing increased secretion of insulin. This islet cell hypertrophy results in non-insulinoma pancreatogenesis hypoglycemia syndrome (NIPHS). More recently, this has been described as a potential cause for patient symptoms following Roux-en-Y gastric bypass surgery [25]. It is unclear why these patients develop this condition, but it may be due to increases in beta-cell trophic factors.

Early on, ASVS was used to localize the site of islet cell proliferation to treat the condition with partial pancreatectomy [26–28]. However, more recently, it has been found that this condition can often be managed medically with diet and lifestyle modifications, rendering surgery resection unnecessary [29, 30]. Thus, this indication for ASVS is now mainly of historical interest.

That is not to say, though, that there is no use for this study in this patient population. Since insulinomas are treated surgically, and nesidioblastosis is treated conservatively, it is important to differentiate the two conditions to manage patients appropriately. There is some evidence to support the use of ASVS in this way, and this will be discussed in more detail later in the chapter.

Other Indications

While most of the published work focuses on the use of the ASVS for patients with either insulinomas or gastrinomas, it has also been used in the evaluation of glucagonomas [31, 32].

Contraindications

ASVS is a safe test to perform, and thus, there are few contraindications. Like all diagnostic angiography, this test should be avoided in patients with uncorrectable coagulopathy. Special consideration should be given to patients with a history of anaphylactic contrast reactions. Finally, this procedure should not be performed in patients with known arterial occlusions that will prevent the successful catheterizations of vessels needed to complete the study.

Technique

Anatomy

The pancreas has a redundant arterial supply with pancreatic branches that arise from both the celiac axis and the superior mesenteric artery [33–38]. When considering the arterial anatomy, it is best to think of this relative to the pancreas' zonal perfusion (Table 10.1). The vascular supply to different regions of the pancreas has been nicely illustrated in a study that combined conventional angiography with CT to show the parenchymal perfusion following injections in the supplied arteries [39]. Based on this study, the pancreas can be divided into five regions: the uncinate process, the superior head, the inferior head, the body, and the tail. The uncinate process receives arterial supply from the superior mesenteric artery (SMA) in nearly all patients. The gastroduodenal artery (GDA) provides blood supply to the superior and inferior head of the pancreas via the pancreato-duodenal branches in most patients, with some patients having arterial supply to

Table 10.1 Arterial supply to pancreatic regions

Pancreatic Region	Usual Arterial Supply
Uncinate process	SMA
Superior head	GDA
Inferior head	GSA/SMA
Body	Splenic SMA in about half of patients
Tail	Splenic

the superior head via the SMA. The body and tail of the pancreas receive their blood supply from branches of the splenic artery. The dorsal pancreatic artery is often the largest artery to the pancreas and typically arises from the proximal common hepatic artery or the proximal splenic artery. Next, the pancreatica magna artery arises from the mid splenic artery. It feeds the pancreatic body, while the caudal pancreatic artery arises from the distal splenic artery and supplies the tail of the pancreas. Between these two vessels runs the transverse pancreatic artery. This artery runs along the long axis of the pancreas between the body and tail and provides collateral blood supply between the pancreatica magna and caudal pancreatic arteries.

Procedure Technique

In preparation for the procedure, it is essential that the patient withhold any medication that can influence insulin secretion since this can result in a false-negative study [40].

As alluded to earlier, this procedure requires both arterial and venous access. Venous access can be obtained nearly anywhere, with the common femoral and internal jugular veins the most common sites. Femoral access does have the advantage of working from a single site if femoral arterial access is also used. After accessing the venous system, a 5–6 French sheath is typically used, though not required. Since the sampling is performed from either the right or the middle hepatic vein, the choice of catheter used to select this vein will depend on the access site location. For internal jugular venous access, a hockey stick-shaped catheter, such as an Multipurpose-A or Multipurpose-B, is often adequate. For femoral venous access, a reverse-curve or Cobra-shaped catheter will allow for the more acute angle at the hepatic vein/IVC confluence. Once in the hepatic vein, the catheter is advanced several centimeters deep, but a wedged position is not required.

On the arterial side, common femoral artery access is the most commonly described technique. However, with the recent popularity of radial access for visceral angiography, using the left wrist is also a viable option. With either approach, a 5–6 French sheath is placed. For femoral access, a Cobra-shaped or reverse-curve catheter will be used to catheterize the celiac and superior mesenteric arteries selectively. A forward-facing catheter is useful to cannulate the celiac and superior mesenteric arteries from the radial approach. Regardless of the access site, a microcatheter is often helpful for more selective catheterizations.

Diagnostic arteriography is performed first with the purpose of identifying any potential hyper-vascular masses and mapping out the relevant anatomy. At a minimum, selective angiograms of the celiac, superior mesenteric, gastroduodenal, proximal splenic (proximal to the pancreatic magna origin), distal splenic, and proper hepatic arteries are performed. The injection of the proper hepatic artery is useful for identifying potential liver metastases that are not visible on cross-sectional imaging. It is not necessary to perform selective angiograms of the pancreatic branches since this is often low yield and can lead to pancreatitis complications [21].

On the diagnostic angiograms, one is looking for hyper-vascular masses. If a lesion is seen, then selective stimulation of the feeding artery will be performed. However, this vessel should be stimulated last to reduce the risk of erroneously elevated insulin levels in other territories. One is also looking for any variant anatomy that may influence the calcium stimulation test results. One of the most common anatomic variants that one may encounter is a replaced dorsal pancreatic artery arising from the proximal SMA, a finding in up to 25% of cases. The dorsal pancreatic artery supplies the body of the pancreas, so a lesion in this location could have a positive result from the SMA injection in up to a quarter of patients. In one report, this variant resulted in a false-negative study when the dorsal pancreatic artery arose close to the origin of the SMA, proximal to the calcium injection site [19].

Another common finding that can affect the ASVS results is celiac stenosis [41, 42]. Celiac stenosis can be due to either extrinsic compression (e.g., by the median arcuate ligament) or intrinsic disease, such as atherosclerosis. Interpreting results in the setting of celiac stenosis or occlusion can be particularly challenging. Severe cases can result in retrograde blood flow through the GDA, a situation that leads to the SMA providing blood supply to the entire pancreas. In this situation, careful angiography and selective catheterization will be essential for an accurate evaluation.

One must also be aware of potential venous variants. One review described a case of anomalous venous drainage through a splenorenal shunt in a patient with underlying liver disease, leading to a false-negative study since the venous drainage did not pass through the hepatic veins [42]. Once recognized, the test was repeated with venous sampling performed from the left renal vein, localizing a lesion in the pancreatic tail.

Following the diagnostic portion of the study is the administration of the stimulating agent. The agent used will be determined by the suspected tumor type. For insulinomas, calcium gluconate is used to stimulate insulin secretion. Many early reports described using a dose adjusted for bodyweight with a formula of 0.025 mEq/kg [4, 40, 41, 43]. As an alternative, some authors have used a fixed dose of 1–2 mL 10% calcium diluted with saline to a total volume of 5 mL, with similar sensitivities and specificities and the added simplicity of not having to calculate the weight-based amount [19, 44]. For gastrinomas, secretin is administered. The administered dose is 30 units of secretin diluted to 5 mL [1].

With the stimulating agents at hand, a baseline venous sample is collected. The catheter or microcatheter is positioned in the specified artery and confirmed with gentle contrast injection. One must be careful not to place the catheter too deep into the artery (beyond the first branch) since this can result in a false-negative study [42]. After the stimulation agent is administered, venous samples are obtained at 30, 60, and 120 s for insulinomas (Fig. 10.1). The same samples are collected for gastrinomas plus an additional sample at 240 s. The samples are placed in a serum gel and sent to the lab on ice. Accurate labeling is essential for each sample.

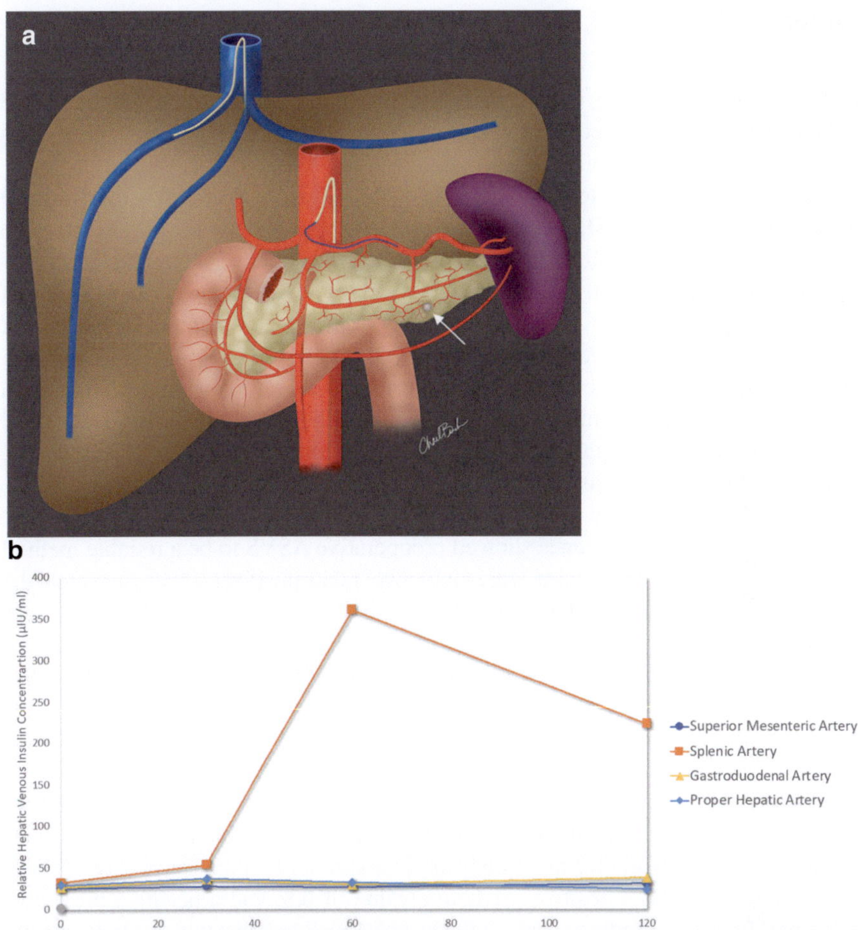

Fig. 10.1 Example of ASVS results for insulinoma in the pancreatic tail. (**a**) Illustration showing small hypervascular mass in the pancreatic tail. (arrow) A calcium gluconate is injected through a microcatheter and venous sampling through a reverse-curve shaped catheter in the hapatic vein (**b**) Graph of results from venous sampling after calcium stimulation. There is marked increase in insulin levels starting at 30 seconds after calcium injection into the splenic artery

After each vessel is sampled, the catheter or microcatheter is repositioned into the next appropriate artery. At least 5 min should elapse between each calcium injection.

When testing for insulinomas, a twofold or higher rise from baseline is the threshold Doppman established and has been used to determine a positive result in most published studies [4]. However, a more recent analysis suggests using a slightly higher threshold of 2.7-fold or higher to consider the test positive for more accurate results [45]. When testing for gastrinomas, a 50% or higher rise at 30 s after injection is the threshold used for a positive result.

Outcomes

Because insulinomas are rare lesions, and many of them may be identified and treated based on cross-sectional imaging alone, there are very few large studies evaluating this test's effectiveness.

In one of the most extensive studies to date, Guettier et al. from the National Institutes of Health (NIH) published a retrospective review of 45 patients who underwent ASVS to localize insulinomas [41]. In this study, 45 patients with suspected insulinomas, based on fasting hypoglycemia, with negative cross-sectional imaging studies underwent ASVS. All patients received 0.0125 mmol Ca/kg, except in obese patients whose dose was reduced to 0.005 mmol Ca/kg. A total of 38/45 (84%) lesions were correctly localized and resected. One interesting finding from this study was the variability in the response. While a twofold threshold was used for a positive test, the mean increase in insulin concentration was 7.9-fold. However, when one looks at the distribution, there was a wide range in responses, likely reflecting the difference in tumor size and/or behavior.

Overall, the NIH experience showed preoperative ASVS to be a reliable method to localize insulinomas. There were only two false positives (4%) in which the tumors were localized to the wrong anatomic area. There were also five false-negative tests (11%). One of these was attributed to a technical error related to the catheter position. The other was associated with the reversal of flow in the GDA from celiac stenosis in a patient with a lesion in the pancreatic head. This case illustrates the importance of ensuring the calcium is delivered to the anatomic region (in this case, the pancreatic head) being studied.

In a recent meta-analysis and systematic review, Wang et al. studied the diagnostic value of ASVS for insulinomas [46]. The authors were able to pool ten studies comprising 337 patients for their analysis. The authors found a sensitivity of 93%, a specificity of 86%, a positive predictive value of 6.8, and a negative predictive value of 0.08. These findings support the use of ASVS as a test with high diagnostic value in localizing the tumor before surgery and exceed the reported sensitivities and specificities of cross-sectional imaging.

Most of the published studies on the value of ASVS have used the 2.0 threshold for a positive test, though this threshold has not been validated in larger studies. One group of investigators applied a decision tree analysis to their data and found a slightly higher threshold of 2.7 times over baseline yielded more accurate results [45]. Sensitivity, specificity, and accuracy improved from 100%, 69%, and 79.1% with a twofold increase threshold to 100%, 91.4%, and 94.2%, respectively, when using the 2.7-fold increase threshold.

As mentioned earlier, there is some evidence to suggest the ASVS may also be useful in distinguishing between occult insulinomas and nesidioblastosis [47]. This distinction has become more critical in recent years as the treatment for nesidioblastosis has changed from a surgical approach to a more conservative management [30, 48, 49]. While these are both rare conditions, researchers at the Mayo Clinic were able to study 116 patients with either insulinoma or nesidioblastosis and underwent ASVS [47]. The investigators were able to compare the two groups to see if the test could reliably differentiate the two conditions. In this study, the researchers derived several conclusions. First, they found that the use of the middle hepatic vein did provide larger differences between the two patient groups than using the right hepatic vein, though both approaches could be used. More importantly, they found patients with insulinomas yielded much higher venous insulin levels than patients with nesidioblastosis. When using the middle hepatic vein, an obtained insulin level of >91.5 µIU/mL resulted in a 95% specificity for insulinoma. When the cutoff was raised to >263.5 µIU/mL, the test was 100% specific.

While most of the reports on ASVS have centered on localizing insulinomas, ASVS also has diagnostic value for gastrinomas. In 1992, Thom et al. published a report that found ASVS to have a sensitivity of 89% in this setting [50]. Other studies have confirmed similar values with sensitivities ranging between 77% and 100% [1, 2].

Complications

The primary risk of the procedure is inducing hypoglycemia in response to the injection of calcium, resulting in a sudden release of insulin. This risk, however, is small due to the small amounts of calcium injected [51]. Other potential complications include pancreatitis from an overzealous injection into an artery directly supplying the pancreas. There are also potential risks that are common to all arteriograms: contrast reaction, vessel dissection, and access site hematomas.

Conclusions

Arterial stimulation venous sampling is a physiologic test that can help identify and localize occult pancreatic endocrine tumors. While it is mostly used for insulinomas, there are other uses, including localizing gastrinomas, differentiating functional from non-functional masses and confirming diagnosis before surgery. While the test is invasive, it is relatively straightforward to perform and has excellent diagnostic results.

References

1. Imamura M, Takahashi K, Adachi H, Minematsu S, Shimada Y, Naito M, et al. Usefulness of selective arterial secretin injection test for localization of gastrinoma in the Zollinger-Ellison syndrome. Ann Surg. 1987;205(3):230–9.
2. Doppman JL, Miller DL, Chang R, Maton PN, London JF, Gardner JD, et al. Gastrinomas: localization by means of selective intraarterial injection of secretin. Radiology. 1990;174(1): 25–9.

3. Norton JA, Doppman JL, Jensen RT. Curative resection in Zollinger-Ellison syndrome. Results of a 10-year prospective study. Ann Surg. 1992;215(1):8–18.
4. Doppman JL, Miller DL, Chang R, Shawker TH, Gorden P, Norton JA. Insulinomas: localization with selective intraarterial injection of calcium. Radiology. 1991;178(1):237–41.
5. Pereira PL, Roche AJ, Maier GW, Huppert PE, Dammann F, Farnsworth CT, et al. Insulinoma and islet cell hyperplasia: value of the calcium intraarterial stimulation test when findings of other preoperative studies are negative. Radiology. 1998;206(3):703–9.
6. Roche A, Raisonnier A, Gillon-Savouret MC. Pancreatic venous sampling and arteriography in localizing insulinomas and gastrinomas: procedure and results in 55 cases. Radiology. 1982;145(3):621–7.
7. Gaeke RF, Kaplan EL, Rubenstein A, Starr J, Burke G. Insulin and proinsulin release during calcium infusion in a patient with islet-cell tumor. Metabolism. 1975;24(9):1029–34.
8. Liu Y, Song Q, Jin HT, Lin XZ, Chen KM. The value of multidetector-row CT in the preoperative detection of pancreatic insulinomas. Radiol Med. 2009;114(8):1232–8.
9. Gouya H, Vignaux O, Augui J, Dousset B, Palazzo L, Louvel A, et al. CT, endoscopic sonography, and a combined protocol for preoperative evaluation of pancreatic insulinomas. AJR Am J Roentgenol. 2003;181(4):987–92.
10. Lin XZ, Wu ZY, Tao R, Guo Y, Li JY, Zhang J, et al. Dual energy spectral CT imaging of insulinoma-value in preoperative diagnosis compared with conventional multi-detector CT. Eur J Radiol. 2012;81(10):2487–94.
11. Stark DD, Moss AA, Goldberg HI, Deveney CW. CT of pancreatic islet cell tumors. Radiology. 1984;150(2):491–4.
12. Rossi P, Baert A, Passariello R, Simonetti G, Pavone P, Tempesta P. CT of functioning tumors of the pancreas. AJR Am J Roentgenol. 1985;144(1):57–60.
13. Günther RW, Klose KJ, Rückert K, Kuhn FP, Beyer J, Klotter HJ, et al. Islet-cell tumors: detection of small lesions with computed tomography and ultrasound. Radiology. 1983;148(2):485–8.
14. Günther RW, Klose KJ, Rückert K, Beyer J, Kuhn FP, Klotter HJ. Localization of small islet-cell tumors. Preoperative and intraoperative ultrasound, computed tomography, arteriography, digital subtraction angiography, and pancreatic venous sampling. Gastrointest Radiol. 1985;10(2):145–52.
15. Kann PH, Rothmund M, Zielke A. Endoscopic ultrasound imaging of insulinomas: limitations and clinical relevance. Exp Clin Endocrinol Diabetes. 2005;113(8):471–4.
16. Kann PH, Moll R, Bartsch D, Pfützner A, Forst T, Tamagno G, et al. Endoscopic ultrasound-guided fine-needle aspiration biopsy (EUS-FNA) in insulinomas: indications and clinical relevance in a single investigator cohort of 47 patients. Endocrine. 2017;56(1):158–63.
17. Wang H, Ba Y, Xing Q, Du JL. Diagnostic value of endoscopic ultrasound for insulinoma localization: a systematic review and meta-analysis. PLoS One. 2018;13(10):e0206099.
18. Kunz PL, Reidy-Lagunes D, Anthony LB, Bertino EM, Brendtro K, Chan JA, et al. Consensus guidelines for the management and treatment of neuroendocrine tumors. Pancreas. 2013;42(4):557–77.
19. Morganstein DL, Lewis DH, Jackson J, Isla A, Lynn J, Devendra D, et al. The role of arterial stimulation and simultaneous venous sampling in addition to cross-sectional imaging for localisation of biochemically proven insulinoma. Eur Radiol. 2009;19(10):2467–73.
20. Lau JH, Drake W, Matson M. The current role of venous sampling in the localization of endocrine disease. Cardiovasc Intervent Radiol. 2007;30(4):555–70.
21. Monroe EJ, Carney BW, Ingraham CR, Johnson GE, Valji K. An interventionist's guide to endocrine consultations. Radiographics. 2017;37(4):1246–67.
22. Harness JK, Geelhoed GW, Thompson NW, Nishiyama RH, Fajans SS, Kraft RO, et al. Nesidioblastosis in adults. A surgical dilemma. Arch Surg. 1981;116(5):575–80.
23. Laidlaw GF. Nesidioblastoma, the islet tumor of the pancreas. Am J Pathol. 1938;14(2):125–34.5.

24. Jabri AL, Bayard C. Nesidioblastosis associated with hyperinsulinemic hypoglycemia in adults: review of the literature. Eur J Intern Med. 2004;15(7):407–10.
25. Service GJ, Thompson GB, Service FJ, Andrews JC, Collazo-Clavell ML, Lloyd RV. Hyperinsulinemic hypoglycemia with nesidioblastosis after gastric-bypass surgery. N Engl J Med. 2005;353(3):249–54.
26. Maeda Y, Yokoyama K, Takeda K, Takada J, Hamada H, Hujioka Y, et al. Adult-onset diffuse nesidioblastosis causing hypoglycemia. Clin J Gastroenterol. 2013;6(1):50–4.
27. Toyomasu Y, Fukuchi M, Yoshida T, Tajima K, Osawa H, Motegi M, et al. Treatment of hyperinsulinemic hypoglycemia due to diffuse nesidioblastosis in adults: a case report. Am Surg. 2009;75(4):331–4.
28. Kenney B, Tormey CA, Qin L, Sosa JA, Jain D, Neto A. Adult nesidioblastosis. Clinicopathologic correlation between pre-operative selective arterial calcium stimulation studies and post-operative pathologic findings. JOP. 2008;9(4):504–11.
29. Malik S, Mitchell JE, Steffen K, Engel S, Wiisanen R, Garcia L, et al. Recognition and management of hyperinsulinemic hypoglycemia after bariatric surgery. Obes Res Clin Pract. 2016;10(1):1–14.
30. Cui Y, Elahi D, Andersen DK. Advances in the etiology and management of hyperinsulinemic hypoglycemia after Roux-en-Y gastric bypass. J Gastrointest Surg. 2011;15(10):1879–88.
31. Okauchi Y, Nammo T, Iwahashi H, Kizu T, Hayashi I, Okita K, et al. Glucagonoma diagnosed by arterial stimulation and venous sampling (ASVS). Intern Med. 2009;48(12):1025–30.
32. Eguchi H, Tanemura M, Marubashi S, Kobayashi S, Wada H, Okita K, et al. Arterial stimulation and venous sampling for glucagonomas of the pancreas. Hepato-Gastroenterology. 2012;59(113):276–9.
33. Bertelli E, Di Gregorio F, Bertelli L, Mosca S. The arterial blood supply of the pancreas: a review. I. The superior pancreaticoduodenal and the anterior superior pancreaticoduodenal arteries. An anatomical and radiological study. Surg Radiol Anat. 1995;17(2):97–106, 1–3.
34. Bertelli E, Di Gregorio F, Bertelli L, Civeli L, Mosca S. The arterial blood supply of the pancreas: a review. II. The posterior superior pancreaticoduodenal artery. An anatomical and radiological study. Surg Radiol Anat. 1996;18(1):1–9.
35. Bertelli E, Di Gregorio F, Bertelli L, Civeli L, Mosca S. The arterial blood supply of the pancreas: a review. III. The inferior pancreaticoduodenal artery. An anatomical review and a radiological study. Surg Radiol Anat. 1996;18(2):67–74.
36. Bertelli E, Di Gregorio F, Bertelli L, Orazioli D, Bastianini A. The arterial blood supply of the pancreas: a review. IV. The anterior inferior and posterior pancreaticoduodenal aa., and minor sources of blood supply for the head of the pancreas. An anatomical review and radiologic study. Surg Radiol Anat. 1997;19(4):203–12.
37. Bertelli E, Di Gregorio F, Mosca S, Bastianini A. The arterial blood supply of the pancreas: a review. V. The dorsal pancreatic artery. An anatomic review and a radiologic study. Surg Radiol Anat. 1998;20(6):445–52.
38. Uflacker R. Atlas of vascular anatomy: an angiographic approach. 2nd ed. Philadelphia: Lippincott Williams & Wilkins; 2007. xiv, 905 p.
39. Sakuhara Y, Kodama Y, Abo D, Hasegawa Y, Shimizu T, Omatsu T, et al. Evaluation of the vascular supply to regions of the pancreas on CT during arteriography. Abdom Imaging. 2008;33(5):563–70.
40. Wiesli P, Brändle M, Schmid C, Krähenbühl L, Furrer J, Keller U, et al. Selective arterial calcium stimulation and hepatic venous sampling in the evaluation of hyperinsulinemic hypoglycemia: potential and limitations. J Vasc Interv Radiol. 2004;15(11):1251–6.
41. Guettier JM, Kam A, Chang R, Skarulis MC, Cochran C, Alexander HR, et al. Localization of insulinomas to regions of the pancreas by intraarterial calcium stimulation: the NIH experience. J Clin Endocrinol Metab. 2009;94(4):1074–80.
42. Thompson SM, Vella A, Service FJ, Grant CS, Thompson GB, Andrews JC. Impact of variant pancreatic arterial anatomy and overlap in regional perfusion on the interpretation of selec-

tive arterial calcium stimulation with hepatic venous sampling for preoperative localization of occult insulinoma. Surgery. 2015;158(1):162–72.

43. Tseng LM, Chen JY, Won JG, Tseng HS, Yang AH, Wang SE, et al. The role of intra-arterial calcium stimulation test with hepatic venous sampling (IACS) in the management of occult insulinomas. Ann Surg Oncol. 2007;14(7):2121–7.

44. Defreyne L, König K, Lerch MM, Hesse UJ, Rottiers R, Feifel G, et al. Modified intra-arterial calcium stimulation with venous sampling test for preoperative localization of insulinomas. Abdom Imaging. 1998;23(3):322–31.

45. Kajiwara K, Yamagami T, Toyota N, Kakizawa H, Urashima M, Hieda M, et al. New diagnostic criteria for the localization of insulinomas with the selective arterial calcium injection test: decision tree analysis. J Vasc Interv Radiol. 2018;29(12):1749–53.

46. Wang H, Ba Y, Xing Q, Cai RC. Diagnostic value of ASVS for insulinoma localization: a systematic review and meta-analysis. PLoS One. 2019;14(11):e0224928.

47. Thompson SM, Vella A, Thompson GB, Rumilla KM, Service FJ, Grant CS, et al. Selective arterial calcium stimulation with hepatic venous sampling differentiates insulinoma from nesidioblastosis. J Clin Endocrinol Metab. 2015;100(11):4189–97.

48. Spanakis E, Gragnoli C. Successful medical management of status post-Roux-en-Y-gastric-bypass hyperinsulinemic hypoglycemia. Obes Surg. 2009;19(9):1333–4.

49. Øhrstrøm CC, Worm D, Hansen DL. Postprandial hyperinsulinemic hypoglycemia after Roux-en-Y gastric bypass: an update. Surg Obes Relat Dis. 2017;13(2):345–51.

50. Thom AK, Norton JA, Doppman JL, Miller DL, Chang R, Jensen RT. Prospective study of the use of intraarterial secretin injection and portal venous sampling to localize duodenal gastrinomas. Surgery. 1992;112(6):1002–8; discussion 8–9.

51. Jackson JE. Angiography and arterial stimulation venous sampling in the localization of pancreatic neuroendocrine tumours. Best Pract Res Clin Endocrinol Metab. 2005;19(2):229–39.

Part III

Medical Treatment of Endocrine Disorders

Chapter 11
Medical Treatment of Hypersecretory Endocrine Disorders

Diana Soliman, Ali Qamar, and Jorge D. Oldan

Hyperaldosteronism

The goals of therapy in hyperaldosteronism are to normalize blood pressure, normalize serum potassium without potassium supplementation and unsuppressed renin, and reverse the adverse cardiovascular and renal effects associated with aldosterone excess.

Surgical/Pharmacological Therapy

For patients with *unilateral* aldosterone-producing adenoma or unilateral hyperplasia, laparoscopic adrenalectomy is recommended. Pharmacological therapy is recommended for patients who cannot undergo surgery or those with *bilateral* hyperaldosteronism [1]. In evaluating patients with hyperaldosteronism, CT imaging is used in conjunction with adrenal vein sampling (AVS) to guide clinical decisions. Although adrenal CT helps detect larger lesions, it may miss microadenomas. Furthermore, nonfunctioning adenomas are common, and CT cannot distinguish these from aldosterone-producing adenomas. Thus, guidelines currently recommend that patients who seek a surgical cure undergo AVS to confirm

D. Soliman (✉) · A. Qamar
Division of Endocrinology, Diabetes and Metabolism, Duke University School of Medicine, Durham, NC, USA
e-mail: diana.botros@duke.edu; ali.qamar@duke.edu

J. D. Oldan
Division of Molecular Imaging and Therapeutics, Department of Radiology, University of North Carolina School of Medicine, Chapel Hill, NC, USA
e-mail: jorge_oldan@med.unc.edu

© The Author(s), under exclusive license to Springer Nature Switzerland AG 2022

H. Yu et al. (eds.), *Diagnosis and Management of Endocrine Disorders in Interventional Radiology*, https://doi.org/10.1007/978-3-030-87189-5_11

unilateral disease. AVS is expensive and invasive, so it should only be performed in patients with primary hyperaldosteronism.

For those who need pharmacological therapy, mineralocorticoid receptor antagonists (MRAs) are the preferred pharmacological agents. Spironolactone is the agent of choice, but eplerenone is an alternative. Both have been shown to reduce blood pressure and increase serum potassium. Spironolactone can cause breast tenderness and menstrual irregularities in women and decreased libido and gynecomastia in men. The starting dose of spironolactone is 12.5–25 mg daily and should be titrated upward gradually to use the lowest effective dose. If side effects of spironolactone limit its use in treating hyperaldosteronism, eplerenone can be trialed. Eplerenone has fewer side effects but is more expensive than spironolactone. Patients with hyperaldosteronism require high doses of MRAs, sometimes exceeding the recommended maximum doses. Serum potassium should be closely monitored when initiating therapy or increasing dosage, especially in patients with chronic kidney disease, due to the risk of hyperkalemia. For patients who can't tolerate MRAs, amiloride or triamterene are second-line therapies. These are potassium-sparing diuretics that block the aldosterone-sensitive sodium channel in the renal collecting tubules. Patients with persistent hypertension, despite upward titration of these medications, should have another antihypertensive medication added to their regimen to normalize their blood pressure.

Nuclear Medicine

At present, there are no commonly used nuclear medicine tests for hyperaldosteronism. A tracer known as NP-59 was used for a short time but is now rarely used due to its poor sensitivity and lack of FDA approval.

Hyperparathyroidism

Management of hyperparathyroidism depends on whether it is primary, secondary, or tertiary hyperparathyroidism and the patient's underlying comorbidities.

Primary Hyperparathyroidism: Surgical/Pharmacological Therapy

Patients with *symptomatic* primary hyperparathyroidism (i.e., symptomatic hypercalcemia, nephrolithiasis, fractures) should have parathyroidectomy. Parathyroid surgery is the only curative treatment for primary hyperparathyroidism. Indications for parathyroidectomy in *asymptomatic* primary hyperparathyroidism are as follows: (1) serum calcium >1 mg/dL higher than the upper limit of normal, (2) osteoporosis as defined by bone mineral density (BMD) on dual-energy X-ray (DXA) or presence of a vertebral fracture on imaging, (3) creatinine clearance of <60 ml/min or nephrolithiasis on imaging, or (4) age less than 50 years [2]. Complications of surgery include hungry bone syndrome, persistent hypoparathyroidism, and recurrent laryngeal nerve injury. Patients who do not undergo surgery require periodic monitoring for worsening hypercalcemia, renal impairment, and bone loss.

For those who meet surgical criteria but have contraindications to surgery or do not want to undergo surgery, medical therapy is recommended [3]. Cinacalcet is a calcimimetic that activates the calcium-sensing receptor and decreases calcium and parathyroid hormone (PTH) levels. Side effects include nausea, diarrhea, arthralgia, myalgia, and paresthesia. Cinacalcet's effects on BMD are unclear. Alendronate is a bisphosphonate that has shown improvement in BMD at the lumbar spine and femoral neck. Bisphosphonates have little to no effect on serum calcium and no significant effect on serum PTH levels. Patients with low BMD and elevated serum calcium may need combination therapy with cinacalcet and bisphosphonate therapy.

Secondary Hyperparathyroidism: Surgical/Pharmacological Therapy

In secondary hyperparathyroidism, treatment is aimed at correcting the causes of hyperparathyroidism. In patients with chronic kidney disease (CKD), serial monitoring of phosphate, calcium, vitamin D, and PTH levels is used to direct treatment [4]. Vitamin D deficiency and insufficiency should be treated. Hyperphosphatemia is managed with dietary phosphate restriction and noncalcium phosphate binders. Phosphate should be lowered toward the normal range while avoiding hypercalcemia. Hypocalcemia can be managed with calcium supplementation. For patients with CKD who are not on dialysis, the optimal PTH level is not known. For those who have severe and progressive secondary hyperparathyroidism, calcitriol and vitamin D analogs may be considered. In patients on dialysis, PTH levels should be maintained at two to nine times the upper limit of normal. In these patients, elevated PTH can be managed with calcimimetics, calcitriol, and/or vitamin D analogs. In patients with CKD stages 3–5 who have severe hyperparathyroidism unresponsive to medical therapy, parathyroidectomy should be considered.

Tertiary Hyperparathyroidism: Surgical/Pharmacological Therapy

In tertiary hyperparathyroidism, the mainstay of treatment is surgery. The most common surgeries are subtotal parathyroidectomy or total parathyroidectomy with autotransplantation. Although calcimimetics are not approved for tertiary hyperparathyroidism, they are sometimes used to reduce serum calcium.

Nuclear Medicine

Technetium-99m sestamibi is used to find occult parathyroid adenomas in hyperparathyroidism; the hypercellular, hypervascular oxyphil cells, common in parathyroid adenomas, take up the tracer in their mitochondria and are described in detail in Chap. 2 [5, 6].

Hyperandrogenism

Treatment of hyperandrogenism is aimed at the underlying etiology. The most common cause of androgen excess is polycystic ovarian syndrome (PCOS). Less commonly, the etiology is idiopathic hyperandrogenism, idiopathic hirsutism, 21-hydroxylase-deficient nonclassic congenital adrenal hyperplasia (NCCAH), hyperandrogenic insulin-resistant acanthosis nigricans (HAIR-AN) syndrome, or an androgen-secreting tumor.

Pharmacological Therapy

First-line therapy for PCOS symptoms is hormonal contraceptives [7]. Oral contraceptives reduce androgens in PCOS and other ovarian causes of hyperandrogenism by suppression of luteinizing hormone (LH) and stimulation of sex hormone-binding globulin (SHBG). For overweight and obese women with PCOS, weight loss is recommended. For women with severe hirsutism, an antiandrogen, such as spironolactone or finasteride, can be added. In addition to its anti-mineralocorticoid properties, spironolactone is an antagonist of the androgen receptor. Finasteride is a 5α-reductase inhibitor that blocks the conversion of testosterone to DHT. Metformin, an insulin-sensitizing agent, can be added in patients with type 2 diabetes mellitus or impaired glucose tolerance. For women with PCOS and anovulatory infertility who are pursuing pregnancy, clomiphene citrate and letrozole are options.

In patients with severe ovarian hyperandrogenism, such as ovarian hyperthecosis, and an inadequate response to hormonal contraceptives and antiandrogens, GnRH agonists can be used. In severe cases, bilateral oophorectomy may be necessary.

In NCCAH, hirsutism and acne can be treated with oral contraceptives, adding an antiandrogen agent if needed [8]. For those who don't respond to these agents or desire fertility, glucocorticoid therapy, such as prednisone or dexamethasone, can be used. Treatment for HAIR-AN syndrome includes weight loss, oral contraceptives, antiandrogens, and metformin. It is recommended that patients who have a virilizing adrenal or ovarian tumor have the tumor surgically excised.

Nuclear Medicine

At present, there are no nuclear medicine tests for hyperandrogenism.

Pancreatic Endocrine Tumors

Pancreatic endocrine tumors or pancreatic neuroendocrine tumors (PNETs) are usually well-differentiated neoplasms. They can occur sporadically or as part of a genetic syndrome. The most common functional PNETs are insulinoma, gastrinoma, VIPoma, glucagonoma, and somatostatinoma.

Surgical/Pharmacological Therapy

It is recommended that functioning PNETs be resected [9, 10]. Medical therapy can be used to control excess hormone secretion, depending on the tumor type. For insulinomas, options include diazoxide, everolimus, or somatostatin analogs (octreotide, lanreotide). Diazoxide use may be limited by the adverse effects of edema, nausea, and hirsutism. When initiating and titrating somatostatin analogs in insulinomas, careful monitoring is required as these agents can paradoxically cause hypoglycemia. For gastrinomas, histamine H2-receptor antagonists and proton pump inhibitors control acid hypersecretion and are first-line agents. For refractory cases, somatostatin analogs can be used. Somatostatin analogs can also be used for the other PNETs, including glucagonomas, VIPomas, and somatostatinomas. Side effects of somatostatin analogs include flatulence, diarrhea/steatorrhea, nausea, gallstones, and glucose intolerance. Options for advanced PNETs are cytoreductive surgery, hepatic artery embolization (for those with liver metastases), and chemotherapy.

Nuclear Medicine

Tracers binding to somatostatin receptors, such as the gamma camera tracer Indium-111 pentetreotide (Octreoscan) and now the positron emission tomography (PET) tracers gallium-68 DOTATATE (Netspot) and DOTATOC, can be used to localize neuroendocrine tumors, including PNETs, carcinoid tumors, gastrinomas, and VIPomas [11, 12]. Pentetreotide has been superseded by DOTATATE and DOTATOC, which has better detection rates (95% vs 43%), PPV (98% vs 84%), and NPV (80% vs 50%), is faster to perform (a few hours vs 24 hours), and results in less radiation dose, but may still be used where PET is not available [13].

Hypercortisolism

Hypercortisolism in Cushing's syndrome can be due to an ACTH-producing pituitary tumor (Cushing's disease), ectopic ACTH production, or excess cortisol production by an adrenal adenoma or carcinoma. The goal of therapy in Cushing's syndrome is to normalize cortisol levels to eliminate the signs and symptoms of Cushing's syndrome and treat comorbidities associated with hypercortisolism [14].

Surgical/Pharmacological Therapy

In Cushing's disease, transsphenoidal selective adenomectomy by an experienced pituitary surgeon is recommended. Before surgery, in the absence of a pituitary lesion on MRI, inferior petrosal sinus sampling (IPSS) can help surgeons identify the correct side of the pituitary tumor. IPSS measures ACTH gradients between the two sinuses during inferior petrosal venous sinus catheterization. After surgery, serum sodium should be measured several times in the first 2 weeks due to the risk of diabetes insipidus. Other risks of surgery include hemorrhage, meningitis, and panhypopituitarism. If surgery is not possible or unsuccessful, second-line therapies include repeat transsphenoidal surgery, radiotherapy, medical treatment, and bilateral adrenalectomy. Repeat transsphenoidal surgery is recommended for patients with incomplete resection or a persistent pituitary lesion on imaging, though it does carry an increased risk of panhypopituitarism. Radiotherapy can be used for patients who are not surgical candidates or have a tumor that is invasive or unresectable. Still, it is more commonly used as a second-line therapy when surgery fails. Pituitary radiation risks include hypopituitarism, optic neuropathy, other cranial neuropathies, and secondary neoplasia. It can take months to years for the full effects of radiation to be achieved, and hypercortisolism will need to be controlled with pharmacological agents in the interim. Pharmacological agents that can be used are adrenal enzyme inhibitors, adrenolytic agents, and glucocorticoid receptor antagonists. Although bilateral total adrenalectomy offers a definitive cure, it requires lifelong glucocorticoid and mineralocorticoid replacement. Given the high likelihood of recurrence in Cushing's disease, patients will need long-term monitoring and should be evaluated for cortisol excess annually.

The preferred therapy for ectopic ACTH-producing tumors is surgical excision of the tumor. For those whom surgery is not an option or have overt metastatic disease, pharmacological therapy or bilateral adrenalectomy are options.

For adrenal adenoma and carcinoma, surgical resection is recommended. Unilateral adrenalectomy is the treatment for adrenal adenomas that cause hypercortisolism. Bilateral adrenalectomy is indicated for bilateral macronodular adrenal hyperplasia and primary pigmented nodular adrenal disease. Patients with adrenocortical carcinoma have a poor prognosis and a high recurrence rate. Initial treatment for adrenocortical carcinoma is surgical resection and adjuvant mitotane therapy. Patients with persistent hypercortisolism will need additional pharmacological therapy.

Though hypercortisolism in Cushing's syndrome is treated surgically, medical therapy is needed if surgery is not possible or unsuccessful. The choice of therapy depends on patient factors and cost. The steroidogenesis inhibitors include ketoconazole, metyrapone, and mitotane. *Ketoconazole* is commonly used and is relatively benign, except for rarely causing idiosyncratic severe hepatic dyscrasia. *Metyrapone* can cause gastrointestinal disturbances and requires monitoring for hypokalemia, edema, and hypertension. By blocking the conversion of 11-deoxycortisol to cortisol, metyrapone causes an elevation of 11-deoxycortisol, which can cross-react with serum and urinary cortisol assays. In severe hypercortisolism, ketoconazole can be used in combination with metyrapone. *Mitotane* has a direct cytotoxic effect on the adrenal cortex and is mainly used as adjuvant therapy to treat adrenocortical carcinoma. Mitotane's side effect profile can limit its tolerability for patients. The most common side effects are nausea, vomiting, fatigue, and anorexia. Mitotane raises the level of cortisol-binding globulin and thus plasma total cortisol. Therefore, urinary free cortisol or salivary cortisol levels are used for monitoring response to therapy.

Pituitary-directed agents are cabergoline and pasireotide. *Cabergoline* is a dopamine agonist. Side effects include nausea, dizziness, and asthenia. *Pasireotide* is a somatostatin receptor agonist that blocks ACTH secretion from the pituitary gland. It can cause diarrhea, nausea, cholelithiasis, hyperglycemia, and transient elevation of liver function tests.

Mifepristone is a glucocorticoid receptor antagonist and antiprogestin. In the United States, it is approved to control hyperglycemia secondary to hypercortisolism. Mifepristone blocks cortisol action, so hormonal measurements cannot be used for monitoring the effectiveness of therapy; instead, clinical parameters must be used. Adverse effects of mifepristone include fatigue, nausea, vomiting, arthralgias, headache, hypertension, hypokalemia, edema, and endometrial thickening.

Nuclear Medicine

At present, there are no nuclear medicine tests specifically for hypercortisolism. However, the somatostatin receptor PET tracer DOTATATE has been used for ectopic ACTH-secreting tumors; overall sensitivity is 64%, while 50% for covert tumors [15].

References

1. Funder JW, Carey RM, Mantero F, Murad MH, Reincke M, Shibata H, et al. The management of primary aldosteronism: case detection, diagnosis, and treatment: an Endocrine Society clinical practice guideline. J Clin Endocrinol Metabol. 2016;101(5):1889–916.
2. Bilezikian JP, Brandi ML, Eastell R, Silverberg SJ, Udelsman R, Marcocci C, et al. Guidelines for the management of asymptomatic primary hyperparathyroidism: summary statement from the fourth international workshop. J Clin Endocrinol Metabol. 2014;99(10):3561–9.

3. Marcocci C, Bollerslev J, Khan AA, Shoback DM. Medical management of primary hyperparathyroidism: proceedings of the fourth international workshop on the management of asymptomatic primary hyperparathyroidism. J Clin Endocrinol Metabol. 2014;99(10):3607–18.

4. Ketteler M, Block GA, Evenepoel P, Fukagawa M, Herzog CA, McCann L, et al. Executive summary of the 2017 KDIGO Chronic Kidney Disease–Mineral and Bone Disorder (CKD-MBD) guideline update: what's changed and why it matters. Kidney Int. 2017;92(1):26–36.

5. Mettler F, Guiberteau M. Thyroid, parathyroid, and salivary glands. Essentials of nuclear medicine and molecular imaging. Elsevier; 2019. p. 85–115.

6. Ziessman H. Endocrine system. In: Nuclear medicine: the requisites. 4th ed. Philadelphia: Elsevier Mosby; 2015. p. 66–97.

7. Legro RS, Arslanian SA, Ehrmann DA, Hoeger KM, Murad MH, Pasquali R, et al. Diagnosis and treatment of polycystic ovary syndrome: an Endocrine Society clinical practice guideline. J Clin Endocrinol Metab. 2013;98(12):4565–92.

8. Martin KA, Anderson RR, Chang RJ, Ehrmann DA, Lobo RA, Murad MH, et al. Evaluation and treatment of hirsutism in premenopausal women: an Endocrine Society clinical practice guideline. J Clin Endocrinol Metab. 2018;103(4):1233–57.

9. Kulke MH, Anthony LB, Bushnell DL, de Herder WW, Goldsmith SJ, Klimstra DS, et al. NANETS treatment guidelines: well-differentiated neuroendocrine tumors of the stomach and pancreas. Pancreas. 2010;39(6):735–52.

10. Kunz PL, Reidy-Lagunes D, Anthony LB, Bertino EM, Brendtro K, Chan JA, et al. Consensus guidelines for the management and treatment of neuroendocrine tumors. Pancreas. 2013;42(4):557–77.

11. Mettler F, Guiberteau M. Non-PET neoplasm imaging and radionuclide therapy. Essentials of nuclear medicine and molecular imaging. Elsevier; 2019. p. 315–27.

12. Young K, Iyer R, Morganstein D, Chau I, Cunningham D, Starling N. Pancreatic neuroendocrine tumors: a review. Future Oncol. 2015;11(5):853–64.

13. Wang R, Zheng-Pywell R, Chen HA, Bibb JA, Chen H, Rose JB. Management of gastrointestinal neuroendocrine tumors. Clin Med Insights Endocrinol Diabetes. 2019;12:1179551419884058.

14. Nieman LK, Biller BMK, Findling JW, Murad MH, Newell-Price J, Savage MO, et al. Treatment of Cushing's syndrome: an Endocrine Society clinical practice guideline. J Clin Endocrinol Metabol. 2015;100(8):2807–31.

15. Varlamov E, Hinojosa-Amaya JM, Stack M, Fleseriu M. Diagnostic utility of Gallium-68-somatostatin receptor PET/CT in ectopic ACTH-secreting tumors: a systematic literature review and single-center clinical experience. Pituitary. 2019;22(5):445–55.

Part IV
Surgical Treatment of Endocrine Disorders

Chapter 12
Surgical Treatment of Primary Aldosteronism

Lawrence Kim and Juan Camilo Mira

Introduction

Primary aldosteronism (PA) is a common cause of secondary hypertension with a prevalence ranging from 5% in uncomplicated hypertension to 20% in resistant hypertension [1, 2]. In PA, aldosterone production is dysregulated and elevated independently of regulation by the renin-angiotensin-aldosterone system leading to inappropriate sodium retention, potassium excretion, and hypertension [3]. Overproduction of aldosterone can occur secondary to bilateral (60% of cases) or unilateral (2%) adrenal hyperplasia, adrenal adenoma (35%), aldosterone-producing carcinoma (<1%), familial hyperaldosteronism (<2%), or ectopic aldosterone production (<0.1%) [4]. Patients with PA are at an increased risk of cardiovascular and cerebrovascular events when compared to patients with essential hypertension [5]. Screening and identification of this increasingly recognized population is imperative as adrenalectomy can cure a subset of this population. Surgical management of PA has proven to be cost-effective and provides long-term improvement in blood pressure, biochemical parameters, and quality of life [6, 7].

Adrenalectomy may be performed via several approaches. The most commonly used techniques are laparoscopic either with or without use of a robotic system. These techniques will be discussed individually in this chapter.

L. Kim (✉) · J. C. Mira
Division of Surgical Oncology and Endocrine Surgery, Department of Surgery, University of North Carolina, Chapel Hill, NC, USA
e-mail: lawrence_kim@med.unc.edu; Juan.Mira@unchealth.unc.edu

© The Author(s), under exclusive license to Springer Nature Switzerland AG 2022

H. Yu et al. (eds.), *Diagnosis and Management of Endocrine Disorders in Interventional Radiology*, https://doi.org/10.1007/978-3-030-87189-5_12

Preoperative Optimization

Patients with PA who have confirmed unilateral disease and are candidates for surgery must be optimized for adrenalectomy. For safe induction of general anesthesia, blood pressure must be controlled and hypokalemia corrected. Spironolactone or eplerenone, a mineralocorticoid receptor antagonist (MRA) in PA, can be used to correct aldosterone-mediated hypokalemia and hypertension. Additional antihypertensives and potassium supplementation may also be necessary [8].

Goal of Surgery: Biochemical and Clinical Remission

Patients with a localized aldosterone-producing adenoma (APA) and unilateral adrenal hyperplasia (UAH) benefit from surgical intervention. When compared to medical treatment in patients with adrenal vein sampling (AVS)-lateralized unilateral PA, adrenalectomy achieves significantly improved systolic and diastolic blood pressure measurements, use of fewer antihypertensive medications, and a complete control rate of hypertension that is 7.75 times higher than is achieved by medication alone [9]. The Primary Aldosteronism Surgical Outcome (PASO) study investigators set to define consensus criteria for the classification of surgical outcomes based on clinical and biochemical outcomes as defined by complete, partial, and absent response to surgery [10]. *Complete biochemical* response was observed on average in 94% of patients undergoing adrenalectomy (normalization of the aldosterone/renin ratio (ARR) and correction of hypokalemia). A *complete clinical* response was noted in 37% (normal blood pressure without medication), and an additional 47% had a *partial clinical* response (either less antihypertensive medication or reduced blood pressure on the same medications) [10]. Importantly, biochemical cure rates of 94% highlight the importance of surgical correction of PA given the known cardiovascular, endothelial, and renal injury associated with prolonged aldosterone hypersecretion [11, 12]. Additionally, adrenalectomy has proven to improve quality-of-life measures in patients with unilateral disease [7, 13]. When counseling patients, it is important to note that certain non-modifiable factors influence rates of remission. Young age, female sex, use of fewer antihypertensives, and the absence of left ventricular hypertrophy are associated with higher rates of clinical and biochemical remission [10]. Race can also impact presentation and outcomes in patients with PA. Despite presenting with similar ARR, Black patients present with a longer duration of hypertension and have a higher mean arterial pressure following adrenalectomy relative to nonblack patients [14].

Given the disparity between clinical and biochemical response rates, several groups have made efforts to predict postoperative hypertensive outcomes (clinical response) for patients with unilateral PA. Examples include the PASO score, nomogram-based preoperative score (NBPS), and aldosteronoma resolution score (ARS) [15–17] (Table 12.1). The predictive factors vary in each group, but all

Table 12.1 Common predictors of postoperative clinical response

Tool	Variables	Favorable score
PASO score	1. Duration of hypertension	1. <10 years
	2. Sex	2. Female
	3. Target organ damage[a]	3. Present
	4. BMI	4. <24
	5. Defined daily dose of antihypertensive medications	5. <3
	6. Largest nodule at imaging	6. >20 mm diameter
NBPS	1. Duration of hypertension	1. ≤5
	2. Sex	2. Female
	3. Target organ damage[a]	3. Present
	4. Aldosterone-to-renin ratio	4. >180 pg.mL–1/mU.L–1
ARS	1. Duration of hypertension	1. ≤6 years
	2. Sex	2. Female
	3. BMI	3. ≤25
	4. Number of antihypertensive medications	4. ≤2 medications

The "favorable score" is noted as the specific values that contribute to increased likelihood of postoperative clinical response as defined by the investigators of the specific predictive tools [15–17]. *PASO* primary aldosteronism surgery outcomes, *NBPS* nomogram-based preoperative score, *ARS* aldosteronoma resolution score, *BMI* body mass index
[a]Defined as presence of left ventricular hypertrophy and/or microalbuminuria

models included sex and duration of hypertension. The developers of the NBPS created their predictive tool using independent predictors of hypertension remission in an Asian cohort and validated it in a Caucasian cohort. Independent predictive variables in this nomogram include sex, duration of hypertension, aldosterone-to-renin ratio, and target organ damage. The nomogram's predictive performance was then compared to the PASO score and ARS in both cohorts. Their findings suggest modest performance in the training and validation populations, with area under the receiver operating characteristic curves (AUCs) in the validation cohort of 0.830 for the NBPS, which was statistically better than the ARS (AUC = 0.745, $P = 0.045$) but equivalent to the PASO score (AUC = 0.825, $P = 0.911$) at predicting postoperative hypertensive outcomes [16].

Adrenalectomy

History of Adrenalectomy

The first successful surgical adrenalectomy was performed in 1889 by K. Thornton, and the procedure became increasingly performed with the discovery of pheochromocytoma (1912), Cushing's disease of adrenal etiology (1949), and primary aldosteronism (1955) [18]. Developments in surgical and anesthetic technique, perioperative blood pressure control, adrenal hormone replacement, and understanding of the pathobiology of these diseases allowed for improved outcomes of a once morbid procedure with mortality approaching 30% [19]. Open surgery was the primary modality employed for adrenalectomy until the development of laparoscopic techniques. The first laparoscopic adrenalectomy was performed in 1992 by M. Gagner [20]. Soon after its inception, laparoscopy was shown to decrease hospital length of stay, diminish narcotic requirement, and cause fewer complications [21]. Importantly, when compared to the open approach, patients with PA undergoing laparoscopic adrenalectomy have equivalent clinical cure rates (improvement in blood pressure and correction of hypokalemia) [22]. While the open approach remains the standard of care for adrenocortical carcinoma, laparoscopic adrenalectomy is the standard for primary aldosteronism from APA and UHA [3, 23].

Surgical Approach

Open Adrenalectomy

Since laparoscopic approaches have become commonplace, open adrenalectomy is seldom performed for hyperaldosteronism. Open adrenalectomy via a transabdominal approach is reserved for patients in whom adrenocortical carcinoma is suspected or in highly selected patients for whom laparoscopic techniques are deemed unadvisable. Adrenocortical carcinoma may be suspected from radiographic findings such as large, lipid poor tumors with irregular borders, heterogeneity, or local invasion [24]. However, isolated hyperaldosteronism is exceedingly rare as a manifestation of adrenocortical carcinoma. Less than 1% of patients with PA have an underlying adrenocortical carcinoma as the primary source [25]. The transabdominal open approach may be performed via a midline or subcostal incision in the supine or lateral position. An open, posterior, retroperitoneal approach via 11th or 12th rib resection was performed by some surgeons until the widespread use of laparoscopy [26]. The open posterior approach is not suitable in cases of malignancy and tends to be a painful incision. It has largely been replaced by laparoscopic approaches.

Laparoscopic Adrenalectomy

As laparoscopy is the standard for benign adrenal lesions; details are described below for the transabdominal and retroperitoneal laparoscopic approaches. Today, there are two main approaches to laparoscopic adrenalectomy: transperitoneal or posterior retroperitoneal.

Transperitoneal (Transabdominal) Adrenalectomy

The laparoscopic transperitoneal adrenalectomy is most commonly performed via a lateral approach [27] though some surgeons perform an anterior approach, especially in cases of other types of adrenal pathology where bilateral adrenalectomy is indicated [28, 29]. One advantage of the lateral position is that gravity allows the viscera to retract away from the surgical field. We prefer the lateral approach.

We prefer to use a beanbag for positioning which is placed on the operating table during room preparation. Draw sheets both below and on top of the beanbag facilitate positioning. The patient is initially placed supine on the operating table and general anesthesia is induced. Secure intravenous access should be assured. In most cases, continuous blood pressure monitoring via arterial access and central venous access is not needed, though may be necessary in some patients due to specific comorbidities. A Foley catheter should be placed. Sequential compression devices are applied. The patient is moved if necessary, so that the space superior to the iliac crest lies over the break point of the table. The patient is then turned into the full lateral position with the appropriate side up. The table is flexed fully to open the space between the costal margin and iliac crest. The beanbag is then deflated. The arms are positioned in neutral positions away from the operative field. The legs are padded and secured in a neutral position.

Transabdominal Approach to the Right Adrenal Gland

The abdomen is entered either via a closed technique and the Veress needle or open technique according to surgeon's preference, and pneumoperitoneum is established to 15 mmHg. The first port is usually positioned just medial to the anterior axillary line. On the right side, usually a total of four ports are required as one will be needed for liver retraction. The right lobe of the liver is retracted cephalad for exposure to the retroperitoneum. Dissection is begun with opening of the posterior peritoneum just inferior to the liver (Fig. 12.1). In thinner patients, the inferior vena cava (IVC) is usually visible just beneath the peritoneum. In larger patients, some dissection may be required before the IVC becomes apparent. Dissection continues along the border of the inferior vena cava to identify the right adrenal vein (Fig. 12.2). The right adrenal vein is a short, sizable vein often located cephalad to the inferior to the edge of the liver. Early identification, dissection, and division of the right adrenal vein are important to avoid surgical complication. The right adrenal vein is clipped and then divided. The adrenal gland can then be dissected away from the IVC (Fig. 12.3). Dissection is carried along the adrenal gland with cautery or an energy device, separating the gland from the retroperitoneal and perirenal adipose tissue. During dissection, it is important not to directly grasp the adrenal gland. This will cause the capsule to rupture resulting in copious bleeding that is difficult to control. Disruption of the tumor may cause seeding of the surrounding space and diffuse

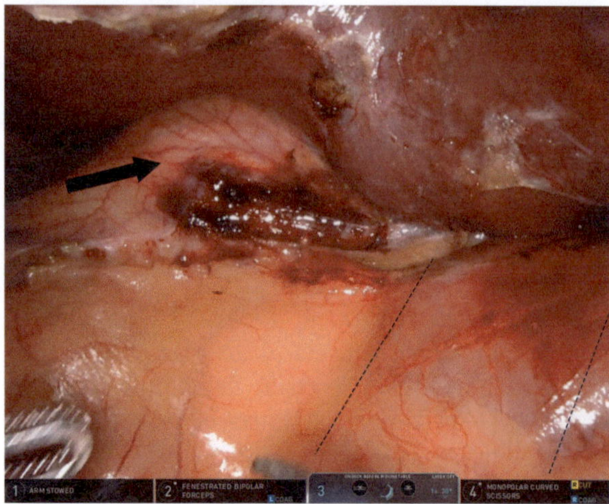

Fig. 12.1 Early view during transabdominal right adrenalectomy. The arrow points to the adrenal gland. The liver is retracted cephalad. Dotted lines indicate the inferior vena cava

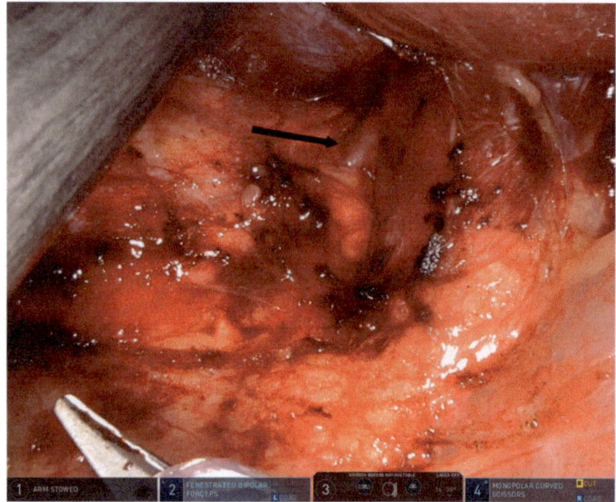

Fig. 12.2 Transabdominal right adrenalectomy. The short adrenal vein has been exposed (arrow)

regrowth of tumor. Usually, the adrenal arterial supply is well controlled with cautery alone, but occasionally, larger vessels may require a clip or an energy device. The superior pole of the kidney will become visible and the pararenal fat is taken along with the adrenal. Care should be taken when dividing the pararenal fat because the irregular shape of the adrenal gland may cause the surgeon to inadvertently leave behind an adrenal limb. Once separated from the retroperitoneum, the adrenal gland is placed in a laparoscopic collection bag and removed. We prefer a strong bag that can tolerate substantial pressure since inadvertent spill of adrenal contents during extraction can be disastrous. The extraction site is closed at the level of the fascia to decrease the risk of incisional hernia. No drains are necessary.

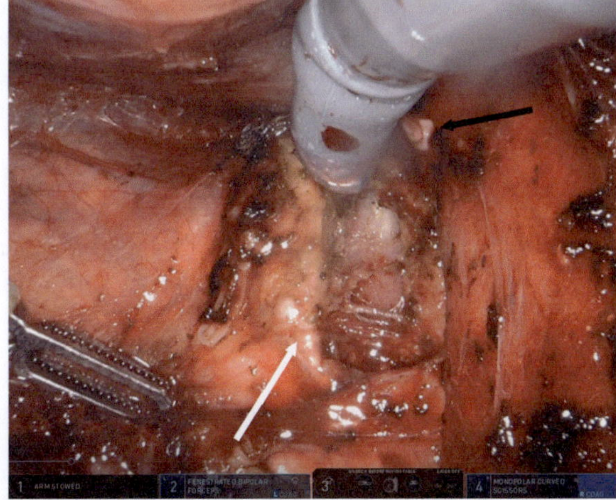

Fig. 12.3 Transabdominal right adrenalectomy. The adrenal gland is being mobilized away from the inferior vena cava. The white arrow points to the edge of the adrenal gland. The black arrow points to the clipped stump of the adrenal vein

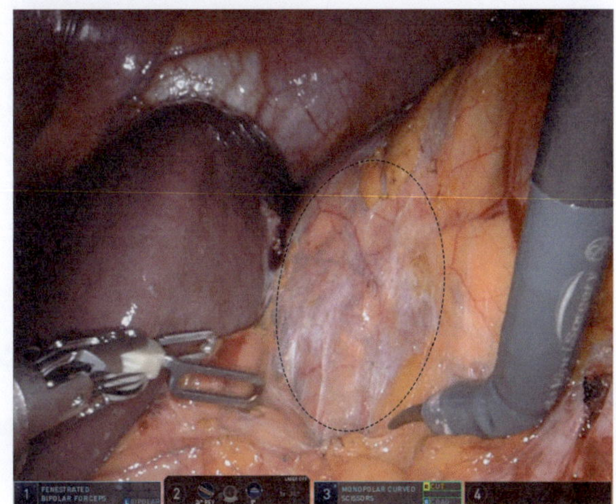

Fig. 12.4 Transabdominal left adrenalectomy. The spleen and pancreas complex have been mobilized anteriorly to expose the left adrenal gland (dotted ellipse)

Transabdominal Approach to the Left Adrenal Gland

The patient is placed in the left lateral decubitus position and the abdomen is entered as described above. Usually, a total of three ports are adequate on the left (a camera port and two working ports). The splenic flexure of the colon is mobilized if necessary to expose the retroperitoneum. Gravity assists on medial retraction of the splenic flexure. The splenorenal and splenophrenic ligaments are divided, and the peritoneum at the inferior edge of the pancreas is incised to allow for medialization of the spleen and tail of the pancreas. Care is taken to avoid inadvertent pancreatic injury. It is critical that the kidney is left undisturbed and the spleen/pancreas complex is mobilized as a unit. This will be an avascular plane that opens with gentle traction and blunt dissection. Gravity will aid in the anterior retraction of the spleen. The left adrenal gland may be visible in thin patients (Fig. 12.4). Gerota's fascia is opened to expose the adrenal gland. Dissection is carried on the inferior border of the adrenal gland to identify the left adrenal vein as it drains into the left renal vein. The left adrenal vein is then identified, clipped, and divided (Fig. 12.5). The inferior phrenic vein may sometimes be seen as it joins the adrenal vein and may be preserved or transected, as necessary. Dissection is carried along the inferior border of the left adrenal gland. Renal vessels will be nearby, and appropriate caution should be taken to avoid their injury. Dissection is carried along the adrenal gland with cautery separating the gland from the retroperitoneal and perirenal adipose tissue. The superior pole of the kidney will become visible (Fig. 12.6). The adrenal gland is placed in a laparoscopic collection bag and the incisions closed as described above.

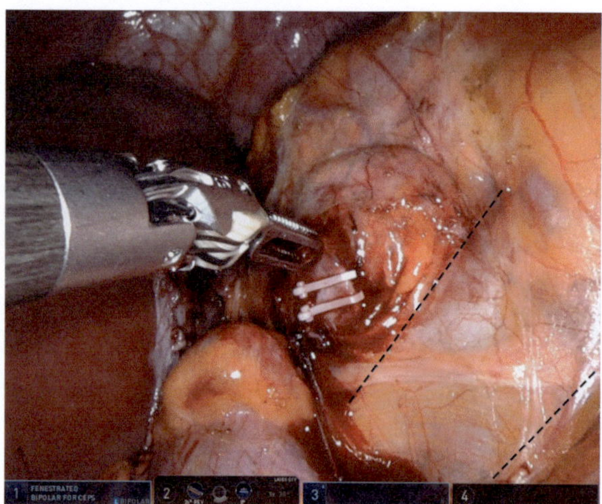

Fig. 12.5 Transabdominal left adrenalectomy. The adrenal vein has been clipped but not yet divided. The left renal vein is outlined by the dotted lines

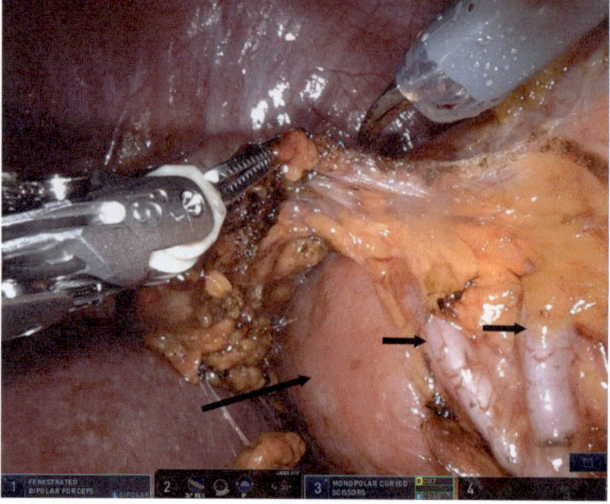

Fig. 12.6 Transabdominal left adrenalectomy. The adrenal gland has been almost completely dissected free. The kidney (long arrow) and renal artery branches (short arrows) are seen

Retroperitoneal Adrenalectomy

Retroperitoneoscopic adrenalectomy was first described in 1995 by MK Walz [30]. This approach may be favored in patients with prior abdominal surgeries and is feasible in the obese [31]. Patients may be positioned in the lateral or prone genuflect position. A large series by Walz of over 500 retroperitoneoscopic adrenalectomies showed excellent outcomes with zero mortality and 1.3% risk of major complications [32]. Several groups have compared laparoscopic transabdominal versus retroperitoneal adrenalectomies [33–35]. While some have favored retroperitoneal adrenalectomies for decreased operative times, blood loss, and hospital length of stay, others have found no significant difference, particularly in terms of complication rates [33–35]. The Society of American Gastrointestinal and Endoscopic Surgeons recommends that surgeons need to perform the approach they are more familiar with and provide the best outcomes in their practice [36].

The patient is placed in the prone genuflect position with all pressure points padded. A 1.5–2 cm incision is made at the tip of the 12th rib, and dissection is carried bluntly to the retroperitoneal space. The initial working space is opened with blunt dissection with the surgeon's finger. Lateral and medial to this incision are two laparoscopic working trocars placed using finger guidance. A sealing balloon or another trocar is placed in the initial incision, and the retroperitoneum is insufflated to 20 mmHg to create a working space. The space is further developed using blunt dissection over the superior pole of the right kidney retracting the kidney caudally and laterally. The inferior aspect of the adrenal gland is identified and completely dissected off the superior pole of the kidney and retracted cephalad (Fig. 12.7). If operating on the right side, the adrenal vein is identified at its insertion to the IVC medially and ventrally. If operating on the left side, the renal vein may be identified and the adrenal vein is recognized as it enters the

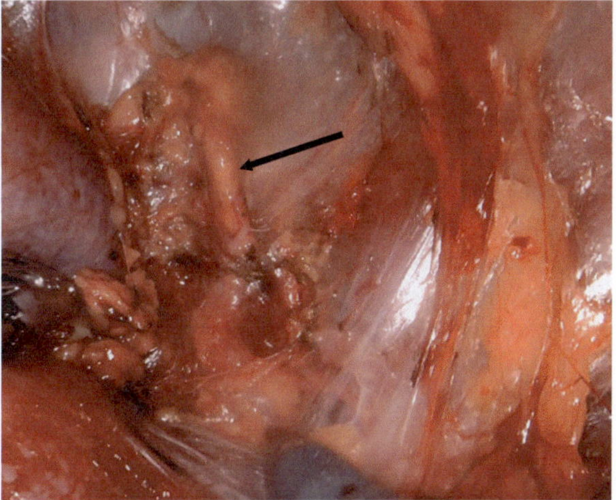

Fig. 12.7 Posterior retroperitoneal left adrenalectomy. Early view of the left adrenal gland (arrow)

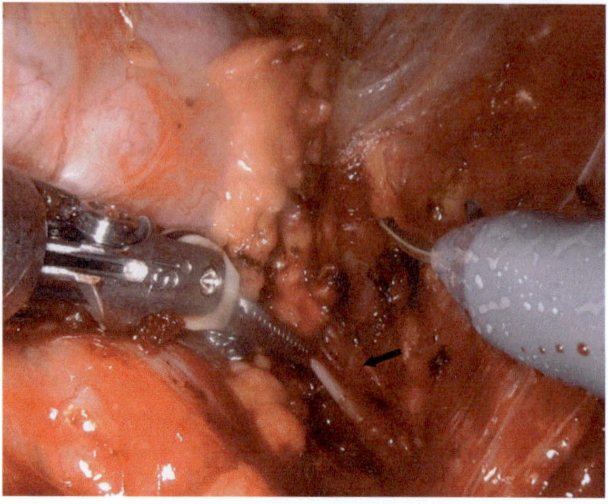

Fig. 12.8 Posterior retroperitoneal left adrenalectomy. The grasper holds the adrenal vein. A left inferior phrenic vein can be seen joining the left adrenal vein (arrow)

renal vein. On the left, the inferior phrenic vein is often seen as it enters the adrenal vein (Fig. 12.8). The adrenal vein is dissected circumferentially, clipped, and divided. The adrenal gland is dissected off its retroperitoneal attachments superiorly and laterally using cautery or an energy device. The gland is removed in a collection bag.

Robotic Adrenalectomy

Robotic surgery has become increasingly common in elective procedures. Adrenalectomy is often performed with robotic assistance, either via the transabdominal or retroperitoneal approach. There is still debate on the benefits of robotic surgery over laparoscopy in adrenal surgery. Overall, there appears to be no difference in overall complications, with some studies favoring decreased blood loss and length of stay for robotic surgery while increasing costs [37, 38]. We prefer to use the robot for the transperitoneal approach because of improved visualization, dexterity, and ability to handle difficult situations such as a vascular injury. However, we agree that the cost is higher and improved patient outcomes have not been clearly shown. We do not use a non-robotic accessory port because of the limited working space, though many surgeons do use an accessory port. With the posterior approach, the available space between ports is very limited. For that reason, the use of a robot may be difficult or impossible. Certainly, older robotic systems are particularly problematic because of bulk. Newer, single-port systems might prove especially useful for the posterior retroperitoneal approach. For now, we prefer not to use the robot for the posterior approach (Fig. 12.9).

Fig. 12.9 Typical aldosteronoma showing the classic golden-yellow color of a cortical adenoma. The specimen has been inked

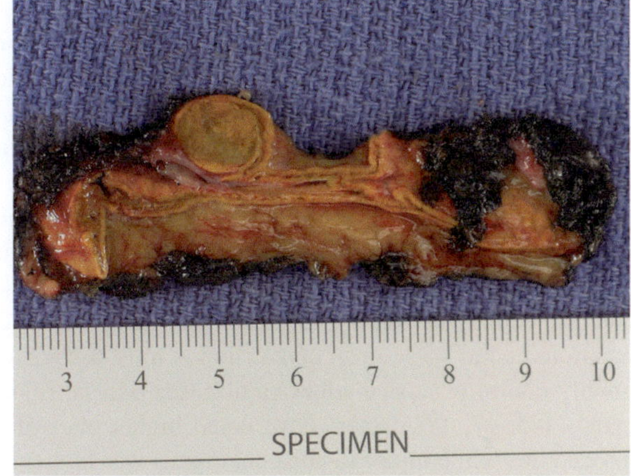

Partial Adrenalectomy

An adrenal sparing approach has been suggested in patients with unilateral APAs detected on imaging studies. Proponents of this approach note decreased risk of adrenal insufficiency with comparable cure rates and no increase in complications [39, 40]. However, results are mixed. Other groups have shown increased rates of persistent aldosteronism after partial adrenalectomy [41–43]. These groups demonstrate two findings: (1) sectioned specimens show hyperplastic nodules at resection margin adjacent to targeted adenoma and (2) nodules detected on imaging studies are not always APAs, even with ipsilateral AVS lateralization, likely secondary to the former. While data has shown improvement in subclinical transient hypocortisolism with partial adrenalectomy when compared to total adrenalectomy (11.5% vs 25%, $p < 0.001$), rates of clinically significant adrenal insufficiency requiring supplementation are equivalent (2.6% vs 1.9%, $p = 0.489$), with no patients developing persistent hypocortisolism in either group [39]. Present guidelines recommend against partial adrenalectomy in PA given the risk of persistent hyperaldosteronism without significant benefit over total adrenalectomy [3].

Complications

Laparoscopic adrenalectomy is a safe procedure with a 30-day mortality of <1% and morbidity of 6.8–14.4% [32, 44, 45]. A granular data with regard to the complication grade and specific type of complications are generally lacking. Surgical morbidity after laparoscopic adrenalectomy can be classified in common complication categories as in other types of abdominal procedures: bleeding, injury to adjacent structures, conversion to open (for minimally invasive approaches), thromboembolic events, infections, cardiac events, pulmonary complications, complications related to anesthesia and positioning, and nerve injuries, among others. Medical complications related to adrenalectomy specific to primary aldosteronism may also be observed: clinically significant hyperkalemia and adrenal insufficiency requiring medical treatment.

Bleeding complications occur <4% in laparoscopic adrenalectomy [46, 47]. Careful dissection along the IVC and left renal veins must be undertaken with careful liver and splenic retraction to minimize events of major hemorrhage from vascular or parenchymal injury. In fact, while rates of conversion from laparoscopy to laparotomy are <5%, open conversion is most associated with bleeding, less commonly due to extensive adhesive disease, visceral injury, and suspicion of malignancy [45, 47, 48]. Others have noted higher rates of bleeding in the right-sided procedures while injury to adjacent organs was higher on the left side [47]. Failure to respect the short right adrenal vein and careless dissection along the IVC on the right or the inferior pancreatic border on the left can account for major bleeding complication. Rates of pulmonary complications, postoperative infections, thromboembolic events, and cardiac events approach 1% or less each [44]. Drains are not placed at the time of adrenalectomy but may be warranted in the event that a pancreatic injury is suspected as this facilitates a control of the pancreatic fistula.

Following adrenalectomy, hyperkalemia has been observed in up to 6.3% of patients secondary to contralateral suppression of aldosterone secretion with about one third of these patients requiring mineralocorticoid replacement therapy [49]. Adrenal insufficiency requiring steroid supplementation may occur in up to 2.6% of patients [39].

Postoperative Care

Following adrenalectomy, electrolytes should be monitored to observe for development of hyperkalemia [3]. To minimize undesired hyperkalemia, potassium supplements and mineralocorticoid receptor antagonists should be stopped, balanced crystalloid solutions without added potassium should be used for intravenous fluid therapy, and a low-potassium and high-sodium diet is recommended [50]. If hyperkalemia does not resolve spontaneously, mineralocorticoid replacement is necessary and continued outpatient monitoring is warranted [50]. Serum aldosterone concentration and renin activity should be measured after surgery to ensure normalization of the aldosterone/renin ratio as evidence of biochemical response [3]. Finally, antihypertensives should be held and stopped if appropriate, keeping in mind that it may require up to 3 months for hypertension to resolve after surgery [51]. Patients should be reassessed annually with measurement of blood pressure and serum potassium levels [10].

References

1. Monticone S, Burrello J, Tizzani D, Bertello C, Viola A, Buffolo F, et al. Prevalence and clinical manifestations of primary Aldosteronism encountered in primary care practice. J Am Coll Cardiol. 2017;69(14):1811–20.
2. Calhoun DA, Nishizaka MK, Zaman MA, Thakkar RB, Weissmann P. Hyperaldosteronism among black and white subjects with resistant hypertension. Hypertension. 2002;40(6):892–6.
3. Funder JW, Carey RM, Mantero F, Murad MH, Reincke M, Shibata H, et al. The management of primary aldosteronism: case detection, diagnosis, and treatment: an Endocrine Society clinical practice guideline. J Clin Endocrinol Metab. 2016;101(5):1889–916.
4. Farrugia FA, Zavras N, Martikos G, Tzanetis P, Charalampopoulos A, Misiakos EP, et al. A short review of primary aldosteronism in a question and answer fashion. Endocr Regul. 2018;52(1):27–40.
5. Mulatero P, Monticone S, Bertello C, Viola A, Tizzani D, Iannaccone A, et al. Long-term cardio- and cerebrovascular events in patients with primary aldosteronism. J Clin Endocrinol Metab. 2013;98(12):4826–33.
6. Sywak M, Pasieka JL. Long-term follow-up and cost benefit of adrenalectomy in patients with primary hyperaldosteronism. Br J Surg. 2002;89(12):1587–93.
7. Sukor N, Kogovsek C, Gordon RD, Robson D, Stowasser M. Improved quality of life, blood pressure, and biochemical status following laparoscopic adrenalectomy for unilateral primary aldosteronism. J Clin Endocrinol Metab. 2010;95(3):1360–4.
8. Young WF Jr. Diagnosis and treatment of primary aldosteronism: practical clinical perspectives. J Intern Med. 2019;285(2):126–48.
9. Meng X, Ma WJ, Jiang XJ, Lu PP, Zhang Y, Fan P, et al. Long-term blood pressure outcomes of patients with adrenal venous sampling-proven unilateral primary aldosteronism. J Hum Hypertens. 2020;34(6):440–7.
10. Williams TA, Lenders JWM, Mulatero P, Burrello J, Rottenkolber M, Adolf C, et al. Outcomes after adrenalectomy for unilateral primary aldosteronism: an international consensus on outcome measures and analysis of remission rates in an international cohort. Lancet Diabetes Endocrinol. 2017;5(9):689–99.
11. Rossi GP, Bernini G, Desideri G, Fabris B, Ferri C, Giacchetti G, et al. Renal damage in primary aldosteronism: results of the PAPY study. Hypertension. 2006;48(2):232–8.
12. Mulatero P, Sechi LA, Williams TA, Lenders JWM, Reincke M, Satoh F, et al. Subtype diagnosis, treatment, complications and outcomes of primary aldosteronism and future direction of research: a position statement and consensus of the Working Group on Endocrine Hypertension of the European Society of Hypertension. J Hypertens. 2020;38(10):1929–36.
13. Velema M, Dekkers T, Hermus A, Timmers H, Lenders J, Groenewoud H, et al. Quality of life in primary aldosteronism: a comparative effectiveness study of adrenalectomy and medical treatment. J Clin Endocrinol Metab. 2018;103(1):16–24.
14. Gershuni VM, Ermer JP, Kelz RR, Roses RE, Cohen DL, Trerotola SO, et al. Clinical presentation and surgical outcomes in primary aldosteronism differ by race. J Surg Oncol. 2020;121(3):456–64.
15. Burrello J, Burrello A, Stowasser M, Nishikawa T, Quinkler M, Prejbisz A, et al. The primary aldosteronism surgical outcome score for the prediction of clinical outcomes after adrenalectomy for unilateral primary aldosteronism. Ann Surg. 2020;272(6):1125–32.
16. Yang Y, Williams TA, Song Y, Yang S, He W, Wang K, et al. Nomogram-based preoperative score for predicting clinical outcome in unilateral primary aldosteronism. J Clin Endocrinol Metab. 2020;105(12):dgaa634.
17. Zarnegar R, Young WF Jr, Lee J, Sweet MP, Kebebew E, Farley DR, et al. The aldosteronoma resolution score: predicting complete resolution of hypertension after adrenalectomy for aldosteronoma. Ann Surg. 2008;247(3):511–8.

18. Harris DA, Wheeler MH. In: Linos D, Van Heerden JA, editors. History of adrenal surgery. Berlin/New York: Springer; 2005.
19. Papadakis M, Manios A, Schoretsanitis G, Trompoukis C. Landmarks in the history of adrenal surgery. Hormones (Athens). 2016;15(1):136–41.
20. Gagner M, Lacroix A, Bolte E. Laparoscopic adrenalectomy in Cushing's syndrome and pheochromocytoma. N Engl J Med. 1992;327(14):1033.
21. Thompson GB, Grant CS, van Heerden JA, Schlinkert RT, Young WF Jr, Farley DR, et al. Laparoscopic versus open posterior adrenalectomy: a case-control study of 100 patients. Surgery. 1997;122(6):1132–6.
22. Shen WT, Lim RC, Siperstein AE, Clark OH, Schecter WP, Hunt TK, et al. Laparoscopic vs open adrenalectomy for the treatment of primary hyperaldosteronism. Arch Surg. 1999;134(6):628–31; discussion 31–2.
23. Dickson PV, Kim L, Yen TWF, Yang A, Grubbs EG, Patel D, et al. Evaluation, staging, and surgical management for adrenocortical carcinoma: an update from the SSO Endocrine and Head and Neck Disease Site Working Group. Ann Surg Oncol. 2018;25(12):3460–8.
24. Fassnacht M, Arlt W, Bancos I, Dralle H, Newell-Price J, Sahdev A, et al. Management of adrenal incidentalomas: European Society of Endocrinology Clinical Practice Guideline in collaboration with the European Network for the Study of Adrenal Tumors. Eur J Endocrinol. 2016;175(2):G1–G34.
25. Seccia TM, Fassina A, Nussdorfer GG, Pessina AC, Rossi GP. Aldosterone-producing adrenocortical carcinoma: an unusual cause of Conn's syndrome with an ominous clinical course. Endocr Relat Cancer. 2005;12(1):149–59.
26. Proye CA, Huart JY, Cuvillier XD, Assez NM, Gambardella B, Carnaille BM. Safety of the posterior approach in adrenal surgery: experience in 105 cases. Surgery. 1993;114(6):1126–31.
27. Raffaelli M, De Crea C, Bellantone R. Laparoscopic adrenalectomy. Gland Surg. 2019;8(Suppl 1):S41–52.
28. Balla A, Ortenzi M, Palmieri L, Corallino D, Meoli F, Ursi P, et al. Laparoscopic bilateral anterior transperitoneal adrenalectomy: 24 years experience. Surg Endosc. 2019;33(11):3718–24.
29. Paganini AM, Balla A, Guerrieri M, Lezoche G, Campagnacci R, D'Ambrosio G, et al. Laparoscopic transperitoneal anterior adrenalectomy in pheochromocytoma: experience in 62 patients. Surg Endosc. 2014;28(9):2683–9.
30. Walz MK, Peitgen K, Krause U, Eigler FW. [Dorsal retroperitoneoscopic adrenalectomy–a new surgical technique]. Zentralbl Chir. 1995;120(1):53–8.
31. Dickson PV, Jimenez C, Chisholm GB, Kennamer DL, Ng C, Grubbs EG, et al. Posterior retroperitoneoscopic adrenalectomy: a contemporary American experience. J Am Coll Surg. 2011;212(4):659–65; discussion 65–7.
32. Walz MK, Alesina PF, Wenger FA, Deligiannis A, Szuczik E, Petersenn S, et al. Posterior retroperitoneoscopic adrenalectomy--results of 560 procedures in 520 patients. Surgery. 2006;140(6):943–8; discussion 8-50.
33. Chai YJ, Kwon H, Yu HW, Kim SJ, Choi JY, Lee KE, et al. Systematic review of surgical approaches for adrenal tumors: lateral transperitoneal versus posterior retroperitoneal and laparoscopic versus robotic adrenalectomy. Int J Endocrinol. 2014;2014:918346.
34. Nigri G, Rosman AS, Petrucciani N, Fancellu A, Pisano M, Zorcolo L, et al. Meta-analysis of trials comparing laparoscopic transperitoneal and retroperitoneal adrenalectomy. Surgery. 2013;153(1):111–9.
35. Conzo G, Tartaglia E, Gambardella C, Esposito D, Sciascia V, Mauriello C, et al. Minimally invasive approach for adrenal lesions: systematic review of laparoscopic versus retroperitoneoscopic adrenalectomy and assessment of risk factors for complications. Int J Surg. 2016;28(Suppl 1):S118–23.
36. Stefanidis D, Goldfarb M, Kercher KW, Hope WW, Richardson W, Fanelli RD, et al. SAGES guidelines for minimally invasive treatment of adrenal pathology. Surg Endosc. 2013;27(11):3960–80.

37. Economopoulos KP, Mylonas KS, Stamou AA, Theocharidis V, Sergentanis TN, Psaltopoulou T, et al. Laparoscopic versus robotic adrenalectomy: a comprehensive meta-analysis. Int J Surg. 2017;38:95–104.
38. Makay O, Erol V, Ozdemir M. Robotic adrenalectomy. Gland Surg. 2019;8(Suppl 1):S10–S6.
39. Billmann F, Billeter A, Thomusch O, Keck T, El Shishtawi S, Langan EA, et al. Minimally invasive partial versus total adrenalectomy for unilateral primary hyperaldosteronism-a retrospective, multicenter matched-pair analysis using the new international consensus on outcome measures. Surgery. 2021;169(6):1361–70.
40. Jeschke K, Janetschek G, Peschel R, Schellander L, Bartsch G, Henning K. Laparoscopic partial adrenalectomy in patients with aldosterone-producing adenomas: indications, technique, and results. Urology. 2003;61(1):69–72; discussion.
41. Ishidoya S, Ito A, Sakai K, Satoh M, Chiba Y, Sato F, et al. Laparoscopic partial versus total adrenalectomy for aldosterone producing adenoma. J Urol. 2005;174(1):40–3.
42. Liu JH, Wei XD, Fu CC, Li QX, Hou JQ, Lv JX, et al. Long-term results of laparoscopic partial versus total adrenalectomy for aldosterone producing adenoma. Urol J. 2020;17(4):4981.
43. Nanba AT, Nanba K, Byrd JB, Shields JJ, Giordano TJ, Miller BS, et al. Discordance between imaging and immunohistochemistry in unilateral primary aldosteronism. Clin Endocrinol. 2017;87(6):665–72.
44. Gupta PK, Natarajan B, Pallati PK, Gupta H, Sainath J, Fitzgibbons RJ Jr. Outcomes after laparoscopic adrenalectomy. Surg Endosc. 2011;25(3):784–94.
45. Sommerey S, Foroghi Y, Chiapponi C, Baumbach SF, Hallfeldt KK, Ladurner R, et al. Laparoscopic adrenalectomy--10-year experience at a teaching hospital. Langenbeck's Arch Surg. 2015;400(3):341–7.
46. Di Buono G, Buscemi S, Lo Monte AI, Geraci G, Sorce V, Citarrella R, et al. Laparoscopic adrenalectomy: preoperative data, surgical technique and clinical outcomes. BMC Surg. 2019;18(Suppl 1):128.
47. Aporowicz M, Domoslawski P, Czopnik P, Sutkowski K, Kaliszewski K. Perioperative complications of adrenalectomy - 12 years of experience from a single center/teaching hospital and literature review. Arch Med Sci. 2018;14(5):1010–9.
48. Gaujoux S, Bonnet S, Leconte M, Zohar S, Bertherat J, Bertagna X, et al. Risk factors for conversion and complications after unilateral laparoscopic adrenalectomy. Br J Surg. 2011;98(10):1392–9.
49. Shariq OA, Bancos I, Cronin PA, Farley DR, Richards ML, Thompson GB, et al. Contralateral suppression of aldosterone at adrenal venous sampling predicts hyperkalemia following adrenalectomy for primary aldosteronism. Surgery. 2018;163(1):183–90.
50. Fischer E, Hanslik G, Pallauf A, Degenhart C, Linsenmaier U, Beuschlein F, et al. Prolonged zona glomerulosa insufficiency causing hyperkalemia in primary aldosteronism after adrenalectomy. J Clin Endocrinol Metab. 2012;97(11):3965–73.
51. Young WF Jr. Minireview: primary aldosteronism--changing concepts in diagnosis and treatment. Endocrinology. 2003;144(6):2208–13.

Chapter 13
Surgical Management of Primary Hyperparathyroidism

Megan Elizabeth Lombardi and Jen Jen Yeh

Preoperative Planning

Initial laboratory evaluation of a patient presenting with either symptoms or a chemical diagnosis of primary hyperparathyroidism should include 25-hydroxyvitamin D, 24-hour urine calcium measurement, DEXA scan, and supplementation of vitamin D deficiency when appropriate. The hallmark biochemical sign of primary hyperparathyroidism is hypercalcemia associated with high or inappropriately normal PTH levels. A 24-hour urine calcium level can be useful to help distinguish familial hypocalciuric hypercalcemia from primary hyperparathyroidism [1, 2].

While parathyroid imaging is not required for diagnosis, it should be used as an adjunct for surgical planning [3]. Most cases of primary hyperparathyroidism are caused by a single adenoma (80%) or multi-gland hyperplastic syndrome (20%), and the type of operation offered to patients is based on the ability of the surgeon to preoperatively localize the diseased gland(s) [4]. Negative or equivocal preoperative imaging may push the surgeon into performing a full bilateral neck exploration which comes with additional risks. Currently, no set imaging guidelines exist, and instead, guidelines depend on several factors including institutional capabilities, radiology expertise, and surgeon preference [5].

M. E. Lombardi · J. J. Yeh (✉)
Department of Surgery, University of North Carolina, Chapel Hill, NC, USA
e-mail: Megan.lombardi@unchealth.unc.edu; jjyeh@med.unc.edu

© The Author(s), under exclusive license to Springer Nature
Switzerland AG 2022

H. Yu et al. (eds.), *Diagnosis and Management of Endocrine Disorders in Interventional Radiology*, https://doi.org/10.1007/978-3-030-87189-5_13

Imaging

Ultrasound Evaluation

Ultrasound is a fast and low-cost method of detecting grossly abnormal parathyroid glands while the patient is in the clinic. It is especially useful for quickly identifying abnormal glands, which are usually vascular hypoechoic oval or bean-shaped structures. Ultrasound can also provide additional anatomic information such as relation to nearby structures [6]. However, ultrasound examinations are limited when the thyroid gland is diffusely enlarged as high-resolution transducers have limited path length through the gland [7].

Nuclear Medicine Imaging Techniques

Preoperative technetium-99m-labeled sestamibi scans accurately localize the hyperactive parathyroid lesion or adenoma in 70–85% of the cases but do not provide detailed anatomic information given that they are two-dimensional planar images. Sestamibi scans are performed by injecting a radiotracer which is initially taken up by both the parathyroid glands as well as the thyroid but is retained by the mitochondrion-rich oxyphil cells of the hyperactive parathyroid gland which persist on delayed phase imaging [8].

SPECT/CT has an advantage over planar sestamibi scintigraphy as it combines the measurement of gamma radiation with anatomic images from multiple angles. SPECT/CT has been shown to have a >94% positive predictive value for the presence of adenoma and correctly showing the laterality of the lesion. The fusion of the SPECT and CT images also allows for better visualization of anatomic structures and ectopic/mediastinal parathyroid adenomas as well as showing the functional status of the glands (Fig. 13.1). However, patients with negative scans or multi-gland disease have higher rates of operative failure, and disease patterns are not as well predicted. Therefore, multiple imaging modalities can be used in combination to achieve an accurate preoperative diagnosis [9].

Dynamic Computed Tomography

Historically, ultrasound and technetium-99m-labeled sestamibi scintigraphy have been the two most used imaging modalities. While studies have shown they have similar sensitivities and specificities in identifying solitary parathyroid adenomas, they struggle at accurately outlining multi-gland disease [4–6]. Recently, this struggle has become more important since minimally invasive surgical techniques have created a need for more precise localization of the parathyroid lesion. This has led to the development of a 4-dimensional (4D) CT which has started to shift the paradigm of preoperative imaging in hyperparathyroidism [4, 10]. 4D CT has emerged

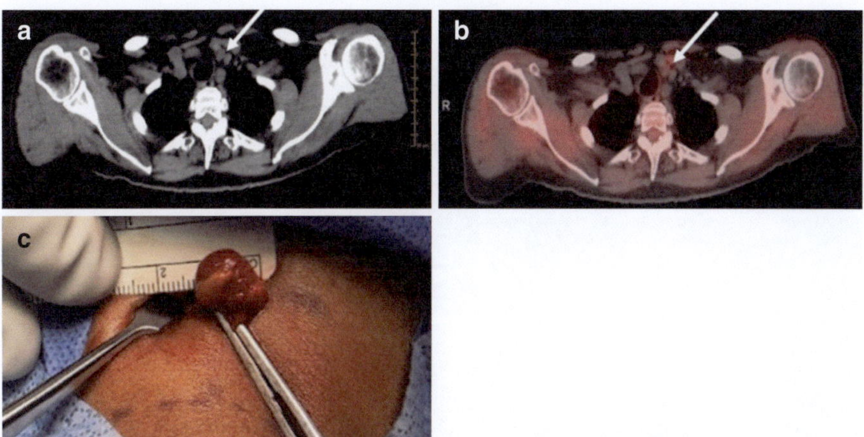

Fig. 13.1 CT (**a**) versus SPECT/CT (**b**) demonstrating the increased localization utility of SPECT/CT over standard CT images. Arrows show the hyperactive parathyroid despite a slight misregistration of the SPECT images. Below (**c**) is the corresponding parathyroid gland being resected using a minimally invasive approach

as an imaging modality to help identify diseased glands in patients with a history of previous neck surgery, mild hyperparathyroidism, and multi-gland disease and in those with negative sestamibi and ultrasound studies (Fig. 13.2). In 4D CT, images are acquired prior to the administration of iodinated contrast and in the arterial and delayed phases. Lesions are identified based on anatomic and attenuation characteristics which are beyond the scope of this chapter. 4D CT has been shown to improve preoperative localization in both single and multi-gland disease when compared to sestamibi SPECT/CT alone [5]. In patients with persistent or recurrent primary hyperparathyroidism after surgical intervention, there may be a role in undergoing both sestamibi SPECT/CT and 4D CT [5].

Fine Needle Aspiration with PTH Wash

In some cases, preoperative imaging may not be able to distinguish parathyroid adenomas from thyroid nodules, which can also concentrate sestamibi. A highly accurate preoperative localization technique that may be especially useful under this circumstance is an US-guided fine needle aspiration (FNA) with PTH wash. This may allow more patients to benefit from minimally invasive techniques, especially at centers without the capability to perform intraoperative PTH monitoring (IPM). FNA with PTH wash has a 91–100% specificity and a 91–100% sensitivity, allowing surgeons to preoperatively characterize the nature of a mass, distinguish parathyroid tissue from lymphoid tissue or thyroid nodules, and plan for directed surgical intervention [11, 12]. An FNA with PTH wash is considered positive when

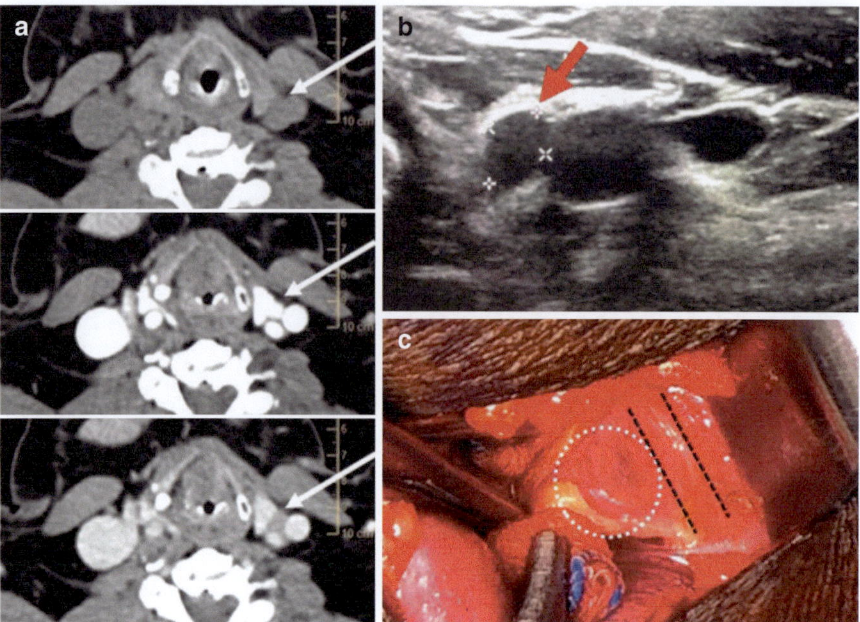

Fig. 13.2 In a patient with a non-localizing SPECT/CT, 4D CT shows the candidate with delayed washout compared to the vasculature on the delayed phase (arrows) (**a**). Top right (**b**) is the corresponding US of the parathyroid candidate adjacent to the carotid sheath (arrow). Bottom right (**c**), operative photograph of the parathyroid candidate (white dashed circle) adjacent to the internal jugular vein (black lines)

the concentration of the PTH in the FNA sample is higher than the serum PTH level [12]. Using this technique, PTH wash successfully identified the lesion in 40 of 45 patients with coexisting nodular thyroid disease, showing its usefulness in this situation [11]. However, FNA with PTH wash continues to be a newer technique and lacks the standardization needed to be studied in randomized controlled trials.

Preoperative Medical Optimization

Besides imaging, the other major portion of preoperative planning for parathyroid surgery involves medical management, specifically vitamin D and calcium optimization. The most basic method of controlling calcium includes adequate hydration to prevent contraction hypercalcemia. Calcium intake does not need to be limited in preoperative patients with primary hyperparathyroidism, but vitamin D levels should be monitored closely as decreased vitamin D can accentuate PTH elevations. Correction of vitamin D levels is the recommended method of reducing bone turnover, fractures, and falls preoperatively as well as preventing hungry bone syndrome postoperatively [13, 14]. Cholecalciferol in weekly doses of 50,000 IU for 1 month followed by monthly doses of 50,000 IU has been shown to lower PTH levels without increasing calcium nor requiring the need for additional calcium supplements [13, 14].

Indications

Parathyroidectomy is the only definitive treatment for primary hyperparathyroidism, and even asymptomatic patients may derive benefit from surgical intervention. Observation and medical therapy are both less effective and less cost-effective due to the potential deleterious effects of long-term hypercalcemia [1].

Indications for parathyroidectomy have been debated over the years but recent guidelines have shown that definitive care should be recommended and carried out in those individuals who meet the following criteria: age < 50 years old, hypercalcemia consistently >1 mg/dL above normal, fractures, renal stones, hypercalciuria, or T-score <−2.5 at any bone site [1, 4]. Surgery may be considered in patients who do not meet the above criteria but have no medical contraindications and have had thorough discussions with their surgeon, primary care provider, and endocrinologist who are all in agreement with an operative plan [4].

Parathyroidectomy should ideally be performed by experienced surgeons at high volume centers as data has shown that the volume of operations inversely correlates with complications, cost, and length of stay [1, 15].

Contraindications

Parathyroidectomy is not recommended in patients in whom the risks of anesthesia and surgery outweigh the benefits. In patients that have significant comorbid diseases, refuse surgery, or simply do not meet the indications, the recommendation is to forego operative intervention and instead pursue medical management [1, 16]. However, patients with even mild disease should understand that their symptoms will possibly progress over time and surgery may be needed at some point in the future [1].

For those who do have contraindications to surgical intervention, 25-hydroxyvitamin D levels should be closely monitored. Cinacalcet, a calcimimetic, is the treatment of choice for those with severe hypercalcemia who cannot undergo parathyroidectomy. Cinacalcet lowers serum calcium with only a modest effect on PTH levels and no change to bone mineral density (BMD). Bisphosphonates are one medication that may be used to improve BMD at the lumbar spine without altering serum calcium concentration [16].

Surgical Interventions

Bilateral Cervical Exploration

While a bilateral cervical exploration (BCE) has historically been the operation of choice for primary hyperparathyroidism with up to a 98% success rate, advancements in imaging and localization techniques have allowed minimally invasive techniques to largely supplant BCE for preoperatively localized glands [1, 17, 18]. BCE now shares the co-gold standard with the targeted parathyroidectomy as single adenomas are routinely identified preoperatively [19]. Long-term cure is defined as a > 50% intraoperative decrease in PTH and a normal-to-low serum calcium level 6 months postoperatively [1, 8, 20]. While minimally invasive techniques have been embraced, all surgeons should be trained to perform a BCE given the propensity for patients with seemingly only a single adenoma to have occult multi-gland disease. In patients with sporadic disease, equivocal preoperative scans, or concurrent thyroid disease, a BCE can be performed with high likelihood for success and cure [16].

Minimally Invasive Techniques

Minimally invasive parathyroidectomy is a feasible operation for patients who have primary hyperparathyroidism secondary to an isolated adenoma, which is the case in approximately 80% of hyperparathyroidism cases [3, 20, 21]. Combining preoperative sestamibi SPECT/CT scans along with intraoperative localization techniques has made minimally invasive techniques safer and more attractive to both surgeons and patients. One study found that complications of BCE and minimally invasive techniques are similar but incision size, operating time, hospital stay, and postoperative analgesia were all significantly reduced in the minimally invasive group, suggesting that minimally invasive approaches should be the operation of choice for patients when possible [21].

Indications for robotic parathyroidectomy are limited. It is considered in patients with single gland disease, a BMI < 30, and an axillary to sternal notch distance of less than 17 cm. Absolute contraindications to robotic surgery include prior neck surgery, significant thyroiditis, or bulky thyroid disease [18]. In this highly selected patient population, robotic surgery has been shown to be equivocal to open surgery in terms of cure [19]. One benefit of the robotic technique is that it allows the patient to avoid a neck scar as most surgeons use an axillary or infraclavicular technique. Avoiding a neck scar can lead to increased patient satisfaction and offer a more appealing operative plan for patients with the propensity to form keloids or hypertrophic scar. Overall, robotic parathyroidectomy will continue to be a niche surgical intervention given its equivocal outcomes with only cosmetic benefits along with a high operative cost and steeper learning curve [19, 22].

Autotransplantation

Autotransplantation, first described in humans by Lahey in 1926, is a preventative measure taken intraoperatively when the parathyroid tissue viability is questioned due to concern for devascularization of the remaining glands in order to minimize postoperative hypoparathyroidism leading to hypocalcemia [1, 23]. Autotransplantation is generally not required when surgical intervention is being done for primary hyperparathyroidism with a single or even double adenoma as there are normal glands left behind. If there is universal hyperplasia of the parathyroid glands, the goal is a subtotal parathyroidectomy where 3.5 glands are removed leaving behind approximately 50 mg of tissue which is either left in its anatomic location or moved to an easier-to-access location. If patients continue to have hyperparathyroidism, a second operation with transplantation of the parathyroid tissue to an area of the body easier to access, such as the arm, is a viable option. If a total parathyroidectomy is being performed, autotransplantation must occur to prevent lifelong hypoparathyroidism [23].

Currently, two methods of autotransplantation exist: immediate and delayed. Delayed autotransplantation is useful in patients who have a substantial risk of postoperative hypoparathyroidism, including those who are undergoing a BCE for parathyroid hyperplasia or those undergoing repeat operative intervention for persistent or recurrent disease [23]. Cryopreservation was first discussed in 1974 and has been extensively researched to improve methods of preservation and therefore increase success rates. Guerrero found that the viability of parathyroid tissue is significantly improved if reimplanted in under 24 months as the parathyroid tissue may have a better ability to promote angiogenesis spontaneously via vascular endothelial growth factor (VEGF) within this time frame [23, 24]. However, Borot found that only 1.6% of patients who had cryopreservation underwent future autotransplantation which allows room for debate of both the practicality and usefulness of routine cryopreservation [23, 25].

Intraoperative PTH Monitoring and Localization

IPM is a technique that allows for increased cure rates (97–99%) and for surgeons to be able to remove a single diseased gland without additional dissection given that PTH has a half-life of only 3.5–4 min. This allows confidence that the pathologic gland or adenoma was completely removed prior to leaving the operating room without the need to visualize all other glands. The Miami criteria requires that the PTH falls by 50% when compared to the highest pre-manipulation or pre-excision blood sample to ensure the lesion was fully removed [3].

As sestamibi is taken up by the parathyroid tissue, it becomes retained in the tissue and allows for the use of an intraoperative gamma probe to identify parathyroid tissue, an alternative form of intraoperative localization. Intraoperative sestamibi gamma probing is able to detect both parathyroid adenomas and hyperplastic parathyroid tissue even in the setting of a negative preoperative sestamibi scan with an accuracy of 90.5% [8, 26]. This allows surgeons to use the most minimally invasive technique as possible while ensuring that the diseased parathyroid tissue is removed to completion. Conventionally, preoperative imaging in conjunction with IPM is the surgical standard for ensuring a successful parathyroidectomy. However, controversies exist when hyperparathyroidism is present alongside concomitant thyroid disease as sestamibi can concentrate in thyroid adenomas or multinodular goiters making preoperative localization of parathyroid adenomas difficult [11, 12]. As discussed above, one highly accurate preoperative localization technique gaining popularity is the ultrasound-guided FNA with PTH wash which has potential to reduce surgical time, decrease complication rates, decrease need for reoperation, and allow more patients to benefit from minimally invasive techniques especially at centers without the capability to perform IPM. With its 91–100% specificity and sensitivity, it allows surgeons to confidently preoperatively characterize the nature of a mass, distinguish parathyroid tissue from lymphoid tissue or thyroid nodules, and plan for directed surgical intervention [11, 12]. A PTH wash is extremely helpful in those patients with both parathyroid and thyroid disease and can help the surgeon ensure all of the diseased gland(s) are being removed [11].

Complications

While complications continue to exist and will always exist for any operative procedure, the complications associated with parathyroidectomy have continued to decrease [15]. Many of the complications of parathyroidectomy are universal to all surgical procedures and include infection, hematoma, and seroma. While wound infections are rare after parathyroidectomy, they can occur especially in the setting of hematoma which occur in approximately 0.5% of cases [27]. If there is any sign of airway compression in the setting of postoperative cervical hematoma formation, the patient should be taken back to the operating room for controlled emergency decompression [1].

Other known morbidities associated with parathyroid surgery include recurrent laryngeal nerve (RLN) injury and transient hypocalcemia [1, 17]. The risk of a RLN injury, which can manifest on a spectrum ranging from voice hoarseness to difficulty breathing due to the paralysis of the ipsilateral posterior cricoarytenoid muscle, is reported to be less than 1% [16]. When a RLN transection or injury is identified intraoperatively, a reinnervation procedure should be attempted [1].

Moderate hypocalcemia is one of the greatest risk factors approaching 15–30% of patients and is generally transient in nature and not a reason for inpatient post-operative care [16]. This may manifest as perioral numbness/tingling, upper extremity paresthesia, prolonged QT interval on EKG, altered mental status, and seizures [1, 23]. Most patients who experience hypocalcemia do so on postoperative day one or two with the majority showing signs and symptoms by postoperative day four [28, 29]. Hypocalcemia is usually easily treated in the outpatient setting with adequate calcium and vitamin D supplementation. Studies show that minimally invasive techniques have a lower incidence of hypocalcemia than BCE [1, 3, 16].

The risk of permanent hypoparathyroidism, defined as permanent when persisting for at least 12 months after parathyroidectomy, continues to be a rare complication affecting up to 3.6% of patients [17]. Operative failure, defined as failure to achieve normocalcemia within 6 months of surgery, is a possibility when the inciting gland is not located or multi-gland disease is present but noted at the time of initial surgery [1].

To accurately record and document complications associated with surgery, patients should be followed for at least 6 months postoperatively and undergo regular blood testing including calcium, PTH, and 25-hydroxyvitamin D levels. Better assessment of prolonged hypoparathyroidism and permanent recurrent laryngeal nerve effects may be made at a 6 month follow up visit [1].

A rarely described but fairly common complication (~30%) of parathyroidectomy performed for primary hyperparathyroidism is transient thyrotoxicosis even without any evidence of underlying thyroid disease [30, 31]. It will generally occur within days to weeks and is clinically mild or even silent but can cause serious arrythmias in some patients [30]. Symptoms most commonly include restlessness, agitation, atrial flutter, or other supraventricular arrythmias, and the mechanism is thought to be related to transient thyroid hormone release due to intraoperative manipulation of the gland [30, 31]. While very few studies and case reports exist on this complication, it appears that few patients require medications. Most patients have full, spontaneous resolution within 2 weeks but occasional reports of symptoms persisting up to 3 months have been seen [30]. The true frequency of this complication however is unknown given that most patients who develop thyrotoxicosis have full resolution within 4–6 weeks and therefore the window of diagnosing in the postoperative period is limited [31].

Postoperative Care

The most common issue regarding postoperative care after parathyroidectomy is symptomatic hypocalcemia which tends to be transient and mild [1, 3]. Many surgeons institute a postoperative calcium supplementation plan for all patients to help eliminate any risk of hypocalcemia [3]. While severe hypocalcemia is rare, many patients may still require calcium and even calcitriol (1,25-dihydroxycholecalciferol) for several weeks to months postoperatively [1].

Managing temporary hypoparathyroidism requires calcium, vitamin D, and occasional magnesium which is slowly tapered as the body recovers [32]. Permanent hypoparathyroidism is much more serious and requires more frequent monitoring to decrease the risk of complications and morbidities. Clinical hypoparathyroidism, defined as a PTH lower than the lower limit of normal (12 pg/mL) accompanied by hypocalcemia and hyperphosphatemia, includes the symptoms discussed above in addition to lower extremity myoclonus, carpopedal spasm, weakness, headache, nausea, and increased bone density.

References

1. Wilhelm S, Wang TS, Ruan DT, Lee JA, Lasa SL, Duh QY, et al. The American Association of Endocrine Surgeons guidelines for definitive management of primary hyperparathyroidism. JAMA Surg. 2016;151(10):959–68. https://doi.org/10.1001/jamasurg.2016.2310.
2. Eastall R, Brandi ML, Costa AG, D'Amour P, Shoback DM, Thakker RV. Diagnosis of asymptomatic primary hyperparathyroidism: proceedings from the fourth international workshop. J Clin Endocrinol Metab. 2014;99(10):3570–9. https://doi.org/10.1210/jc.2014-1414.
3. Bergenfelz A, Lindblom P, Tibblin S, Westerdahl J. Unilateral versus bilateral neck exploration for primary hyperparathyroidism: a prospective randomized controlled trial. Ann Surg. 2002;236(5):543–51. https://doi.org/10.1097/00000658-200211000-00001.
4. Bilezikian JP. Primary hyperparathyroidism. J Clin Endocrinol Metab. 2018;103(11):3993–4004.
5. Yeh R, Tay YD, Tabacco G, Dercle L, Kuo JH, Bandeira L, et al. Diagnostic performance of 4D CT and sestamibi SPECT/CT in localizing parathyroid adenomas in primary hyperparathyroidism. Radiology. 2019;291(2):469–76. https://doi.org/10.1148/radiol.2019182122.
6. Sung JY. Parathyroid ultrasonography: the evolving role of the radiologist. Ultrasonography. 2015;34(4):268–74. https://doi.org/10.14366/usg.14071.
7. Ishibashi M, Nishida H, Hiromatsu Y, Kojima K, Tabuchi E, Hayabuchi N. Comparison of technetium-99m-MIBI, technetium-99m-tetrofosmin, ultrasound, and MRI for localization of abnormal parathyroid glands. J Nucl Med. 1998;39(2):320–4.
8. Buicko JL, Kichler KM, Amundson JR, Scurci S, Kozol R. The sestamibi paradox: improving intraoperative localization of parathyroid adenomas. Am Surg. 2017;83(8):832–5.
9. Taubman ML, Goldfarb M, Lew JI. Role of SPECT and SPECT/CT in the surgical treatment of primary hyperparathyroidism. Int J Mol Imaging. 2011; https://doi.org/10.1155/2011/141593.
10. Kuzminski SJ, Sosa JA, Hoang JK. Update in parathyroid imaging. Magn Reson Imaging Clin N Am. 2018;26(1):151–66. https://doi.org/10.1016/j.mric.2017.08.009.
11. Kuzu F, Arpaci D, Cakmak GK, Emre AU, Elri T, Ilikhan SU, et al. Focused parathyroidectomy without intra-operative parathormone monitoring: the value of PTH assay in preoperative ultrasound guided fine needle aspiration washout. Ann Med Surg. 2016;6:64–7. https://doi.org/10.1016/j.amsu.2015.12.065.
12. Ozderya A, Temizkan S, Cetin K, Ozugur S, Gul AE, Aydin K. The results of parathyroid hormone assay in parathyroid aspirates in pre-operative localization of parathyroid adenomas for focused parathyroidectomy in patients with negative or suspicious technetium-99m-sestamibi scans. Endocr Pract. 2017;23(9):1101–6. https://doi.org/10.4158/EP171921.OR.
13. Khan A. Medical management of primary hyperparathyroidism. J Clin Densitom. 2013;16(1):60–3. https://doi.org/10.1016/j.jocd.2012.11.010.
14. Grey A, Lucas J, Horne A, Gamble G, Davidson JS, Reid IR. Vitamin D repletion in patients with primary hyperparathyroidism and coexistent vitamin D insufficiency. J Clin Endocrinol Metab. 2005;90(4):2122–6. https://doi.org/10.1210/jc.2004-1772.
15. Abdulla AG, Ituarte PHG, Harari A, Wu JX, Yeh MW. Trends in the frequency and quality of parathyroid surgery: analysis of 17,082 cases over 10 years. Ann Surg. 2015;261(4):746–50. https://doi.org/10.1097/SLA.0000000000000812.
16. Marcocci C, Bollerslev J, Khan AA, Shoback DM. Medical management of primary hyperparathyroidism: proceedings of the fourth international workshop on the management of

asymptomatic primary hyperparathyroidism. J Clin Endocrinol Metab. 2014;99(10):3607–18. https://doi.org/10.1210/jc.2014-1417.

17. Allendorf J, DiGorgi M, Spanknebel K, Inabnet W, Chabot J, Logerfo P. 1112 consecutive bilateral neck explorations for primary hyperparathyroidism. World J Surg. 2007;31(11):2075–80. https://doi.org/10.1007/s00268-007-9068-5.

18. Okoh AK, Sound S, Berber E. Robotic parathyroidectomy. J Surg Oncol. 2015;112(3):240–2. https://doi.org/10.1002/jso.23911.

19. Garas G, Holsinger FC, Grant DG, Athanasiou T, Arora A, Tolley N. Is robotic parathyroidectomy a feasible and safe alternative to targeted open parathyroidectomy for the treatment of primary hyperparathyroidism? Int J Surg. 2015;15:55–60. https://doi.org/10.1016/j.ijsu.2015.01.109.

20. Chen H. Surgery for primary hyperparathyroidism: what is the best approach? Ann Surg. 2002;236(5):552–3. https://doi.org/10.1097/00000658-200211000-00002.

21. Sadik KW, Kell M, Gorey T. Minimally invasive parathyroidectomy using surgical sonography. Int J Med Sci. 2011;8(4):283–6. https://doi.org/10.7150/ijms.8.283.

22. Tolley N, Garas G, Palazzo F, Prichard A, Chaidas K, Cox J, et al. Long-term prospective evaluation comparing robotic parathyroidectomy with minimally invasive open parathyroidectomy for primary hyperparathyroidism. Head Neck. 2016;38(1):300–6. https://doi.org/10.1002/hed.23990.

23. Moffett JM, Suliburk JW. Parathyroid autotransplantation. Endocr Pract. 2011;17:83–9. https://doi.org/10.4158/EP10377.RA.

24. Guerrero MA, Evans DB, Lee JE, Bao R, Bereket A, Gantela S, et al. Viability of cryopreserved parathyroid tissue: when is continued storage versus disposal indicated? World J Surg. 2008;32:836–9. https://doi.org/10.1007/s00268-007-9437-0.

25. Borot S, Lapierre V, Carnaille B, Goudet P, Penfornis A. Results of cryopreserved parathyroid autografts: a retrospective multicenter study. Surgery. 2010;147:529–35. https://doi.org/10.1016/j.surg.2009.10.010.

26. Chen H, Sippel RS, Schaefer S. The effectiveness of radioguided parathyroidectomy in patients with negative technetium tc-99-m sestamibi scans. JAMA Surg. 2009;144(7):643–8. https://doi.org/10.1001/archsurg.2009.104.

27. Farndon JR. Post-operative complications of parathyroidectomy. In: Holzheimer RG, Mannick JA, editors. Surgical treatment: evidence-based and problem-oriented. Munich: Academic; 2001.

28. Tredici P, Grosso E, Gibelli B, Massaro MA, Arrigoni C, Tradati N. Identification of patients at high risk for hypocalcemia after total thyroidectomy. Acta Otorhinolaryngol Ital. 2011;31(3):144–8.

29. Westerdahl J, Lindblom P, Valdemarsson S, Tibblin S, Bergenfelz A. Risk factors for postoperative hypocalcemia after surgery for primary hyperparathyroidism. JAMA Surg. 2000;135(2):142–7. https://doi.org/10.1001/archsurg.135.2.142.

30. Asmar A, Ross E. Post-parathyroidectomy thyrotoxicosis and atrial flutter: a case for caution. NDT Plus. 2011;4(2):117–9. https://doi.org/10.1093/ndtplus/sfq200.

31. Rudofsky G, Grafe IA, Metzner C, Leowardi C, Fohr B. Transient post-operative thyrotoxicosis after parathyroidectomy. Med Sci Monit. 2009;15(3):CS41–3.

32. Stack BC, Bimston DN, Bodenner DL, Brett EM, Dralle H, Orloff LA, et al. American Association of Clinical Endocrinologists and American College of Endocrinology disease state clinical review: postoperative hypoparathyroidism – definitions and management. Endocr Pract. 2015;21(6):674–85. https://doi.org/10.4158/EP14462.DSC.

Chapter 14
Surgical Management of Hypercortisolism from ACTH-Secreting Pituitary Adenomas

Justin C. Morse, Brian D. Thorp, and Adam J. Kimple

Introduction

Cushing syndrome (CS) is the constellation of findings that are noted from prolonged exposure to glucocorticoids. Typical findings include obesity, hypertension, diabetes mellitus, and osteoporosis. CS may result from multiple causes including immunosuppression with corticosteroids and adrenal tumors or form Cushing's disease. Cushing's disease (CD) results from a benign monomorphic pituitary corticotroph adenoma that secretes excessive adrenocorticotropic hormone (ACTH). Increased ACTH stimulates secretion of cortisol by the adrenal glands, resulting in supraphysiological levels of endogenous steroid resulting in the combination of symptomatology and findings characteristic of CS.

CD is rare with an incidence estimated at one to two per million which limits large studies of these patients [1]. These tumors remain challenging to treat for both the surgeon and endocrinologist. Transsphenoidal adenomectomy (TSS) remains the treatment of choice for the vast majority of patients with the concurrent goals of biochemical remission and maintenance of pituitary function; however, remission rates after TSS range from 65% to 80% [2, 3]. Unsuccessful treatment results in reduced quality of life and increased mortality [4]. This chapter seeks to (1) discuss the preoperative planning for surgical resection of ACTH-secreting pituitary adenomas, (2) describe the endoscopic surgical technique for transsphenoidal resection of sellar tumors, and (3) discuss the postoperative care of patients after resection of an ACTH-secreting pituitary adenoma. For readers interested in a nuanced discussion

J. C. Morse · B. D. Thorp · A. J. Kimple (✉)
Department of Otolaryngology-Head and Neck Surgery, University of North Carolina
Medical Center, Chapel Hill, NC, USA
e-mail: adam_kimple@med.unc.edu

© The Author(s), under exclusive license to Springer Nature Switzerland AG 2022

199

H. Yu et al. (eds.), *Diagnosis and Management of Endocrine Disorders in Interventional Radiology*, https://doi.org/10.1007/978-3-030-87189-5_14

of the pros and cons of different surgical and reconstructive techniques, we recommend the text by Drs. Snyderman and Gardner entitled *Master Techniques in Otolaryngology – Head and Neck Surgery: Skull Base Surgery* [5].

Diagnosis and Preoperative Planning

Patients with suspected CD presenting to a surgeon have usually already undergone an extensive diagnostic workup including demonstration of elevated ACTH and cortisol in combination with imaging evidence of a pituitary adenoma. However, several diagnostic dilemmas exist that deserve special attention. ACTH-secreting pituitary tumors are often discovered when they are quite small because of their potent biological/clinical effects. In fact, large case series indicate that over 90% of ACTH adenomas are microadenomas with a mean diameter of 6 mm at the time of diagnosis [6, 7]. As such it is not uncommon to have negative imaging or discordant biochemical and radiological studies leading to diagnostic uncertainty. Furthermore, the small size and the lack of contrast between the adenoma and the surrounding pituitary gland result in a negative magnetic resonance imaging (MRI) scan nearly 50% of the time at diagnosis. New imaging techniques have sought to improve visualization of these small lesions, and some have advocated for spoiled gradient recalled (SPGR) acquisition MRI sequences. This imaging sequence has been suggested to increase identification of adenomas to 65–80% at the time of diagnosis [8, 9].

Unfortunately, even with advanced imaging techniques, negative imaging remains relatively common. Moreover, peripheral ACTH levels can be nondiagnostic or discordant. To address these issues, inferior petrosal sinus venous sampling (IPSS) has been advocated to help confirm a diagnosis and has been reported to help localize laterality of the tumor at some centers [10, 11]. IPSS is based on anatomic venous drainage of the pituitary gland which occurs laterally into the cavernous sinuses and subsequently into the inferior petrosal sinuses. The short half-life of ACTH leads to an ACTH concentration difference between the inferior petrosal veins and the peripheral blood. As such, more concentrated blood can be sampled from the direct venous drainage of the pituitary compared with sampling from the systemic venous system. Furthermore, corticotropin-releasing hormone (CRH) stimulation during inferior petrosal sinus sampling allows for improved diagnostic confirmation of an ACTH adenoma [12]. Because cavernous sinus blood generally enters the petrosal venous system unilaterally, bilateral sampling is recommended [10]. Furthermore, because of the frequent ipsilateral lateralization of the pituitary gland drainage, lateralization of ACTH concentration in the inferior petrosal sinuses identified by bilateral assessment can also assist in the lateralization of adenoma within the pituitary gland in some cases [10, 13]. It is important to note that in order to avoid false-positive results, IPSS must be performed while the patient is hypercortisolemic. If IPSS is performed in the absence of sustained hypercortisolism, the normal corticotrophs are not suppressed and will respond to CRH leading to an inferior petrosal sinus-to-peripheral ACTH gradient suggestive of CD, when in fact it should be normal [14]. While IPSS remains a successful tool in the diagnosis of CD, its success remains quite operator dependent and varies substantially from center to center [11, 15]. Ultimately IPPS has a diagnostic accuracy around 95% in institutions with broad experience [11, 14, 16].

Indications for IPSS vary between centers; however, most institutions with expertise in CS use this technique only in patients with ACTH-dependent CD that has conflicting results of noninvasive endocrine evaluation, discordant biochemical and radiological studies, or negative pituitary MR imaging [6].

Once the diagnosis is confirmed, further preoperative planning for any suspected pituitary tumor including those with ACTH secretion is approached in a similar fashion. A multidisciplinary approach remains paramount to achieving a successful surgical outcome. While imaging has been obtained for the identification of tumor location, separate imaging should be performed for preoperative planning to be utilized with intraoperative image guidance systems. Specifically, thin-slice MRI with and without contrast as well as thin-slice (~0.6 mm) computed tomography of the sinuses provides adequate visualization of the surrounding anatomic structures and tumor location while further allowing utilization of image guidance surgical systems. Preoperative pituitary hormone labs including cortisol, TSH, IGF-1, and prolactin are drawn for baseline values if not already obtained.

Indications and Contraindications

Apart from prolactinomas and a subset of growth hormone-secreting tumors, surgery remains the first-line therapy for pituitary tumors, including ACTH-secreting adenomas [17]. Few surgical contraindications exist and can be generalized as comorbidities preventing safe administration of anesthesia or increased risk of surgical bleeding. These include but are not limited to bleeding diatheses or anticoagulation that cannot be safely stopped, uncontrolled hypertension, or significant comorbidities that increase anesthetic risk to the point that risks of surgery outweigh any potential benefit. Reducing intraoperative and postoperative bleeding risk is particularly important in these cases as hematoma development can result in significant morbidity including rapid vision loss, seizures, or other neurologic decline.

Surgical Technique

The origins of pituitary surgery have been reported as early as the seventeenth century [18]. Modern resection of sellar masses is usually accomplished via the transnasal approach as opposed to transcranial or transfacial approaches. Historically these transnasal approaches were performed with a microscope, but contemporary management generally consists of endoscopic transnasal resection [6]. Equivalency of the transnasal endoscopic approach compared to the transnasal microscopic approach is well documented [19]. Furthermore, current evidence appears to favor the endoscopic approach for multiple reasons including improved visualization and improved access and some reports detailing improved resection outcomes/lower recurrences [20]. ACTH-secreting pituitary adenomas are effectively managed with endoscopic techniques, and the authors herein describe this surgical approach.

Approach

An understanding of endoscopic transsphenoidal surgical resection of sellar tumors including ACTH-secreting tumors relies on an intricate understanding of both nasal and sellar anatomy. We describe a brief overview of the endoscopic/intranasal anatomic landmarks utilized for this approach and the surgical technique. Resection of these tumors remains a team-based approach with both the otolaryngologist, specifically those subspecializing in rhinology and endoscopic skull base surgery, and a neurosurgeon. We will focus specifically on two key components of this surgery: (1) the intranasal approach and (2) the sella and its corresponding anatomy to a transsphenoidal approach for resection of an ACTH adenoma.

The intranasal cavity is the space between the vestibule of the nose and the choanae. The nasal passages are separated in the midline by the nasal septum. This passageway provides access to several adjacent corridors including the surrounding sinuses, anterior, middle, and posterior cranial fossa, craniocervical junction, and the sella.

Herein we describe an overview of the endoscopic approach to the sella. A 0-degree endoscope is utilized to perform nasal endoscopy. The middle turbinates are lateralized or removed thereby allowing visualization and access to the sphenoethmoidal recess and superior turbinate. The inferior 1/3 of the superior turbinate is removed with cutting instrumentation allowing visualization of the natural os of the sphenoid sinus which is medial to the superior turbinate approximately 1.5–2 cm from the superior aspect of the choanae. If a nasoseptal flap reconstruction is planned, the flap is raised at this point in the surgery and placed into the nasopharynx (see sellar reconstruction techniques below). The os is entered and widened to the planum of the sphenoid bone superiorly and laterally to the orbital apex (Fig. 14.1). Opening of posterior ethmoid cells increases visualization. If a nasal septal flap or rescue flap is going to be used for reconstruction, the inferior mucoperiosteum of the sphenoid face must be preserved to avoid injury of the posterior septal branch of the sphenopalatine artery which courses 1 cm superior above the top of the choanae and is the vascular pedicle for the nasoseptal flap that remains the main workhorse for reconstruction.

With the skull base identified on one side, a superior septectomy of the posterior nasal septum is performed to allow access to the contralateral sphenoid os. Bilateral sphenoid access is obtained, and the contralateral face of the sphenoid is opened resulting in a common sphenoid cavity. At this point the sphenoid intersinus septum

Fig. 14.1 Endoscopic transsphenoidal visualization of the sella and labeled osteologic landmarks prior to the opening of sella dura for resection of ACTH-secreting adenoma

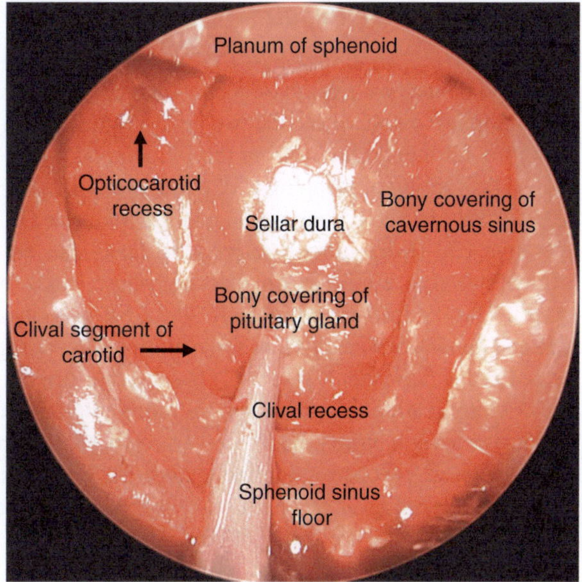

is removed allowing wide visualization of the sellar osteology. Visualization of the clival recess, sella, clival carotids, and lateral opticocarotid recesses is important prior to performing any osteotomy (Fig. 14.1). With the surrounding anatomy visualized, an osteotomy of the anterior face of the sella is performed to expose the dura of the anterior pituitary gland. This exposure allows for transnasal instrumentation and easy visualization of the surrounding anatomy to facilitate a safe tumor resection.

Tumor Resection

Tumor resection requires a complete understanding of the sellar and parasellar regions. This is a complex anatomic region that contains critical neurovascular structures. A midline durotomy allows visualization of the tumor and pituitary gland. Care should be taken to avoid entering the cavernous sinus. At times, a pseudocapsule surrounding the tumor can allow an extracapsular dissection, particularly in ACTH-secreting tumors. A combination of curettes, suction, and grasping instruments is used to remove the adenoma. Direct transsellar endoscopic visualization facilitates gross total resection. In the setting of lateral dural invasion, the dura of the cavernous sinus wall can be resected for removal of the entirety of an invasive tumor. Further dissection may need to occur into the retro cavernous carotid space as this is a common area for tumor to be missed. Once tumor resection is complete, attention is turned toward the reconstruction of the skull base/sellar defect.

Skull Base/Sellar Repair

While the nuances of skull base reconstruction are outside the scope of this chapter, it is important to understand the two primary goals of sellar reconstruction: (1) separating the intranasal cavity from the intracranial cavity for prevention of infection and (2) preventing or stopping CSF extravasation. Sellar reconstruction can broadly be thought of in two scenarios: (1) no intraoperative CSF leak and (2) with an intraoperative CSF leak. Intraoperative CSF leaks can be classified as low-flow (not originating from a CSF basin) and high-flow leaks (originating from a cisternal space). The reconstruction of high-flow CSF leaks has higher complication rates [21] and generally warrants a multilayer repair including an inlay graft and a vascularized onlay nasoseptal flap. ACTH-secreting tumors have been shown to have higher complication rates than non-secreting pituitary adenomas [6], and we generally advocate for a more robust reconstruction, such as the nasoseptal flap. If no leak is encountered, reconstruction techniques are highly variable and surgeon dependent. Several common reconstruction practices include abdominal fat graft [22], synthetic dural inlay, an overlay mucosal graft, pedicled flap, or dissolvable packing material alone [23].

Surgical Challenges

For ACTH-secreting pituitary adenomas, surgery can be complicated by negative preoperative imaging, small adenoma size, complicating intraoperative localization, or dural invasion. Preoperative identification of the tumor results in increased chances of intraoperative identification and postoperative biochemical remission [24]. If not identified preoperatively on MRI, systematic exploration of the pituitary gland is often efficacious in identifying the tumor [25]. Interestingly, adenomas of ~3 mm or greater often develop a surrounding microscopic pseudocapsule that can be used for tumor identification and facilitate selective enucleation [25, 26]. When applicable, selective adenomectomy using the histological pseudocapsule to define the boundaries achieves immediate and lasting remission in the majority of both adult and pediatric CD patients [7].

When adenomas cannot be identified, a partial hypophysectomy or total hypophysectomy may be performed. Partial hypophysectomy involves either removal of 70–80% of the anterior pituitary lobe, leaving 20–30% attached to the pituitary stalk, or removal of half of the anterior lobe corresponding to IPSS lateralization. Partial and total hypophysectomies have similar biochemical remission rates with the clear advantage of partial hypophysectomy as it allows most patients to retain normal pituitary function and not require lifelong pituitary supplementation [27].

Dural invasion can result in non-curative outcomes. If dural invasion is limited to partial thickness invasion of the cavernous sinus wall, invaded portions of dura can be removed safely, resulting in biochemical remission [28]. Unfortunately, if the adenoma extends through the dural wall leading to subsequent cavernous sinus invasion, surgery is unlikely to be curative, even with gross total removal of the tumor from the cavernous sinus [7].

Postoperative Care

Postoperative care varies between institutions; however, in patients with CD, we advocate for at least 24 h in the neurointensive care unit postoperatively. This allows improved management of blood pressure and glucose. Urine output and osmolarity are assessed for diabetes insipidus. In our practice, a lumbar drain is not routinely utilized. Postoperative cortisol is measured on postoperative day 2 to confirm successful resection. Nasal saline sprays are initiated on postoperative day 1, and nasal saline irrigations are typically initiated after the first postoperative appointment. During the surgical admission, a postsurgical MRI is obtained to serve as a new baseline. Clinical follow-up is scheduled with otolaryngology at 1, 4, and 12 weeks postoperatively for nasal debridement. Neurosurgical follow-up is recommended at approximately 1 month postoperatively and endocrinology follow-up at 1–2 weeks. Continuous positive airway pressure is avoided for 4 weeks following surgery.

Postsurgical endocrinological management deserves special attention. A successful surgery results in postoperative hypocortisolism secondary to suppression of the normal pituitary corticotrophs by long-standing hypercortisolism. Recovery of the suppressed normal pituitary gland corticotrophs occurs over 6–12 months. During recovery, it is crucial that patients receive physiological glucocorticoid replacement. Restoration of function of the hypothalamic-pituitary-adrenal axis is confirmed with a normal morning cortisol level and/or a normal cortisol response to ACTH stimulation. At this point, steroid supplementation is discontinued.

While the goal of adenoma resection is to preserve normal pituitary tissue and function, hypopituitarism occurs approximately 5% of the time [7, 27, 29]. Management of postoperative hypopituitarism includes pituitary functional assessment with T4 and prolactin measurements 2 weeks after surgery. The pituitary is considered functional if preoperative T4 and postoperative T4 are similar, and prolactin is greater than 4 ng/ml. Treatment for CS-associated hypogonadism, relative hypothyroidism, and low growth hormone is individualized to the patient and is expected to resolve gradually over 6–12 months.

Surgical Complications, Unsuccessful Surgical Resection, and Non-remission

Morbidity from transsphenoidal surgery has been estimated at 2–10% and mortality at <2% which align with the rates seen in all pituitary surgery [29]. Complications from surgery can broadly be divided into (1) rhinologic, (2) neurologic, and (3) endocrinologic.

Rhinologic complications include intranasal bleeding and infection. Postoperative bleeding is rare and with a reported incidence of 0.6–3.3% [30]. In most cases, postoperative bleeding can be stopped with the use of an intranasal hemostatic agents and/or a vasoconstrictive nasal spray such as oxymetazoline. Bleeding refractory to medical management or high-volume hemorrhage requires endoscopic control in the operating room. The most severe form of postoperative infection is meningitis, and it is estimated to occur <1% of the time [19, 31, 32]. Culture-directed antibiotics are the primary treatment.

Neurologic complications include intraoperative damage to surrounding structures and postoperative CSF leak. Management of postoperative leak can be managed using either with a revision skull base reconstruction or more conservative methods depending on surgeon preference. Initial treatment with CSF diversion using a lumbar drain can be successful [21]. If CSF extravasation persists despite a lumbar drain, head of bed elevation and bed rest and additional surgical repair are required. Additionally, neurologic complications primarily include carotid injury, vision loss, or stroke [31].

Finally, endocrinologic complications result from manipulation and/or resection of the normal pituitary gland. As discussed above, postoperative pan-hypopituitarism occurs in <5% of patients. Berker et al. report endocrinologic complication rates of 570 pituitary adenomas with a rate of transient diabetes insipidus (DI) of 4.6%, permanent DI in 0.4%, and inappropriate antidiuretic hormone secretion syndrome occurred in 1.1% [6, 31].

Unsuccessful surgical resection is suspected in the absence of hypocortisolism postoperatively. Most patients in remission from CD develop a glucocorticoid withdrawal syndrome within 48 h of resection. Lonser et al. describe several reasons that influence incomplete tumor removal: (1) the removal of an incidental adenomas rather than the actual corticotroph tumor [33], (2) the removal of a site that appears abnormal at surgery but proves to be a normal gland on histological inspection, and (3) the incomplete removal of an ACTH-secreting adenoma due to inadequate resection or invasion into surrounding structures [6, 7].

When the actual tumor is not resected, revision surgery can be attempted to remove the adenoma or remove additional anterior pituitary gland if no tumor is identifiable. If pathology from the initial surgery demonstrates an ACTH-staining adenoma, repeat surgery offers an excellent chance of complete resection [6, 34]. It is important to note that if the gland is completely explored at the initial surgery or there is invasion into the cavernous sinus, achieving remission with a revision surgery is unlikely [6]. As such, medical therapy remains second-line treatment in the scenario of unsuccessful surgery or when surgery cannot be performed. Medical therapies include steroidogenesis inhibitors, corticotroph-directed agents, and glucocorticoid receptor blockers [6]. Discussion of the use of each of these therapies is outside of the scope of this chapter.

Another adjuvant treatment in the setting of unsuccessful surgical remission is radiation therapy and can include either stereotactic radiosurgery or standard fractionated irradiation [27, 35, 36]. Studies have demonstrated that both modalities are equally efficacious in treating CD [27, 36, 37]. The major risk with radiation therapy is long-term pituitary hypofunction with reported rates of up to 40% 10 years posttreatment [36].

Conclusion

ACTH-secreting pituitary tumors resulting in CD are generally small. Diagnosis relies on imaging and lab workup. While diagnostic challenges exist, IPSS has significantly improved the ability of confirmatory diagnosis and can assist with localization of tumors not seen on imaging. Surgical management via an endonasal transsphenoidal approach of ACTH-secreting pituitary adenomas resulting in CD remains first-line therapy with excellent success at experienced centers. Surgical complications are rare. The goals of surgery remain gross total resection resulting in biochemical remission of hypercortisolism with simultaneous maintenance of pituitary function. Non-remission remains a challenge, and options to treat this include revision surgery, medical therapies, and radiation therapy.

References

1. Lindholm J, Juul S, Jørgensen JOL, Astrup J, Bjerre P, Feldt-Rasmussen U, et al. Incidence and late prognosis of Cushing's syndrome: a population-based study. J Clin Endocrinol Metab. 2001;86(1):117–23. Available from: https://pubmed-ncbi-nlm-nih-gov.proxy.library.vanderbilt.edu/11231987/
2. Alwani RA, De Herder WW, Van Aken MO, Van Den Berge JH, Delwel EJ, Dallenga AHG, et al. Biochemical predictors of outcome of pituitary surgery for cushing's disease. Neuroendocrinology. 2010;91(2):169–78. Available from: https://pubmed-ncbi-nlm-nih-gov.proxy.library.vanderbilt.edu/19907141/.
3. Alexandraki KI, Kaltsas GA, Isidori AM, Storr HL, Afshar F, Sabin I, et al. Long-term remission and recurrence rates in Cushing's disease: predictive factors in a single-centre study. Eur J Endocrinol. 2013;168(4):639–48.
4. Clayton RN, Raskauskiene D, Reulen RC, Jones PW. Mortality and morbidity in Cushing's disease over 50 years in stoke-on-Trent, UK: audit and meta-analysis of literature. J Clin Endocrinol Metab. 2011;96(3):632–42. Available from: https://pubmed-ncbi-nlm-nih-gov.proxy.library.vanderbilt.edu/21193542/.
5. Snyderman C, Gardner P. Master techniques in otolaryngology—head and neck surgery: skull base surgery. Google Books [Internet]. [cited 2020 Nov 9]. Available from: https://books.google.com/books?hl=en&lr=&id=ZzSmBAAAQBAJ&oi=fnd&pg=PT29&dq=master+techniques+in+skull+base+surgery&ots=mB_RRxqikN&sig=VX8t_xN2XSOjaDAInagejGtv0k#v=onepage&q=master%20techniques%20in%20skull%20base%20surgery&f=false.
6. Lonser RR, Nieman L, Oldfield EH. Cushing's disease: pathobiology, diagnosis, and management. J Neurosurg. 2017;126(2):404–17. Available from: http://thejns.org/doi/abs/10.3171/2016.1.JNS152119

7. Lonser RR, Wind JJ, Nieman LK, Weil RJ, DeVroom HL, Oldfield EH. Outcome of surgical treatment of 200 children with cushing's disease. J Clin Endocrinol Metab. 2013;98(3):892–901. Available from: https://pubmed-ncbi-nlm-nih-gov.proxy.library.vanderbilt.edu/23372173/.

8. Patronas N, Bulakbasi N, Stratakis CA, Lafferty A, Oldfield EH, Doppman J, et al. Spoiled gradient recalled acquisition in the steady state technique is superior to conventional postcontrast spin echo technique for magnetic resonance imaging detection of adrenocorticotropin-secreting pituitary tumors. J Clin Endocrinol Metab. 2003;88(4):1565–9. Available from: https://pubmed-ncbi-nlm-nih-gov.proxy.library.vanderbilt.edu/12679440/.

9. Batista D, Courkoutsakis NA, Oldfield EH, Griffin KJ, Keil M, Patronas NJ, et al. Detection of adrenocorticotropin-secreting pituitary adenomas by magnetic resonance imaging in children and adolescents with Cushing disease. J Clin Endocrinol Metab. 2005;90(9):5134–40. Available from: https://pubmed-ncbi-nlm-nih-gov.proxy.library.vanderbilt.edu/15941871/.

10. Oldfield EH, Doppman JL, Miller D, Nieman LK, Chrousos GP, Cutler GB, et al. Petrosal sinus sampling with and without corticotropin-releasing hormone for the differential diagnosis of cushing's syndrome. N Engl J Med. 1991;325(13):897–905. Available from: https://pubmed-ncbi-nlm-nih-gov.proxy.library.vanderbilt.edu/1652686/.

11. Findling JW, Kehoe ME, Raff H. Identification of patients with cushing's disease with negative pituitary adrenocorticotropin gradients during inferior petrosal sinus sampling: Prolactin as an index of pituitary venous effluent. J Clin Endocrinol Metab. 2004;89(12):6005–9. Available from: https://pubmed-ncbi-nlm-nih-gov.proxy.library.vanderbilt.edu/15579751/.

12. Nieman LK, Cutler GB, Oldfield EH, Loriaux DL, Chrousos GP. The Ovine Corticotropin-Releasing Hormone (CRH) stimulation test is superior to the human CRH stimulation test for the diagnosis of Cushing's disease. J Clin Endocrinol Metab. 1989;69(1):165–9. Available from: https://academic.oup.com/jcem/article-lookup/doi/10.1210/jcem-69-1-165.

13. Findling JW, Kehoe ME, Shaker JL, Raff H. Routine inferior petrosal sinus sampling in the differential diagnosis of adrenocorticotropin (ACTH)-dependent Cushing's syndrome: early recognition of the occult ectopic ACTH syndrome. J Clin Endocrinol Metab. 1991;73(2):408–13. Available from: https://pubmed-ncbi-nlm-nih-gov.proxy.library.vanderbilt.edu/1649842/.

14. Patil CG, Prevedello DM, Lad SP, Vance ML, Thorner MO, Katznelson L, et al. Late recurrences of Cushing's disease after initial successful transsphenoidal surgery. J Clin Endocrinol Metab. 2008;93(2):358–62. Available from: https://pubmed-ncbi-nlm-nih-gov.proxy.library.vanderbilt.edu/18056770/.

15. Gandhi CD, Meyer SA, Patel AB, Johnson DM, Post KD. Neurologic complications of inferior petrosal sinus sampling. Am J Neuroradiol. 2008;29(4):760–5. Available from: https://pubmed-ncbi-nlm-nih-gov.proxy.library.vanderbilt.edu/18238844/.

16. Sharma ST, Raff H, Nieman LK. Prolactin as a marker of successful catheterization during IPSS in patients with ACTH-dependent Cushing's syndrome. J Clin Endocrinol Metab. 2011;96(12):3687–94. Available from: https://pubmed-ncbi-nlm-nih-gov.proxy.library.vanderbilt.edu/22031511/.

17. Biller BMK, Grossman AB, Stewart PM, Melmed S, Bertagna X, Bertherat J, et al. Treatment of adrenocorticotropin-dependent cushing's syndrome: a consensus statement. J Clin Endocrinol Metab. 2008;93(7):2454–62. Available from: https://pubmed-ncbi-nlm-nih-gov.proxy.library.vanderbilt.edu/18413427/.

18. Artico M, Pastore FS, Fraioli B, Giuffrè R. The contribution of Davide Giordano (1864–1954) to pituitary surgery: the transglabellar-nasal approach. Neurosurgery. 1998;42(4):909–11. Available from: https://academic.oup.com/neurosurgery/article/42/4/909/2846930.

19. Kabil MS, Eby JB, Shahinian HK. Fully endoscopic endonasal vs. transseptal transsphenoidal pituitary surgery. Minim Invasive Neurosurg. 2005;48(6):348–54. Available from: https://pubmed-ncbi-nlm-nih-gov.proxy.library.vanderbilt.edu/16432784/.

20. Sindwani R, Woodard TD, Recinos PF. Endoscopic cranial base and pituitary surgery [Internet]. Otolaryngol Clin N Am. W.B. Saunders. 2016;49:xix–xx. Available from: https://pubmed-ncbi-nlm-nih-gov.proxy.library.vanderbilt.edu/26614843/.

21. Patel PN, Stafford AM, Patrinely JR, Smith DK, Turner JH, Russell PT, et al. Risk factors for intraoperative and postoperative cerebrospinal fluid leaks in endoscopic transsphenoidal sellar surgery. Otolaryngol Head Neck Surg. 2018;158(5):952–60. Available from: https://pubmed-ncbi-nlm-nih-gov.proxy.library.vanderbilt.edu/29405885/.
22. Roca E, Penn DL, Safain MG, Burke WT, Castlen JP, Laws ER. Abdominal fat graft for sellar reconstruction: retrospective outcomes review and technical note. Oper Neurosurg. 2019;16(6):667–74. Available from: https://pubmed-ncbi-nlm-nih-gov.proxy.library.vanderbilt.edu/30124966/.
23. Scagnelli RJ, Patel V, Peris-Celda M, Kenning TJ, Pinheiro-Neto CD. Implementation of free mucosal graft technique for sellar reconstruction after pituitary surgery: outcomes of 158 consecutive patients. World Neurosurg. 2019;122:e506–11. Available from: https://pubmed-ncbi-nlm-nih-gov.proxy.library.vanderbilt.edu/30368014/.
24. Chrousos GP, Schulte HM, Oldfield EH, Gold PW, Cutler GB, Loriaux DL. The corticotropin-releasing factor stimulation test: an aid in the evaluation of patients with Cushing's syndrome. N Engl J Med. 1984;310(10):622–6. Available from: https://pubmed-ncbi-nlm-nih-gov.proxy.library.vanderbilt.edu/6319991/.
25. Jagannathan J, Smith R, DeVroom HL, Vortmeyer AO, Stratakis CA, Nieman LK, et al. Outcome of using the histological pseudocapsule as a surgical capsule in Cushing disease: clinical article. J Neurosurg. 2009;111(3):531–9. Available from: https://pubmed-ncbi-nlm-nih-gov.proxy.library.vanderbilt.edu/19267526/.
26. Oldfield EH, Vortmeyer AO. Development of a histological pseudocapsule and its use as a surgical capsule in the excision of pituitary tumors. J Neurosurg. 2006;104(1):7–19. Available from: https://pubmed-ncbi-nlm-nih-gov.proxy.library.vanderbilt.edu/16509142/.
27. Pouratian N, Prevedello DM, Jagannathan J, Lopes MB, Vance ML, Laws ER. Outcomes and management of patients with Cushing's disease without pathological confirmation of tumor resection after transsphenoidal surgery. J Clin Endocrinol Metab. 2007;92(9):3383–8. Available from: https://pubmed-ncbi-nlm-nih-gov.proxy.library.vanderbilt.edu/17595252/.
28. Lonser RR, Ksendzovsky A, Wind JJ, Vortmeyer AO, Oldfield EH. Prospective evaluation of the characteristics and incidence of adenoma-associated dural invasion in Cushing disease. J Neurosurg. 2012;116(2):272–9. Available from: https://pubmed-ncbi-nlm-nih-gov.proxy.library.vanderbilt.edu/21923247/.
29. Ciric I, Zhao JC, Du H, Findling JW, Molitch ME, Weiss RE, et al. Transsphenoidal surgery for cushing disease: experience with 136 patients. Neurosurgery. 2012;70(1):70–80. Available from: https://pubmed-ncbi-nlm-nih-gov.proxy.library.vanderbilt.edu/21772221/.
30. Alzhrani G, Sivakumar W, Park MS, Taussky P, Couldwell WT. Delayed complications after transsphenoidal surgery for pituitary adenomas. World Neurosurg (Elsevier Inc). 2018;109:233–41. Available from: https://pubmed-ncbi-nlm-nih-gov.proxy.library.vanderbilt.edu/28989047/.
31. Berker M, Hazer DB, Yücel T, Gürlek A, Cila A, Aldur M, et al. Complications of endoscopic surgery of the pituitary adenomas: analysis of 570 patients and review of the literature. Pituitary. 2012;15:288–300. Available from: https://pubmed-ncbi-nlm-nih-gov.proxy.library.vanderbilt.edu/22161543/.
32. Karsy M, Bowers CA, Scoville J, Kundu B, Azab MA, Gee JM, et al. Evaluation of complications and costs during overlapping Transsphenoidal surgery in the treatment of pituitary adenoma. Neurosurgery. 2019;84(5):1104–11. Available from: https://pubmed-ncbi-nlm-nih-gov.proxy.library.vanderbilt.edu/29897572/.
33. Machado MC, De Sa SV, Domenice S, Fragoso MCBV, Puglia P, Pereira MAA, et al. The role of desmopressin in bilateral and simultaneous inferior petrosal sinus sampling for differential diagnosis of ACTH-dependent Cushing's syndrome. Clin Endocrinol. 2007;66(1):136–42. Available from: https://pubmed-ncbi-nlm-nih-gov.proxy.library.vanderbilt.edu/17201813/.
34. Starke RM, Reames DL, Chen CJ, Laws ER, Jane JA. Endoscopic transsphenoidal surgery for cushing disease: techniques, outcomes, and predictors of remission. Clin Neurosurg.

2013;72(2):240–7. Available from: https://pubmed-ncbi-nlm-nih-gov.proxy.library.vanderbilt.edu/23149974/.

35. Tritos NA, Biller BMK. Update on radiation therapy in patients with Cushing's disease. Pituitary (Springer New York LLC). 2015;18:263–8. Available from: https://pubmed-ncbi-nlm-nih-gov.proxy.library.vanderbilt.edu/25359445/.

36. Starke RM, Williams BJ, Vance ML, Sheehan JP. Radiation therapy and stereotactic radiosurgery for the treatment of Cushings disease: an evidence-based review. Curr Opin Endocrinol Diabetes Obes. 2010;17:356–64. Available from: https://pubmed-ncbi-nlm-nih-gov.proxy.library.vanderbilt.edu/20531182/.

37. Wilson PJ, Williams JR, Smee RI. Cushing's disease: a single centre's experience using the linear accelerator (LINAC) for stereotactic radiosurgery and fractionated stereotactic radiotherapy. J Clin Neurosci. 2014;21(1):100–6. Available from: https://pubmed-ncbi-nlm-nih-gov.proxy.library.vanderbilt.edu/24074805/.

Chapter 15
Surgical Treatment of Pancreatic Islet Cell Tumors

Joseph Kearney, Jeffrey Johnson, and Hong Jin Kim

Introduction

The surgical management of functional pancreatic neuroendocrine tumors (PNETs) involves a multidisciplinary approach, including the patient, surgeon, medical and radiation oncologists, radiologist, and endocrinologist. The goal of this chapter is to provide an understanding of the evidence-based approach to the decisions regarding surgical management of functional PNETs.

PNETs arise from the endocrine tissues of the pancreas, known as the islets of Langerhans, although there is evidence of derivation from precursors arising within the ductal/acinar system [1]. The neuroendocrine cells of the pancreas, along with the exocrine acinar cells, ductal epithelium, and all other gut endocrine cells, are derived from the endoderm as opposed to the neural crest or other ectodermal tissues [2, 3]. PNETs account for 7% of all neuroendocrine tumors that originate within the GI tract and 2% of all tumors arising from the pancreas. They are rare, with an annual incidence of less than 1/100,000 [4]. The incidence of PNETs has been increasing over the last decade, likely secondary to the increased use of cross-sectional abdominal imaging identifying small, nonfunctional tumors. This belief is reinforced by postmortem autopsy studies showing an incidence of 0.8% to 10% [5].

J. Kearney
Department of Surgery, University of North Carolina at Chapel Hill, Chapel Hill, NC, USA
e-mail: joseph.kearney@unchealth.unc.edu

J. Johnson (✉) · H. J. Kim
Division of Surgical Oncology and Endocrine Surgery, University of North Carolina at Chapel Hill, Chapel Hill, NC, USA
e-mail: jeffrey_johnson@med.unc.edu; kimhj@med.unc.edu

© The Author(s), under exclusive license to Springer Nature Switzerland AG 2022

H. Yu et al. (eds.), *Diagnosis and Management of Endocrine Disorders in Interventional Radiology*, https://doi.org/10.1007/978-3-030-87189-5_15

Diagnosis and Surgical Evaluation

Rationale for Surgery

Considerations guiding surgical resection of functional PNETs fall into two categories: oncologic and endocrine. Oncologic considerations depend on balancing the long-term benefits of resection with the risks of surgery; these considerations depend on tumor-specific factors that inform the risk of metastatic spread (phenotype, stage, grade, size, location), anatomy, and patient-specific factors including age and comorbidities. This is tempered in some cases of genetic predisposition to tumors where recurrent or multifocal disease diminishes the benefits of local resection (see below). In many patients with localized disease, complete resection is curative. In patients with locoregional or metastatic disease, debulking surgery may prolong life and provide local control of the tumor in anatomic areas that may be compromised by a bulky lesion, e.g., porta hepatis, duodenum, and root of the mesentery [6–8]. Pancreatic surgery carries significant risks of morbidity and complication, and oncologic goals must be weighed against the functional status of the patient and the perceived benefit of resecting tumors that may have an indolent course.

Outside of oncologic considerations, resection may be used to manage the endocrine symptoms of secretory tumors. Even small lesions may produce morbid clinical syndromes. In this case, surgery is the definitive management of local disease. Again, the risks and benefits of surgery must be weighed against alternative treatments, such as medical control of a hypersecretory syndrome, and patient factors. In general, given both the oncologic and endocrine benefits, localized functional PNETs should be resected in all patients who can tolerate surgery.

WHO 2017 Histological Classification

PNETs are categorized by histology into three broad categories: well-differentiated neuroendocrine neoplasms (NEN), poorly differentiated neuroendocrine neoplasms, and mixed neuroendocrine neoplasms [9, 10]. Functional neuroendocrine neoplasms all fall within the category of well-differentiated NEN. Well-differentiated NEN are subcategorized into grades 1–3, which are defined by measures of proliferation (mitoses or Ki-67). Ki-67 represents the most important prognostic pathologic factor. Poorly differentiated NEN, or neuroendocrine carcinoma (NEC), has an aggressive course marked by frequent metastases at presentation and median survival of less than 1 year despite therapy. Surgery is not considered beneficial for this group of patients [11, 12]. High-grade, well-differentiated NEN have higher rates of metastases and limited survival compared with grades 1 and 2. Previous WHO classification had grouped grade 3 well-differentiated NEN with NEC; however, mounting evidence suggests distinct biology and behavior between the two

diagnoses. The most recent classification distinguishes the two into separate categories [5, 10]. For treatment planning, high-grade well-differentiated NEN should be
considered on a spectrum with the other well-differentiated neoplasms, although the
poorer prognosis should be weighed when considering aggressive surgical therapies
[11, 13, 14].

Functional PNET

The physiologic aberrances from functional PNETs are driven by the hormones
normally produced by islet cells, including insulin and glucagon, as well as gastrin,
somatostatin, and vasoactive intestinal peptide (VIP) [15] (Table 15.1). Functional
PNETs are classified by the hormones they produce, as they are associated with
discrete clinical syndromes and exhibit different anatomic distributions, natural history, and malignant potential. These factors affect the decision to proceed with
resection. Tumors with high malignant potential require anatomic resections and
consideration for lymphadenectomy. Benign tumors (insulinoma) and multifocal
tumors are more likely to be managed with enucleation. The specific diagnostic
workup for these tumors has been covered earlier in this book.

Insulinoma

Insulinomas are the most common hormone-secreting tumors, accounting for about
40–55% of functional PNETs. They are most often sporadic and benign, with fewer
than 10% being malignant. Insulinomas are distributed throughout the pancreas and
often small at the time of diagnosis, as the classic hypoglycemic symptoms (tachy-
cardia, light-headedness, fainting) lead to early presentation and diagnosis.

Table 15.1 Clinical characteristics of the hypersecretory syndromes associated with
functional PNETs

	Insulinoma	Gastrinoma	Glucagonoma	VIPoma	Somatostatinoma
Occurance rate	40–55% of PNETs	25–50% of PNETS	Rare	Rare	Rare (4% of PNETS)
Typical location	Throughout	Gastrinoma triangle	Body/tail	Body/tail	Ampulla of Vater, head/tail
Typical size at diagnosis	Small	Small	Large	Large	Large
Malignancy rate	10%	>50%	80%	70%	80%
Common symptoms	Hypoglycemia	Zollinger-Ellison syndrome	Dermatitis, diabetes, stomatitis, glossitis, cheilosis	Watery, secretory diarrhea	Diabetes, gallstones, diarrhea, weight loss

Gastrinoma

Gastrinomas are the second most common, accounting for about 25–50% of functional PNETs. Patients may present with Zollinger-Ellison syndrome, consisting of abdominal pain, gastroesophageal reflux disease, refractory ulcers throughout the small intestine, and diarrhea. In contrast to insulinomas, gastrinomas are more often malignant (>50%) and can be multiple at presentation. Gastrinomas are frequently small and difficult to localize; anatomically, most occur in the gastrinoma triangle, whose points are defined by the second/third portions of the duodenum, the neck/body of the pancreas, and the confluence of the cystic and common bile ducts. This helps guide operative exploration when preoperative imaging is inconclusive. Gastrinomas not located here are most often found in the body and tail of the pancreas or duodenum but have been found in various sites, including the ovaries.

Glucagonoma

Glucagonomas are malignant in 80% of cases. They are often large at presentation and generally occur within the body or tail of the pancreas. They present with migratory dermatitis, new-onset type II diabetes mellitus, and superficial oral symptoms, such as stomatitis, glossitis, and cheilosis.

VIPoma

VIPomas usually present as large tumors. They occur in the body and tail of the pancreas and carry high malignant potential. Patients classically present with watery secretory diarrhea that persists with fasting.

Somatostatinoma

Somatostatinomas are most often found in the head and tail of the pancreas. Metastatic disease, commonly in the liver and peripancreatic lymph nodes, is present in up to 80% of patients at diagnosis. Patients typically present with new-onset diabetes mellitus, gallstones (from cholecystokinin inhibition), and diarrhea. Some patients also show weight loss and hypochlorhydria (from gastric acid inhibition) [16].

Nonfunctional PNET

Management is different for functioning and nonfunctioning tumors in weighing the benefits of nonoperative management. For nonfunctional tumors that do not require resection to alleviate the effects of hormone hypersecretion, the oncologic benefit of resection is weighed against the risks of surgery. Many nonfunctional tumors are incidentally identified and indolent, with only rare progression and disease-specific mortality [17–21]. Observation for nonfunctional tumors is then considered in select cases, where the risks of surgery are presumed to outweigh benefits. In the setting of small, well-differentiated, incidentally discovered tumors, surgical and patient factors may favor observation rather than resection. Rare functioning tumors that produce hormones without an associated clinical syndrome (pancreatic polypeptide, human chorionic gonadotropin subunits, calcitonin, neurotensin) are considered as nonfunctional PNETs in this regard [22]. Current guidelines recommend observation for nonfunctional lesions smaller than 1 cm, individualized risk and benefit assessment for intermediate lesions 1–2 cm, and resection for lesions greater than 2 cm [13, 23].

Hereditary Syndromes

Ten percent of PNETs arise within the context of a broader hereditary syndrome [5, 24]. The most common genetic syndromes associated with PNETs are multiple endocrine neoplasia type 1 (MEN-1) and von Hippel-Lindau disease (VHL) (Table 15.2).

MEN-1

MEN-1 results from an autosomal dominant mutation in the menin gene, which has multiple roles in tumor suppression [25]. Patients with MEN-1 present with Wermer syndrome, which consists of parathyroid gland hyperplasia (95% prevalence), pituitary tumors (30% prevalence), and PNETs (80–100% prevalence). In distinction to sporadic tumors, patients with MEN-1 will develop multiple pancreatic lesions, most of which will be nonfunctional NETs. While total pancreatectomy would be effectively curative in this population and may in some cases be necessary if there are multiple masses concerning for neoplasm or unmanageable functional syndromes, the loss of pancreatic exocrine and endocrine function carries significant morbidity and diminished quality of life and is generally avoided. The surgical approach is more conservative for nonfunctional tumors, with active surveillance for tumors smaller than 2 cm and medical management attempted for many

Table 15.2 Genetic syndromes predisposing to the development of PNETs

	Multiple endocrine neoplasia type I	Von Hippel-Lindau syndrome
Gene	Menin	VHL
Primary neoplasms involved	Parathyroid gland hyperplasia, pituitary tumors, pancreatic neuroendocrine tumors	CNS hemangioblastomas, clear cell renal cell carcinoma, pheochromocytoma, pancreatic neuroendocrine tumors

functional tumors. In the setting of suspicious imaging features, rapid growth, size over 2 cm, or functional tumors refractory to medical management, surgery is recommended [23, 26, 27]. This requires preoperative localization to plan parenchyma-sparing approaches as opposed to anatomic resections.

About 80–100% of patients with MEN-1 will develop multifocal and nonfunctional PNETS; however, roughly half of these patients also develop functional PNETs [28]. Insulinomas and gastrinomas are the most frequently occurring functional PNETs, and these are often small and multifocal. In most cases, enucleation is the preferred approach for both functional and nonfunctional PNETS that are small, superficial, and easily localized. Anatomic resections are required for multifocal disease not amenable to enucleation or in the setting of concern of malignancy. Pancreatic resection for gastrinemia without a discrete, localized mass is controversial as gastrinomas are multifocal and often arise in the duodenum, rendering pancreatic resection nonbeneficial. These patients are managed more aggressively with medical management, with surgery reserved for concern for malignancy or refractory medical symptoms [13].

Von Hippel-Lindau Syndrome

Von Hippel-Lindau syndrome (VHL) results from an autosomal dominant mutation in the *VHL* tumor suppressor gene and is associated with hemangioblastomas in the central nervous system (60–80% prevalence), clear cell renal cell carcinoma (30% prevalence), pheochromocytomas (20% prevalence), and PNETs (9–17% prevalence) [29]. Patients with VHL frequently develop benign pancreatic lesions, most frequently cysts, serous cystadenomas, and hemangioblastomas [30]. PNETs in VHL are most frequently solitary and nonfunctional and have a better prognosis than sporadic PNETs. Studies have demonstrated that specific mutations of *VHL* may prognosticate which patients will develop metastatic PNETs and require operative intervention [31]. Reflecting this, the approach to surgery is more conservative, with observation considered for masses smaller than 3 cm that exhibit slow growth or low-risk mutations [13].

Preoperative Workup

Preoperative evaluation is necessary to determine whether surgery is indicated and the specific surgery to be performed. This depends on the type of tumor, presence of a genetic syndrome, anatomic location and local extent of the tumor, and presence of regional and/or distant metastatic disease. For functional tumors, medical and clinical workup and diagnoses have been covered in previous chapters. Patients with a history concerning for MEN-1 should undergo genetic testing prior to surgery.

The anatomic location and local extent of the tumor are best defined with multiphasic, contrast-enhanced cross-sectional imaging of the abdomen, including either CT or MRI. Intravenous contrast timing is essential when there is a question of vascular involvement and critical to assess the liver with arterial and portal venous phase imaging. Functional imaging with somatostatin receptor-based methods (e.g., 68 Ga-DOTATATE PET/CT or MRI) is useful to resolve diagnostic uncertainty on cross-sectional imaging studies, to identify nodal involvement in normal or borderline enlarged nodes, to localize occult tumors, and to identify metastatic disease and serves as a useful adjunct to standard cross-sectional imaging in the preoperative workup. It has particular utility in MEN-1 in identifying multifocal disease and extrapancreatic tumors [32, 33] (Fig. 15.1).

Endoscopic ultrasound (EUS) with or without biopsy may be used in cases where the information gained would alter the management of the patient. Cross-sectional imaging with CT or MRI is usually sufficient to determine resectability with respect to vascular structures. EUS and biopsy may aid in determining the extent of resection in the presence of multiple masses on cross-sectional imaging or to confirm the diagnosis in equivocal cases. As regional lymph nodes will be resected at the time of surgery, there is likely no benefit to sampling nodes prior to resection. EUS may be useful as an adjunct to cross-sectional imaging in MEN-1 for identifying multifocal disease [34].

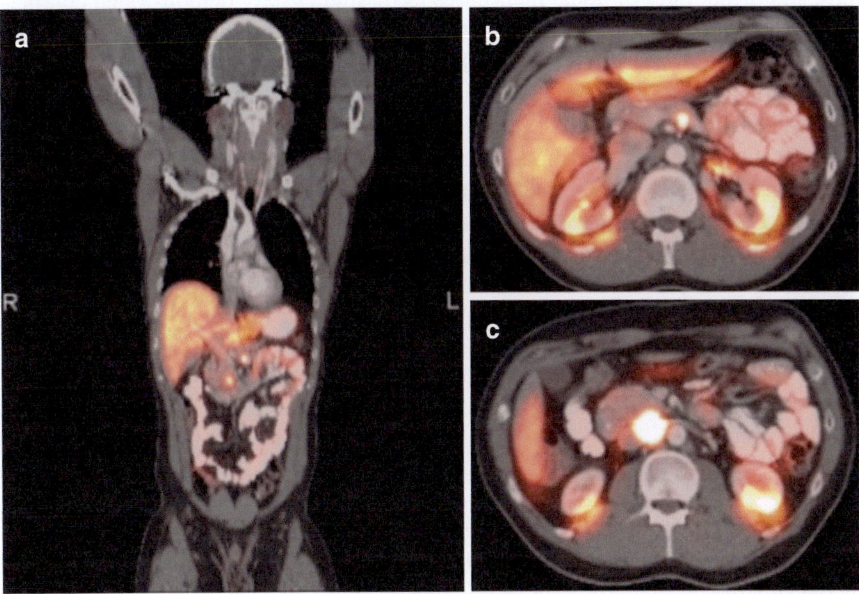

Fig. 15.1 DOTATATE PET CT scan for a 28-year-old man with MEN-1 with multiple pancreatic neuroendocrine tumors. The patient had multifocal PNET with involved peripancreatic lymph nodes (**a** and **b**), and underwent pancreaticoduodenectomy for a dominant 3 cm mass in the uncinate process (best seen in **c**), with final pathology demonstrating a well-differentiated, grade 2 neuroendocrine tumor with 5/26 lymph nodes positive

Operative Approaches

Curative Intent

Resection of functional PNETs serves the dual purposes of diminishing risks associated with malignancy and definitively treating morbid endocrine syndromes. For localized disease, the goal of surgery is removing the tumor with an R0 resection, i.e., negative margins with no residual microscopic disease [8]. For patients with MEN-1, the surgical techniques and principles are the same, but the risk/benefit analysis of surgery is different and is considered separately in section "MEN-1" above. For most neuroendocrine tumors, an additional margin of normal soft tissue is not required as the tumors are focal or discrete entities without the extensive infiltration seen in other malignancies such as pancreatic adenocarcinoma. The extent of resection is then determined by the lesion's malignant potential and, moreover, by the anatomic location. The extent of resection is considered below.

The data is mixed for the value of regional lymphadenectomy. The prognostic significance of lymph node metastases is unclear, although most surgeons would remove suspicious nodes or nodes with biopsy-confirmed disease. Further, as the risk of nodal metastases increases with the size of the primary lesion, lymphadenectomy is recommended for tumors over 1.5 cm in size, although smaller tumors also have significant rates of nodal metastases [35]. Studies have demonstrated conflicting conclusions such as the presence of metastatic disease within lymph nodes is not associated with overall survival [36–38], is associated with diminished disease free survival [35, 39, 40], is associated with survival in T1-T2 disease with no benefit seen with lymphadenectomy [41], or is associated with diminished overall survival [35, 42]. Overall, formal lymphadenectomy should be considered in the case of suspicion for nodal disease, in the setting of primary tumors larger than 1.5 cm or with other high-risk features, and in the setting of formal pancreatic resections. This may ultimately diminish later complications from tumor burden, although evidence supporting an impact on survival is lacking.

Pancreatic Resections

Pancreaticoduodenectomy

More commonly referred to as the Whipple procedure, this is the standard of care for tumors in the head and uncinate process of the pancreas, which are to the right of the superior mesenteric vein (SMV)/portal vein (PV) confluence as it courses posterior to the pancreas. The approach (open, laparoscopic, or robotic) is determined on a case-by-case basis and by the surgeon's preference and experience. The surgery includes en bloc resection of the pancreatic head and uncinate process, distal stomach and pylorus (classic pancreaticoduodenectomy), duodenum, proximal jejunum, distal common bile duct, and gallbladder. Reconstruction involves the creation of several anastomoses, including gastrojejunostomy, hepaticojejunostomy, and pancreaticojejunostomy. This surgery requires patency of the celiac trunk with antegrade flow through the hepatic artery since the gastroduodenal artery (GDA), which may provide collateral flow retrograde from the superior mesenteric artery (SMA) through the plexus of pancreaticoduodenal vessels, is ligated. Masses in the pancreatic head and uncinate process must be confirmed not to involve the celiac trunk or common hepatic artery or aberrant arterial variants, potentially precluding resection. Pancreaticoduodenectomy is a morbid procedure with a relatively high rate of perioperative complications, including most commonly pancreatic fistula, delayed gastric emptying, wound infection, hemorrhage, pancreatic endocrine or exocrine insufficiency, and pneumonia. Perioperative mortality is low in experienced centers, with rates less than 3% [43].

Distal Pancreatectomy

Distal pancreatectomy or left-sided pancreatectomy is the preferred procedure for patients with tumors to the left of the SMV/PV confluence in the body or tail of the pancreas. If the tumor is not apparent on gross examination, intraoperative ultrasound is a useful adjunct to physical examination to assist with localization of the tumor. The resection begins with dissection and delineation of the splenic artery after its takeoff from the celiac trunk and splenic vein before the confluence with the SMV. This is followed by dissection of the distal pancreas with ligation of the pancreas proximal to the tumor. Splenectomy is often performed in cases with bulky masses or concern for malignancy necessitating regional lymphadenectomy and must be accompanied by vaccination against encapsulated organisms to reduce the risk of overwhelming post-splenectomy infections [44, 45].

Total Pancreatectomy

Complete resection of the pancreas is rarely seen in the surgical treatment of pancreatic neuroendocrine tumors and is almost exclusively employed for the management of the multifocal disease in conjunction with a hereditary syndrome [46]. Patients undergoing this operation need counseling on the risks of labile insulin-dependent diabetes that ensues following this operation. The resection consists of removing the pancreatic head/body/tail distal common bile duct, duodenum, and often the spleen. The reconstruction involves mobilization of the proximal jejunum and two anastomoses: a hepaticojejunostomy and a gastrojejunostomy. There are variations to this procedure, including duodenal and spleen preserving techniques, which are beyond the scope of this text.

Enucleation

Excision of a mass along its capsule within the pancreatic parenchyma is a common approach to small nonfunctional tumors in the head of the pancreas, insulinomas, and multifocal disease in the setting of MEN-1. Larger tumors, tumors with concern for malignancy or nodal involvement, or tumors within 2–3 mm of the pancreatic duct are not suitable for enucleation. These anatomic features are often determined preoperatively with cross-sectional imaging but also verified intraoperatively with ultrasound guidance. If a tumor is not amenable to enucleation, formal anatomic resections are performed. Enucleation offers the benefit of preserved pancreatic parenchyma at the risk of a higher rate of postoperative pancreatic fistulas [47].

Transduodenal Approach

Duodenotomy and local resection was investigated in the early 2000s for the management of small duodenal neuroendocrine tumors with some surgeons successfully resecting these lesions with endoscopic mucosal resections and laparoscopic transduodenal resections. These approaches fell out of favor due to the prevalence of lymph node metastases occurring in greater than 50% in patients with duodenal NETs < 2 cm. At present, the standard of care for these lesions is a pancreaticoduodenectomy [48].

Nonlocalized Lesions

Exploration without preoperative localization almost exclusively occurs in the setting of Zollinger-Ellison syndrome due to the need for swift control of the gastrin secreting tumor, which may be small and/or multifocal. In other tumors, patients can often be medically managed and followed with serial imaging until their primary tumors are visualized on imaging. Experienced surgeons are able to locate a nonlocalized gastrinoma nearly 100% of the time using palpation, ultrasound, and, if warranted, duodenotomy [49].

Intraoperative ultrasound is also used to identify masses that are not readily palpated or identified on the surface of the pancreas. This modality helps to identify and characterize small and/or multiple tumors and evaluate distance to the pancreatic duct in cases being considered for enucleation. This is particularly useful in the setting of insulinoma, where the use of intraoperative ultrasound in combination with preoperative modalities raises the probability of successfully identifying and resecting small, solitary tumors to near 100% [50].

Contraindications and the Management of Advanced and Inoperable Disease

Surgery for Advanced Disease

Resection is contraindicated when the anatomic distribution of metastatic disease or advanced local disease precludes surgery or when a patient is unable to tolerate surgery due to medical risks. For pancreatic tumor resections in general, intraoperative ultrasound can be employed to assist surgeons in defining key anatomical relationships to vessels throughout the progression of the surgery [51]. Locally advanced tumors are inoperable if there is direct involvement of the celiac axis, SMA, and/or common hepatic artery. However, unlike pancreatic adenocarcinoma, PNETs are more likely to abut vessels without directly invading them, allowing resection even in cases where masses appear to encroach on critical vessels [52]. Invasion of the splenic artery and/or vein does not preclude surgery, and splenectomy may be a necessary addition to pancreatic resection. Tumor involvement of the PV, SMV, or adjacent organs (e.g., colon and stomach) also does not preclude resection, and venous resection and reconstruction have comparable outcomes when performed at an experienced center [53, 54]. Neoadjuvant therapies, including chemotherapy, peptide receptor radionuclide therapy (PRRT), somatostatin analogues (SSA), and radiation, have been employed to attempt to downstage tumors and facilitate resection with mixed success [55].

Numerous multimodal therapies may also be used outside the context of neoadjuvant therapy to treat metastatic disease. The choice of therapy necessarily involves a multidisciplinary discussion involving surgery, medical oncology, gastroenterology, and interventional radiology. The decision on a specific therapy depends on a number of factors: prior therapies and surgeries, patient functional status and comorbidities, extent and location of disease, health and volume of liver, and patient and provider preference. Systemic therapies include SSA, cytotoxic chemotherapy, molecular targeted therapies (everolimus, small molecule tyrosine kinase inhibitors, and bevacizumab), and PRRT. For liver-dominant metastatic disease, a number of transarterial embolization approaches may be used to limit tumor growth, including bland embolization, transarterial chemoembolization (TACE), and transarterial radioembolization (TARE). Percutaneous or surgical-assisted ablation (radiofrequency ablation, microwave ablation, cryoablation) may also be used to manage smaller lesions, generally <3 cm, that may be unresectable or in patients unable to undergo liver resection. Liver transplantation is not generally considered an available option for patients with unresectable metastatic NET.

Debulking and Palliative Resections

Metastases from PNETs typically involve regional lymph nodes and the liver. Bulky primary lesions of the pancreas or regional lymph nodes are often symptomatic and can lead to acute or subacute life-threatening complications in patients who may otherwise live for years with metastatic disease. Such complications include gastric outlet and bowel obstructions, bowel perforations, biliary obstructions and cholangitis, pancreatitis, and hemorrhage. Palliative resection of the primary tumor may increase survival through local control [8, 56–58]. Debulking may prolong life not only by preventing anatomic complications but may decrease the rate of future metastasis and increase the sensitivity to systemic therapies, including PRRT [59].

For metastatic functional tumors, effective debulking, generally greater than 70% of tumor load, may offer symptomatic relief from medically refractory hypersecretion syndromes and improve survival. Patient selection in this setting is difficult as patient factors, rate of disease progression, number and size of liver lesions, anatomic distribution, prior therapies, and sites of extrahepatic disease may influence the decision to proceed with therapy. In addition, other local and regional therapies must be considered in addition to or instead of surgery.

Other Operative Considerations

Cholecystectomy

Cholecystectomy should be considered at the time of resection in all patients and should be performed in patients anticipated to receive somatostatin analogue therapy unless there exists a specific contraindication. Somatostatin analogues are associated with a significant increase in the risk of cholelithiasis and related complications [60]. Additionally, patients who may undergo hepatic artery-directed therapies also have a significant risk of cholecystitis [61]. Cholecystectomy at the time of PNET resection is associated with a significant decrease in the rate of subsequent biliary complications [60]. There are no data to support prophylactic cholecystectomy as a separate operation in otherwise asymptomatic patients.

Perioperative Somatostatin Analogues

Somatostatin analogues are more frequently used during surgery for small bowel NETs to prevent carcinoid crisis. Serotonin secretion has been reported during resection of both functional and nonfunctional PNETs, and there are case reports of carcinoid syndrome in PNET, but there is no unambiguous evidence of surgery prompting carcinoid crisis in PNETs [62–64]. For functional PNETs, it is more critical to manage the clinical hypersecretory syndromes to optimize patients for surgery, which may include the use of SSAs in addition to syndrome-specific management (discussed in a prior chapter). There is no role for perioperative SSAs for the prevention of carcinoid crisis.

Postoperative Care and Complications after Pancreatic Resections

Postoperative Care

Over the past decade, there has been a nationwide trend among institutions toward the adoption of enhanced recovery after surgery (ERAS) pathways after abdominal surgery, including pancreatic resections. ERAS is a multipronged, evidence-based approach to optimize patient care before, during, and after surgery to optimize outcomes for patients, including shorter lengths of stay, lower complication rates, and better symptomatic management. These pathways often vary between institutions but typically involve several core components [65]. In the preoperative period, attention is given to identifying and optimizing comorbidities, functional status, and nutrition using objective, validated tools. Patients are also counseled on what to expect with their perioperative course so that patient expectations are in line with both the expected postoperative course as well as potential complications. Perioperative care includes utilizing objective measures to guide fluid resuscitation, using of multimodal analgesia including neuraxial techniques, and pursuing minimally invasive operative techniques as a given procedure allows. Postoperative care focuses on expediting a return to functional recovery including early removal of drains and tubes, reinstitution of enteral nutrition, early ambulation, and multidisciplinary discharge planning to ensure an optimal transition out of the hospital that may prevent the need for readmission [65, 66].

Although the evidence supporting drain placement after pancreaticoduodenectomy is mixed, recent retrospective studies support drain placement and following drain amylase levels for the early detection of clinically relevant postoperative pancreatic fistula (CR-POPF) [67, 68]. In a recent retrospective analysis, postoperative hemorrhage requiring either reoperation or endovascular repair occurred in 3.3% of cases in the postoperative period. The complications most commonly requiring re-intervention include GI complications from anastomotic issues and incisional hernias [69].

Postoperative Complications

Complications after complex resections involving the liver, biliary tree, and pancreas are not unexpected and frequently result after what would be considered a technically optimal procedure. Complications in this setting are anticipated and proactively managed. The use of ERAS protocols and consolidation of technically challenging procedures in high-volume centers helps to diminish rates of complications and improve outcomes [70].

Pancreatic Fistula

A common complication after pancreatic resection, with an average preoperative risk of 15%, although varying greatly depending on operative risk factors, is the development of clinically relevant postoperative pancreatic fistula [71, 72]. After pancreatic resection, including both anatomic resection and enucleation, there is a risk of failure of the transected pancreatic ducts to seal, allowing pancreatic fluid with digestive proteases to leak. These leaks delay healing of the pancreas, impair initiation of adequate nutrition, and may also result in prolonged drainage of pancreatic fluid. Factors associated with pancreatic leak include intraoperative blood loss, gland texture (firm/soft), history of pancreatitis, and main pancreatic duct size [71, 73]. Risks of pancreatic leak after enucleation approach those of pancreaticoduodenectomy and distal pancreatectomy in some series [74, 75].

Leaks are categorized by clinical severity and range from asymptomatic (grade A; detected on biochemical analysis of drain fluid), to involving escalation of postoperative care (grade B; requiring drainage and medical management), to requiring reoperation or resulting in single or multisystem organ failure (grade C) [76]. Grades B and C leaks may cause infected intra-abdominal fluid collections, hemorrhage, ileus and delayed gastric emptying, malnutrition, and wound complications. Pancreatic fistula is most commonly managed with percutaneous drain placement, if a drain was not left at the time of surgery; nutritional management with an effort to reduce stimulation of pancreatic secretion through low-fat and low-protein diets or total parenteral nutrition; and use of somatostatin analogues to decrease pancreatic fluid production [77, 78]. Additional care, such as antibiotics, gastric drainage, and wound management, is frequently required. Drain placement at the time of surgery is a controversial topic; drains are typically left at the time of surgery in an effort to mitigate the effects of a pancreatic leak, particularly in high-risk patients, although the absolute benefit of this approach has not been demonstrated [79]. Uncommonly, refractory leaks that continue after a period of weeks may be managed with further intervention, including pancreatic duct stent placement or additional surgery.

Pancreatic Insufficiency

Following pancreatic resection, patients may develop exocrine pancreatic insufficiency and/or endocrine pancreatic insufficiency. The risk of pancreatic insufficiency is related to the preoperative function of the pancreas, which may be diminished in the setting of prior pancreatitis, metabolic syndrome, and/or resection, and the extent of pancreatic resection. Concern for pancreatic insufficiency contributes to the decision for parenchyma-sparing enucleation in tumors at a low risk of malignancy or in patients at high risk of multiple surgical resections (MEN-1).

Exocrine pancreatic insufficiency, defined by inadequate production of pancreatic juice containing alkaline fluid and digestive enzymes in response to a food bolus, may occur in up to three-fourths of patients after pancreaticoduodenectomy or distal pancreatectomy [80]. This typically results in malabsorption manifest by bloating, cramping, steatorrhea, and, in severe cases, malnutrition and vitamin deficiency. Management includes dietary modification with low-fat meals, administration of exogenous pancreatic enzymes, supplementation of fat-soluble vitamins, and consideration for supplementation with medium-chain triglycerides. Inadequate endocrine pancreatic function results in pancreatogenic diabetes mellitus (type 3c) and is managed with treatment of concomitant exocrine insufficiency, dietary modification, close blood glucose monitoring, and exogenous insulin. Treatment with metformin, insulin sensitizers, secretagogues, incretin-based therapies, or other specific medications should be considered by endocrinologists in the appropriate setting [81]. In one series, the risk of developing insufficiency is approximately 16% after pancreaticoduodenectomy and 21% after distal pancreatectomy [82].

Conclusion

The surgical management of PNETs is dependent on the tumor's functional status, location, histology/grade, and genetic predisposition. The approach chosen is dependent on both the tumor type and predisposition for malignancy, as well as the location of the tumor. All of these procedures have risks and potential complications that need to be weighed against patient's comorbidities and the goals of resection (i.e., curative or palliative). These patients are best managed and treated in coordination with a multidisciplinary team at high-volume centers.

References

1. Vortmeyer AO, Huang S, Lubensky I, Zhuang Z. Non-islet origin of pancreatic islet cell tumors. J Clin Endocrinol Metab. 2004;89(4):1934–8.
2. Pictet RL, Rall LB, Phelps P, Rutter WJ. The neural crest and the origin of the insulin-producing and other gastrointestinal hormone-producing cells. Science. 1976;191(4223):191–2.
3. Andrew A, Kramer B, Rawdon BB. The origin of gut and pancreatic neuroendocrine (APUD) cells – the last word? J Pathol. 1998;186(2):117–8.
4. Dasari A, Shen C, Halperin D, Zhao B, Zhou S, Xu Y, et al. Trends in the incidence, prevalence, and survival outcomes in patients with neuroendocrine tumors in the United States. JAMA Oncol. 2017;3(10):1335–42.
5. Singhi AD, Klimstra DS. Well-differentiated pancreatic neuroendocrine tumours (PanNETs) and poorly differentiated pancreatic neuroendocrine carcinomas (PanNECs): concepts, issues and a practical diagnostic approach to high-grade (G3) cases. Histopathology. 2018;72(1):168–77.

6. Hodul PJ, Strosberg JR, Kvols LK. Aggressive surgical resection in the management of pancreatic neuroendocrine tumors: when is it indicated? Cancer Control. 2008;15(4):314–21.

7. Hill JS, McPhee JT, McDade TP, Zhou Z, Sullivan ME, Whalen GF, et al. Pancreatic neuroendocrine tumors: the impact of surgical resection on survival. Cancer. 2009;115(4):741–51.

8. Schurr PG, Strate T, Rese K, Kaifi JT, Reichelt U, Petri S, et al. Aggressive surgery improves long-term survival in neuroendocrine pancreatic tumors: an institutional experience. Ann Surg. 2007;245(2):273–81.

9. Lloyd RV, Osamura RY, Klöppel G, Rosai J, World Health O, International Agency for Research on C, et al. WHO classification of tumours of endocrine organs. Lyon: International Agency for Research on Cancer; 2017.

10. Choe J, Kim KW, Kim HJ, Kim DW, Kim KP, Hong SM, et al. What is new in the 2017 World Health Organization classification and 8th American joint committee on cancer staging system for pancreatic neuroendocrine neoplasms? Korean J Radiol. 2019;20(1):5–17.

11. Basturk O, Yang Z, Tang LH, Hruban RH, Adsay V, McCall CM, et al. The high-grade (WHO G3) pancreatic neuroendocrine tumor category is morphologically and biologically heterogenous and includes both well differentiated and poorly differentiated neoplasms. Am J Surg Pathol. 2015;39(5):683–90.

12. Basturk O, Tang L, Hruban RH, Adsay V, Yang Z, Krasinskas AM, et al. Poorly differentiated neuroendocrine carcinomas of the pancreas: a clinicopathologic analysis of 44 cases. Am J Surg Pathol. 2014;38(4):437–47.

13. Howe JR, Merchant NB, Conrad C, Keutgen XM, Hallet J, Drebin JA, et al. The North American Neuroendocrine Tumor Society consensus paper on the surgical management of pancreatic neuroendocrine tumors. Pancreas. 2020;49(1):1–33.

14. Nuñez-Valdovinos B, Carmona-Bayonas A, Jimenez-Fonseca P, Capdevila J, Castaño-Pascual Á, Benavent M, et al. Neuroendocrine tumor heterogeneity adds uncertainty to the World Health Organization 2010 classification: real-world data from the Spanish Tumor Registry (R-GETNE). Oncologist. 2018;23(4):422–32.

15. Da Silva Xavier G. The cells of the Islets of Langerhans. J Clin Med. 2018;7(3):54.

16. Feingold KR, Anawalt B, Boyce A, Chrousos G, de Herder WW, Dungan K, et al. Endotext. South Dartmouth: MDText.com, Inc; 2000.

17. Sadot E, Reidy-Lagunes DL, Tang LH, Do RK, Gonen M, D'Angelica MI, et al. Observation versus resection for small asymptomatic pancreatic neuroendocrine tumors: a matched case-control study. Ann Surg Oncol. 2016;23(4):1361–70.

18. Lee LC, Grant CS, Salomao DR, Fletcher JG, Takahashi N, Fidler JL, et al. Small, nonfunctioning, asymptomatic pancreatic neuroendocrine tumors (PNETs): role for nonoperative management. Surgery. 2012;152(6):965–74.

19. Gaujoux S, Partelli S, Maire F, D'Onofrio M, Larroque B, Tamburrino D, et al. Observational study of natural history of small sporadic nonfunctioning pancreatic neuroendocrine tumors. J Clin Endocrinol Metab. 2013;98(12):4784–9.

20. Toste PA, Kadera BE, Tatishchev SF, Dawson DW, Clerkin BM, Muthusamy R, et al. Nonfunctional pancreatic neuroendocrine tumors <2 cm on preoperative imaging are associated with a low incidence of nodal metastasis and an excellent overall survival. J Gastrointest Surg. 2013;17(12):2105–13.

21. Finkelstein P, Sharma R, Picado O, Gadde R, Stuart H, Ripat C, et al. Pancreatic neuroendocrine tumors (panNETs): analysis of overall survival of nonsurgical management versus surgical resection. J Gastrointest Surg. 2017;21(5):855–66.

22. O'Toole D, Salazar R, Falconi M, Kaltsas G, Couvelard A, de Herder WW, et al. Rare functioning pancreatic endocrine tumors. Neuroendocrinology. 2006;84(3):189–95.

23. National Comprehensive Cancer Network. Neuroendocrine and adrenal tumors (Version 2.2020). 2020. Available from: https://www.nccn.org/professionals/physician_gls/pdf/neuroendocrine.pdf.

24. Katabathina VS, Rikhtehgar OY, Dasyam AK, Manickam R, Prasad SR. Genetics of pancreatic neoplasms and role of screening. Magn Reson Imaging Clin N Am. 2018;26(3):375–89.

25. Ehrlich L, Hall C, Meng F, Lairmore T, Alpini G, Glaser S. A review of the scaffold protein Menin and its role in hepatobiliary pathology. Gene Expr. 2017;17(3):251–63.
26. Yates CJ, Newey PJ, Thakker RV. Challenges and controversies in management of pancreatic neuroendocrine tumours in patients with MEN1. Lancet Diabetes Endocrinol. 2015;3(11):895–905.
27. Frost M, Lines KE, Thakker RV. Current and emerging therapies for PNETs in patients with or without MEN1. Nat Rev Endocrinol. 2018;14(4):216–27.
28. Jensen RT, Norton JA. Treatment of pancreatic neuroendocrine tumors in multiple endocrine neoplasia type 1: some clarity but continued controversy. Pancreas. 2017;46(5):589–94.
29. Varshney N, Kebede AA, Owusu-Dapaah H, Lather J, Kaushik M, Bhullar JS. A review of Von Hippel-Lindau syndrome. J Kidney Cancer VHL. 2017;4(3):20–9.
30. Keutgen XM, Hammel P, Choyke PL, Libutti SK, Jonasch E, Kebebew E. Evaluation and management of pancreatic lesions in patients with von Hippel-Lindau disease. Nat Rev Clin Oncol. 2016;13(9):537–49.
31. Tirosh A, Sadowski SM, Linehan WM, Libutti SK, Patel D, Nilubol N, et al. Association of VHL genotype with pancreatic neuroendocrine tumor phenotype in patients with von Hippel-Lindau disease. JAMA Oncol. 2018;4(1):124–6.
32. Morgat C, Vélayoudom-Céphise FL, Schwartz P, Guyot M, Gaye D, Vimont D, et al. Evaluation of (68)Ga-DOTA-TOC PET/CT for the detection of duodenopancreatic neuroendocrine tumors in patients with MEN1. Eur J Nucl Med Mol Imaging. 2016;43(7):1258–66.
33. van Asselt SJ, Brouwers AH, van Dullemen HM, van der Jagt EJ, Bongaerts AH, Kema IP, et al. EUS is superior for detection of pancreatic lesions compared with standard imaging in patients with multiple endocrine neoplasia type 1. Gastrointest Endosc. 2015;81(1):159–67.e2.
34. Barbe C, Murat A, Dupas B, Ruszniewski P, Tabarin A, Vullierme MP, et al. Magnetic resonance imaging versus endoscopic ultrasonography for the detection of pancreatic tumours in multiple endocrine neoplasia type 1. Dig Liver Dis. 2012;44(3):228–34.
35. Hashim YM, Trinkaus KM, Linehan DC, Strasberg SS, Fields RC, Cao D, et al. Regional lymphadenectomy is indicated in the surgical treatment of pancreatic neuroendocrine tumors (PNETs). Ann Surg. 2014;259(2):197–203.
36. Bilimoria KY, Talamonti MS, Tomlinson JS, Stewart AK, Winchester DP, Ko CY, et al. Prognostic score predicting survival after resection of pancreatic neuroendocrine tumors: analysis of 3851 patients. Ann Surg. 2008;247(3):490–500.
37. Roland CL, Bian A, Mansour JC, Yopp AC, Balch GC, Sharma R, et al. Survival impact of malignant pancreatic neuroendocrine and islet cell neoplasm phenotypes. J Surg Oncol. 2012;105(6):595–600.
38. Ekeblad S, Skogseid B, Dunder K, Oberg K, Eriksson B. Prognostic factors and survival in 324 patients with pancreatic endocrine tumor treated at a single institution. Clin Cancer Res. 2008;14(23):7798–803.
39. Postlewait LM, Ethun CG, Baptiste GG, Le N, McInnis MR, Cardona K, et al. Pancreatic neuroendocrine tumors: preoperative factors that predict lymph node metastases to guide operative strategy. J Surg Oncol. 2016;114(4):440–5.
40. Ballian N, Loeffler AG, Rajamanickam V, Norstedt PA, Weber SM, Cho CS. A simplified prognostic system for resected pancreatic neuroendocrine neoplasms. HPB (Oxford). 2009;11(5):422–8.
41. Conrad C, Kutlu OC, Dasari A, Chan JA, Vauthey JN, Adams DB, et al. Prognostic value of lymph node status and extent of lymphadenectomy in pancreatic neuroendocrine tumors confined to and extending beyond the pancreas. J Gastrointest Surg. 2016;20(12):1966–74.
42. Tomassetti P, Campana D, Piscitelli L, Casadei R, Santini D, Nori F, et al. Endocrine pancreatic tumors: factors correlated with survival. Ann Oncol. 2005;16(11):1806–10.
43. DeOliveira ML, Winter JM, Schafer M, Cunningham SC, Cameron JL, Yeo CJ, et al. Assessment of complications after pancreatic surgery: a novel grading system applied to 633 patients undergoing pancreaticoduodenectomy. Ann Surg. 2006;244(6):931–7; discussion 7–9.

44. Di Sabatino A, Carsetti R, Corazza GR. Post-splenectomy and hyposplenic states. Lancet. 2011;378(9785):86–97.
45. Hernandez MC, Khasawneh M, Contreras-Peraza N, Lohse C, Stephens D, Kim BD, et al. Vaccination and splenectomy in Olmsted County. Surgery. 2019;166(4):556–63.
46. Senthinathan P, Jankar SV, Sabnis SC, Kaje V, Srivatsan Gurumurthy S, Anand Vijai N, et al. Laparoscopic total pancreatectomy for multiple endocrine neoplasia type 1 syndrome-associated multifocal, non-functioning pancreatic neuroendocrine tumor: a case report. Asian J Endosc Surg. 2017;10(4):434–7.
47. Hüttner FJ, Koessler-Ebs J, Hackert T, Ulrich A, Büchler MW, Diener MK. Meta-analysis of surgical outcome after enucleation versus standard resection for pancreatic neoplasms. Br J Surg. 2015;102(9):1026–36.
48. Huang LC, Poultsides GA, Norton JA. Surgical management of neuroendocrine tumors of the gastrointestinal tract. Oncology (Williston Park). 2011;25(9):794–803.
49. Zogakis TG, Gibril F, Libutti SK, Norton JA, White DE, Jensen RT, et al. Management and outcome of patients with sporadic gastrinoma arising in the duodenum. Ann Surg. 2003;238(1):42–8.
50. Burghardt L, Meier JJ, Uhl W, Kahle-Stefan M, Schmidt WE, Nauck MA. Importance of localization of insulinomas: a systematic analysis. J Hepatobiliary Pancreat Sci. 2019;26(9):383–92.
51. Spinelli A, Del Fabbro D, Sacchi M, Zerbi A, Torzilli G, Lutman FR, et al. Intraoperative ultrasound with contrast medium in resective pancreatic surgery: a pilot study. World J Surg. 2011;35(11):2521–7.
52. Norton JA, Harris EJ, Chen Y, Visser BC, Poultsides GA, Kunz PC, et al. Pancreatic endocrine tumors with major vascular abutment, involvement, or encasement and indication for resection. Arch Surg. 2011;146(6):724–32.
53. Thiels CA, Bergquist JR, Laan DV, Croome KP, Smoot RL, Nagorney DM, et al. Outcomes of pancreaticoduodenectomy for pancreatic neuroendocrine tumors: are combined procedures justified? J Gastrointest Surg. 2016;20(5):891–8.
54. Prakash L, Lee JE, Yao J, Bhosale P, Balachandran A, Wang H, et al. Role and operative technique of portal venous tumor thrombectomy in patients with pancreatic neuroendocrine tumors. J Gastrointest Surg. 2015;19(11):2011–8.
55. Prakash L, Bhosale P, Cloyd J, Kim M, Parker N, Yao J, et al. Role of fluorouracil, doxorubicin, and streptozocin therapy in the preoperative treatment of localized pancreatic neuroendocrine tumors. J Gastrointest Surg. 2017;21(1):155–63.
56. Hüttner FJ, Schneider L, Tarantino I, Warschkow R, Schmied BM, Hackert T, et al. Palliative resection of the primary tumor in 442 metastasized neuroendocrine tumors of the pancreas: a population-based, propensity score-matched survival analysis. Langenbeck's Arch Surg. 2015;400(6):715–23.
57. Bertani E, Fazio N, Radice D, Zardini C, Spinoglio G, Chiappa A, et al. Assessing the role of primary tumour resection in patients with synchronous unresectable liver metastases from pancreatic neuroendocrine tumour of the body and tail. A propensity score survival evaluation. Eur J Surg Oncol. 2017;43(2):372–9.
58. Starr JS, Sonbol MB, Hobday TJ, Sharma A, Kendi AT, Halfdanarson TR. Peptide receptor radionuclide therapy for the treatment of pancreatic neuroendocrine tumors: recent insights. Onco Targets Ther. 2020;13:3545–55.
59. Bertani E, Fazio N, Radice D, Zardini C, Grana C, Bodei L, et al. Resection of the primary tumor followed by peptide receptor radionuclide therapy as upfront strategy for the treatment of G1-G2 pancreatic neuroendocrine tumors with unresectable liver metastases. Ann Surg Oncol. 2016;23(Suppl 5):981–9.
60. Brighi N, Lamberti G, Maggio I, Manuzzi L, Ricci C, Casadei R, et al. Biliary stone disease in patients receiving somatostatin analogs for neuroendocrine neoplasms. A retrospective observational study. Dig Liver Dis. 2019;51(5):689–94.

61. Jayakrishnan TT, Groeschl RT, George B, Thomas JP, Clark Gamblin T, Turaga KK. Review of the impact of antineoplastic therapies on the risk for cholelithiasis and acute cholecystitis. Ann Surg Oncol. 2014;21(1):240–7.
62. Mirakhur B, Pavel ME, Pommier RF, Fisher GA, Phan AT, Massien C, et al. Biochemical responses in symptomatic and asymptomatic patients with neuroendocrine tumors: pooled analysis of 2 phase 3 trials. Endocr Pract. 2018;24(11):948–62.
63. Gerson JN, Witteles RM, Chang DT, Beygui RE, Iagaru AH, Kunz PL. Carcinoid syndrome complicating a pancreatic neuroendocrine tumor: a case report. Pancreas. 2017;46(10):1381–5.
64. Tsoukalas N, Chatzellis E, Rontogianni D, Alexandraki KI, Boutzios G, Angelousi A, et al. Pancreatic carcinoids (serotonin-producing pancreatic neuroendocrine neoplasms): report of 5 cases and review of the literature. Medicine (Baltimore). 2017;96(16):e6201.
65. Lillemoe HA, Aloia TA. Enhanced recovery after surgery: hepatobiliary. Surg Clin North Am. 2018;98(6):1251–64.
66. Lavu H, McCall NS, Winter JM, Burkhart RA, Pucci M, Leiby BE, et al. Enhancing patient outcomes while containing costs after complex abdominal operation: a randomized controlled trial of the Whipple accelerated recovery pathway. J Am Coll Surg. 2019;228(4):415–24.
67. Linnemann RJA, Patijn GA, van Rijssen LB, Besselink MG, Mungroop TH, de Hingh IH, et al. The role of abdominal drainage in pancreatic resection - a multicenter validation study for early drain removal. Pancreatology. 2019;19(6):888–96.
68. Zaghal A, Tamim H, Habib S, Jaafar R, Mukherji D, Khalife M, et al. Drain or no drain following pancreaticoduodenectomy: the unsolved dilemma. Scand J Surg. 2020;109(3):228–37.
69. Narayanan S, Martin AN, Turrentine FE, Bauer TW, Adams RB, Zaydfudim VM. Mortality after pancreaticoduodenectomy: assessing early and late causes of patient death. J Surg Res. 2018;231:304–8.
70. Kagedan DJ, Ahmed M, Devitt KS, Wei AC. Enhanced recovery after pancreatic surgery: a systematic review of the evidence. HPB (Oxford). 2015;17(1):11–6.
71. Callery MP, Pratt WB, Kent TS, Chaikof EL, Vollmer CM Jr. A prospectively validated clinical risk score accurately predicts pancreatic fistula after pancreatoduodenectomy. J Am Coll Surg. 2013;216(1):1–14.
72. Trudeau MT, Casciani F, Ecker BL, Maggino L, Seykora TF, Puri P, et al. The fistula risk score catalog: toward precision medicine for pancreatic fistula after pancreatoduodenectomy. Ann Surg. 2020; https://doi.org/10.1097/SLA.0000000000004068.
73. Søreide K, Healey AJ, Mole DJ, Parks RW. Pre-, peri- and post-operative factors for the development of pancreatic fistula after pancreatic surgery. HPB (Oxford). 2019;21(12):1621–31.
74. Strobel O, Cherrez A, Hinz U, Mayer P, Kaiser J, Fritz S, et al. Risk of pancreatic fistula after enucleation of pancreatic tumours. Br J Surg. 2015;102(10):1258–66.
75. Chua TC, Yang TX, Gill AJ, Samra JS. Systematic review and meta-analysis of enucleation versus standardized resection for small pancreatic lesions. Ann Surg Oncol. 2016;23(2):592–9.
76. Bassi C, Marchegiani G, Dervenis C, Sarr M, Abu Hilal M, Adham M, et al. The 2016 update of the international study group (ISGPS) definition and grading of postoperative pancreatic fistula: 11 years after. Surgery. 2017;161(3):584–91.
77. Malleo G, Pulvirenti A, Marchegiani G, Butturini G, Salvia R, Bassi C. Diagnosis and management of postoperative pancreatic fistula. Langenbeck's Arch Surg. 2014;399(7):801–10.
78. Callery MP, Pratt WB, Vollmer CM Jr. Prevention and management of pancreatic fistula. J Gastrointest Surg. 2009;13(1):163–73.
79. McMillan MT, Fisher WE, Van Buren G 2nd, McElhany A, Bloomston M, Hughes SJ, et al. The value of drains as a fistula mitigation strategy for pancreatoduodenectomy: something for everyone? Results of a randomized prospective multi-institutional study. J Gastrointest Surg. 2015;19(1):21–30; discussion −1.
80. Tseng DS, Molenaar IQ, Besselink MG, van Eijck CH, Borel Rinkes IH, van Santvoort HC. Pancreatic exocrine insufficiency in patients with pancreatic or periampullary cancer: a systematic review. Pancreas. 2016;45(3):325–30.

81. Rickels MR, Bellin M, Toledo FG, Robertson RP, Andersen DK, Chari ST, et al. Detection, evaluation and treatment of diabetes mellitus in chronic pancreatitis: recommendations from PancreasFest 2012. Pancreatology. 2013;13(4):336–42.
82. Wu L, Nahm CB, Jamieson NB, Samra J, Clifton-Bligh R, Mittal A, et al. Risk factors for development of diabetes mellitus (Type 3c) after partial pancreatectomy: a systematic review. Clin Endocrinol. 2020;92(5):396–406.

Part V
Interventional Treatment of Endocrine Disorders

Chapter 16
Interventional Treatment of Primary Aldosteronism

Christos Georgiades, Panagiotis Liasides, and Kelvin Hong

Introduction

Primary aldosteronism (PA) is the excessive production of aldosterone by one or both adrenal glands resulting in related clinical signs and symptoms. It is an underappreciated cause of hypertension with a reported prevalence between 2.7% and 10% among the hypertensive population [1–3]. Considering there are more than 65 million Americans diagnosed with hypertension (HTN) [4], PA is the causative factor in two to seven million patients who are mislabeled as "essential" hypertensives. In approximately one-third of these, PA is due to a unilateral functioning adrenal adenoma, while the rest are due to bilateral hyperplasia or bilateral adenomas [5]. It is staggering then to consider that one to two million Americans are suffering from a more virulent form of HTN compared to its "essential" counterpart one that can potentially be cured if diagnosed and treated. Indeed, it has been shown that PA is associated with accelerated and worse cardiovascular outcomes compared to those from primary hypertension, including the risk of coronary artery disease and cerebrovascular stroke [6].

Unilateral total, or when feasible partial, adrenalectomy is the standard of care for a functioning adrenal adenoma causing medication-resistant PA. Minimally invasive, image-guided treatments have recently become available to the wider

C. Georgiades (✉) · K. Hong
Department of Radiology & Radiological Sciences, Johns Hopkins University,
Baltimore, MD, USA
e-mail: Khong1@jhmi.edu

P. Liasides
USC Medical Center, Los Angeles, CA, USA

Division of Trauma and Surgical Critical Care, University of Southern California Keck
School of Medicine, Los Angeles, CA, USA

© The Author(s), under exclusive license to Springer Nature
Switzerland AG 2022

H. Yu et al. (eds.), *Diagnosis and Management of Endocrine Disorders in
Interventional Radiology*, https://doi.org/10.1007/978-3-030-87189-5_16

public, and accumulating evidence points to high efficacy and an excellent safety profile. These image-guided treatments include percutaneous ablation and endovascular embolization of the unilateral functioning adrenal adenoma.

Adrenal Vein Sampling

Prior to any non-pharmaceutical definitive treatment, confirmation of a unilateral source of independent and excessive aldosterone production as well as lateralization is necessary [7]. This is achieved with adrenal vein sampling (AVS). Rarely, unilateral adrenal hyperplasia and contralateral nonfunctioning adenoma can coexist. If resection of the adenoma is performed without prior AVS confirmation, the patient will continue to suffer from PA and miss the opportunity for curative resection. There exist different technical protocols on how to perform AVS. The most rigorous, sensitive, and specific one includes pre- and post-adrenocorticotropic hormone (ACTH) stimulation sampling and the use of C-arm CT to confirm selectivity in order to render biochemical lateralization reliable [3, 8]. Briefly, both adrenal veins are selected with catheters from a common femoral vein approach (Fig. 16.1c and d). A C-arm CT is performed during contrast injection to confirm selectivity (Fig. 16.1c and d). Venous blood sampling is performed, followed by ACTH administration. Sampling is repeated 30 min post-ACTH stimulation. Cortisol adrenal vein levels are compared to that from inferior vena cava (IVC) levels to confirm catheter selectivity. Once selectivity is confirmed, aldosterone levels are compared between adrenal vein samples to confirm lateralization. If both catheter selectivity and biochemical lateralization are confirmed, surgical or image-guided treatment can be undertaken. Less rigorous protocols sample the adrenal veins only post-ACTH stimulation. Though less time-consuming, this protocol can result in false-negative results in approximately 22% of patients tested [8].

Ablation

Ablation refers to the destruction of targeted tissue by way of heating (radiofrequency ablation [RFA] or microwave ablation [MWA]) or freezing (cryoablation). Current technology allows effective ablation for lesions up to around 3–4 cm in diameter, which is inclusive of the majority of functioning adrenal adenomas. The technical objective of ablation is to kill the entire targeted functioning adrenal tissue without damaging nearby collateral structures such as the bowel, pancreas, kidney, etc. The clinical objective is to significantly reduce the patient's blood pressure, eliminate/reduce the number of antihypertensive medications, and eliminate hypokalemia and the need for potassium supplementation.

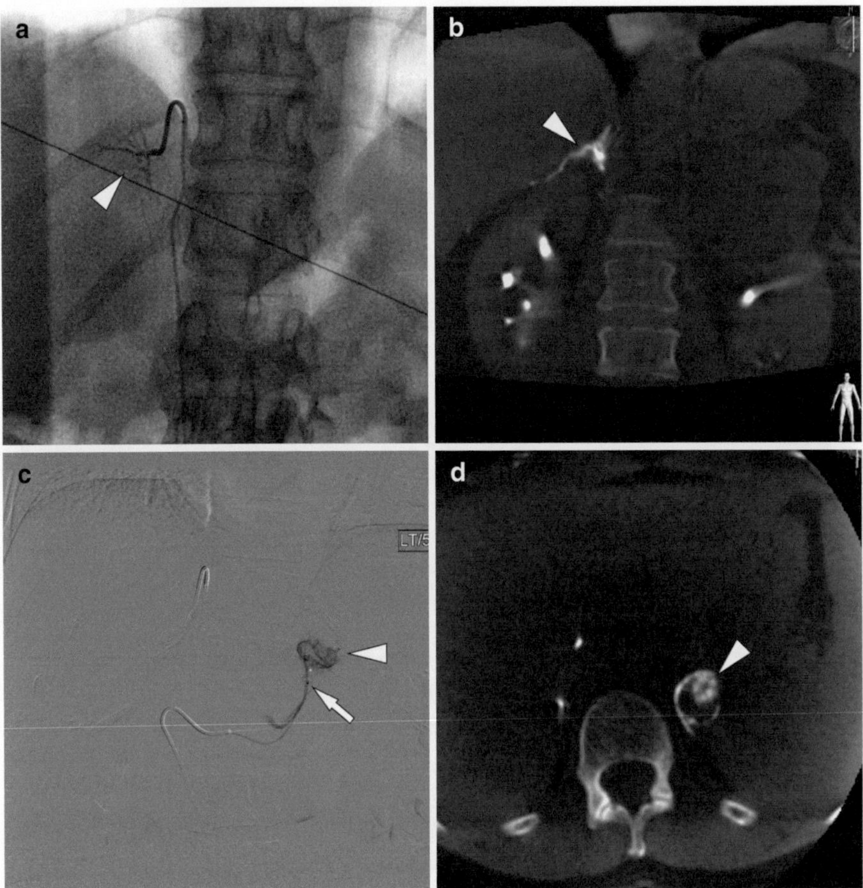

Fig. 16.1 Adrenal vein sampling in a patient with PA and a left adrenal adenoma noted on diagnostic MRI. Right adrenal venogram (**a**) via a catheter shows the classic "feathery" appearance of the adrenal gland (white arrowhead). Coronal C-arm CT during the venogram (**b**) shows diffuse parenchymal enhancement of the right adrenal gland (white arrowhead), confirming catheter selectivity. Digital subtraction venogram of the left adrenal gland (**c**) via a super-selective microcatheter (white arrow) shows enhancement of the left adrenal nodule (white arrowhead). Axial C-arm CT during the left adrenal venogram (**d**) shows enhancement of the left adrenal adenoma (white arrowhead), confirming catheter selectivity

Patient Preparation

Unilateral functioning aldosteronoma is confirmed by AVS. A cross-sectional imaging study (CT or MRI, Fig. 16.2a) is reviewed to ensure there is a safe ablation window. Eight-hour fasting is required as the procedure is performed with the patient under conscious sedation or possibly general anesthesia. One of the perioperative risks is catecholamine shock, which manifests as severe hypertension and/or arrhythmia and can be life-threatening. To reduce this risk, a 5-day premedication

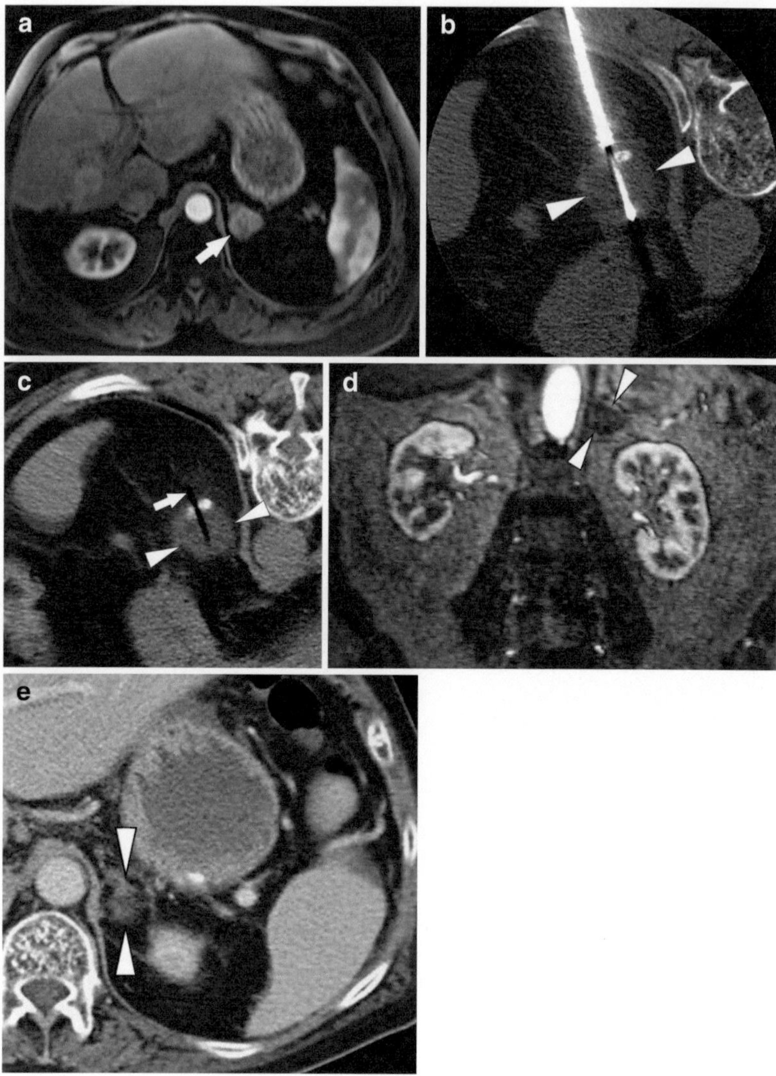

Fig. 16.2 A 55-year-old male with severe chronic hypertension resistant to five antihypertensive medications and with hypokalemia. The plasma aldosterone-to-renin ratio was elevated. The patient had a prior AVS, which confirmed a functioning aldosteronoma in the left adrenal gland. Contrast-enhanced, T1-weighted, fat-suppressed MR image (**a**) shows a 2.5 cm hyper-vascular left adrenal mass (white arrow). Axial CT image during cryoablation (**b**) shows the cryo-needle penetrating the left adrenal mass (white arrowheads). Post-cryoablation CT (**c**) shows the still frozen left adrenal mass (white arrowheads) and the "ghost" trajectory of the removed cryo-needle (white arrow). Within days post-cryoablation, the patient's blood pressure showed a significant reduction, the number of antihypertensive medications dropped from 5 to 2, and the patient no longer required potassium supplementation. One-month post-cryoablation, coronal, contrast-enhanced MR image (**d**) shows a complete devascularization (lack of contrast enhancement) of the ablated adrenal nodule (white arrowheads). One-year, axial, post-ablation, contrast-enhanced CT image (**e**) shows size reduction and persistent devascularization (lack of enhancement) of the left adrenal nodule (white arrowheads)

with both alpha- and beta-blockers is strongly recommended. Ablation is performed with the patient in the prone position and in the CT scanner. In addition, if cryoablation is chosen, it should be remembered that in case of emergency, the cryoprobes will take 2–3 min to be adequately thawed for removal. To further reduce the risk of adverse outcomes from possible arrhythmia, the placement of external pacing pads is also recommended.

Procedure

The procedure is performed under continuous patient monitoring. After sedation induction and aseptic preparation, a baseline CT is obtained to plan probe access/ trajectory. The probe is inserted into the targeted lesion (Fig. 16.2b). After ablation is completed, the probe is removed, and a repeat non-contrast CT is obtained to exclude immediate complications, such as hemorrhage or pneumothorax (Fig. 16.2c). The patient is recovered, observed for a minimum of 3 h, and discharged to home.

Follow-Up

Because of the possibility of the post-ablation precipitous blood pressure drop as aldosterone levels drop, the patient is advised to monitor blood pressure at home and consult his/her primary care or interventionalist for a possible reduction of the number or dosages of his/her antihypertensive medications. Long-term follow-up relies solely on the stability or recurrence of symptoms and/or signs of hyperaldosteronism and not on imaging response, though the latter can be confirmatory for complete tissue ablation (Fig. 16.2d and e).

Outcomes

An important meta-analysis by Liang et al. included a total of 89 patients (7 studies) with clinical symptoms from PA who were treated with thermal ablation. During the nearly 4-year follow-up, 75% of patients saw significant and sustained improvement or the resolution of their HTN with a mean systolic blood pressure reduction of 29.06 mm Hg (95% confidence interval [CI], −33.93 to −24.19) and mean diastolic blood pressure reduction of 16.03 mm Hg (95% CI, −18.33 to −13.73). All patients saw a reduction in the number of antihypertensives used and potassium levels normalized in all seven studies [9]. Though not as important as clinical follow-up, imaging response can also provide evidence as to the efficacy of percutaneous ablation. In a prospective study, Nunes TF et al. reported a 94% (16/17) complete and sustained imaging response rate [10]. Early data on the biochemical response after ablation are equally promising, with a reported normalization of aldosterone levels in nearly 90% of patients treated. Aldosterone levels decreased from a baseline of 63.3 ng/dL ± 28.0 to 13.3 ng/dL ± 13.5 post-ablation (P = 0.008), with a concomitant decrease in systolic, diastolic, and mean blood pressures [11].

Embolization

During embolization, the operator seeks to select the arterial supply to the adrenal adenoma and effect ischemic necrosis. Vascular anatomy knowledge and experience with embolization are both key factors for optimum outcomes. Arterial supply to the right adrenal gland is usually from the proximal right renal artery, while to the left adrenal gland directly from the aorta. Frequently, however, there can be normal variants complicating adrenal artery identification and selection. Embolization can be achieved with a variety of methods, and the specific choice is operator dependent. Choices include bland particles (ischemic necrosis), alcohol (ischemia and direct cytotoxicity) or lipiodol (ischemia and direct cytotoxicity), or any combination of the above. The use of embolization coils alone is discouraged as the target adenoma may develop collateral vascular supply and survive.

Patient Preparation

Patient preparation is identical to that for ablation, except that no external pacing pads are necessary since the patient is supine during the procedure. Again, a review of the baseline cross-sectional imaging is important in treatment planning (Fig. 16.3a).

Procedure

Vascular access can be a common femoral or radial artery. A pigtail catheter is used to perform a juxta-renal aortogram to identify the arterial supply to the targeted adrenal artery (Fig. 16.3b). A long sheath or reverse curve catheter alone is used to select the ostium of the adrenal or renal artery (Fig. 16.3c). A coaxially placed microcatheter is then used to super-select the adrenal artery (Fig. 16.3d). The optimum location of the catheter is one from which the entire adenoma can be embolized and avoids nontarget embolization. From this location, embolization is performed using the operator's choice of embolic agent to complete stasis. A minimum of 6-h observation post-embolization is recommended, both for vitals and arterial puncture site monitoring.

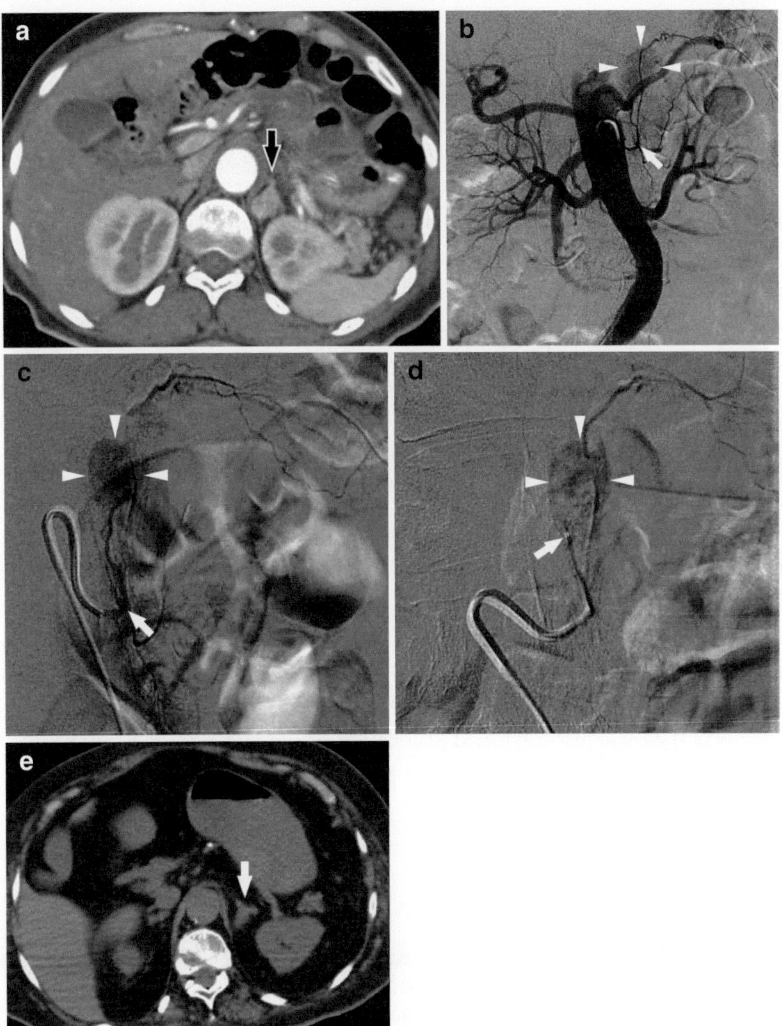

Fig. 16.3 A 60-year-old female with progressive bulbar palsy (PBP), severe uncontrolled hypertension, and hypokalemia. An elevated aldosterone-to-renin ratio prompted AVS, which was selective and biochemically lateralized to the left adrenal gland. Because of her PBP she was not a surgical candidate and referred for endovascular embolization of the functioning adenoma. Axial, contrast-enhanced CT image (**a**) shows a 2 cm enhancing nodule in the left adrenal gland. Digitally subtracted, abdominal aortogram (**b**) shows a left adrenal artery (white arrow) supplying a hypervascular mass in the left adrenal gland (white arrows). Digital subtraction left adrenal arteriogram (**c**) via a reverse curve catheter with its tip in the ostium of the left adrenal artery (white arrow) shows the hyper-vascular mass to better advantage (white arrowheads). Digital subtraction, selective adrenal arteriogram (**d**) via a coaxially placed microcatheter with its tip in the distal left adrenal artery (white arrow) was used to deliver 2 cc of ethanol into the targeted mass (white arrowheads). The patient's hypertension resolved within 1 week of the procedure, and the patient required no antihypertensive medications or further potassium supplementation. Axial, nonenhanced CT, 6-month post-embolization (**e**) shows near resolution of the left adrenal nodule (white arrow)

Follow-Up

Follow-up is identical to that of ablation (Fig. 16.3e).

Outcomes

A review of the literature suggests that ethanol embolization is the preferred method. In a study with 33 patients with PA, Octoate et al. reported a significant reduction in blood pressure after embolization. Interestingly, the author reported blood pressure reduction in all (100%) of patients younger than 45 years old and only in half of those older than 45 years old [12]. This likely reflects the fact that older patients have essential hypertension in addition to PA.

Conclusion

Though still sparse, there is accumulating evidence that interventional treatments of clinically evident primary aldosteronism can be viable alternatives in nonsurgical patients. For patients with AVS-confirmed, unilateral hyperfunctioning adrenal adenomas, early data suggest a clinical efficacy of around 75% with a low procedure-related (ablation or embolization) risk profile.

References

1. Brown MA, Cramp HA, Zammit VC, Whitworth JA. Primary hyperaldosteronism: a missed diagnosis in "essential hypertensives"? Aust NZ J Med. 1996;26:533–8.
2. Nadar S, Lip GY, Beevers DG. Primary hyperaldosteronism. Ann Clin Biochem. 2003;40:439–52.
3. Georgiades CS, Hong K, Geschwind JF, et al. Adjunctive use of C-arm CT may eliminate technical failure in adrenal vein sampling. J Vasc Interv Radiol. 2007;18(9):1102–5.
4. Wang TJ, Vasan RS. Epidemiology of uncontrolled hypertension in the United States. Circulation. 2005;112:1651–62.
5. Mattsson C, Young WF Jr. Primary aldosteronism: diagnostic and treatment strategies. Nat Clin Pract Nephrol. 2006;2:198–208.
6. Chen ZW, Tsai CH, Pan CT, Chou CH, Liao CW, Hung CS, Wu VC, Lin YH, TAIPAI Study Group. Endothelial dysfunction in primary aldosteronism. Int J Mol Sci. 2019;20(20):5214–39.
7. Gordon RD, Stowasser M, Rutherford JC. Primary aldosteronism: are we diagnosing and operating on too few patients? World J Surg. 2001;25(7):941–7.
8. Violari EG, Arici M, Singh CK, et al. Adrenal vein sampling with and without cosyntropin stimulation for detection of surgically remediable aldosteronism. Endocrinol Diabetes Metab. 2019;2(2):e00066.

 9. Liang KW, Jahangiri Y, Tsao TF, Tyan YS, Huang HH. Effectiveness of thermal ablation for aldosterone-producing adrenal adenoma: a systematic review and meta-analysis of clinical and biochemical parameters. J Vasc Interv Radiol. 2019;30(9):1335–42.
10. Nunes TF, Szejnfeld D, Szejnfeld J, et al. Assessment of early treatment response with DWI after CT-guided radiofrequency ablation of functioning adrenal adenomas. AJR Am J Roentgenol. 2016;207(4):804–10.
11. Szejnfeld D, Nunes TF, Giordano EE, et al. Radiofrequency ablation of functioning adrenal adenomas: preliminary clinical and laboratory findings. J Vasc Interv Radiol. 2015;26(10):1459–64.
12. Octoate H, Inoue H, Baba Y, Tsuchimochi S, Nakajo M. Aldosteronomas: experience with superselective adrenal arterial embolization in 33 cases. Radiology. 2003;227(2):401–6.

Chapter 17
Interventional Treatment of Hyperparathyroidism

Chengzhong Peng and Qian Yang

Percutaneous chemical and thermal ablations are two main techniques for the interventional treatment of parathyroid diseases. For chemical ablation, ultrasonographic-guided percutaneous access of the parathyroid gland is performed using a needle, and the target tissue is destroyed by injecting either ethanol or calcitriol. For thermal ablation, an electrode is inserted percutaneously into the parathyroid gland under ultrasound guidance, and the target tissue is ablated using either radiofrequency, microwave, or laser technique. Currently, thermal ablation is the most used percutaneous method for hyperparathyroidism.

History of Interventional Treatment of Hyperparathyroidism

In 1984, Solbiati et al. first described percutaneous injection of ethanol into the parathyroid gland under ultrasound guidance to treat secondary hyperparathyroidism (SHPT) [1]. The technique, however, has not been widely adopted due to difficulty in localization and multiple complications.

Later in 1992, Giangrande et al. reported a successful reduction of parathyroid hormone (PTH) concentration in 50 uremic patients who underwent percutaneous injection of ethanol into 4 parathyroid glands simultaneously [2]. The treatment subsequently improved hypercalcemia, making it possible for the patients to start or to increase daily vitamin D treatment.

The original version of the book has been revised. The correction to this book can be found at https://doi.org/10.1007/978-3-030-87189-5_22

C. Peng (✉)
Department of Ultrasound, Zhejiang Provincial People's Hospital, and Hangzhou Medical College, Hangzhou, Zhejiang, China

Q. Yang
Laboratory for Investigatory Imaging, School of Health and Rehabilitation Sciences, The Ohio State University, Columbus, USA

© The Author(s), under exclusive license to Springer Nature Switzerland AG 2022, corrected publication 2022

243

H. Yu et al. (eds.), *Diagnosis and Management of Endocrine Disorders in Interventional Radiology*, https://doi.org/10.1007/978-3-030-87189-5_17

The percutaneous injection technique evolved in 1994 by Japanese researchers, Fukagawa et al., who reported interventional treatment of parathyroid hyperplasia in chronic dialysis patients [3]. Using color Doppler ultrasonography, they could optimize the site and volume of ethanol injection with better detection of the recurrence of parathyroid cell growth and lower risk of complications.

Despite promising data from previous studies, in most cases, SHPT may not be treated entirely by percutaneous ethanol injection alone due to a rebound of PTH. Also, injection-related complications frequently occur from extravasation of ethanol, including local pain and recurrent laryngeal nerve injury. Therefore, ethanol injection is used only for additional treatment after surgery or thermal ablation.

The local injection of calcitriol has been proposed by Fukagawa et al. as an alternative method for treating secondary hyperparathyroidism [4]. Direct injection of calcitriol in the parathyroid gland results in high local concentration and, therefore, maximizes the effect on the vitamin D receptors and avoids adverse reactions from hypercalcemia commonly encountered after systemic administration. This method is considered safer with less risk for pain and recurrent laryngeal nerve injury than ethanol injection. However, the actual therapeutic effect is only temporary due to the resecretion of PTH from the hyperplastic parathyroid gland shortly after the injection as the local concentration of calcitriol decreases. Therefore, local injection of calcitriol is used only for palliative treatment in a patient who is not a candidate for either surgery or thermal ablation.

While the applications of various thermal ablation technologies to the liver, lung, kidney, bone, and other soft tissues have been well established, data for the parathyroid gland are relatively limited [5–10]. In 2001, Bennedbaek et al. first reported a laser ablation in the parathyroid gland and showed its safety and effectiveness in primary hyperparathyroidism (PHPT) [11]. Since then, the thermal ablation technique has been gradually adopted for patients with PHPT [12–14]. However, the method was not widely accepted for patients with SHPT until 2012, when Kovatcheva et al. reported successful application of thermal ablation in treating SHPT [15]. Later in 2013, Zhang et al. reported more favorable outcomes with detailed follow-ups in Chinese patients who underwent thermal ablation for SHPT [16]. The data were also supported by a similar study by Peng et al. who further expanded the application to SHPT [17–19]. More data show thermal ablation as a safe and reliable method for treating SHPT, especially for patients who are not a surgical candidate or have relapsed after surgery. Thermal ablation is considered an essential supplementary treatment method for intractable SHPT [20–22].

Percutaneous Thermal Ablation of Parathyroid Glands

Under ultrasound guidance, an electrode is percutaneously advanced into the parathyroid gland. Radiofrequency, microwave, or laser is then used to generate heat and destroy the target tissue thus reducing PTH secretion. Irreversible coagulation necrosis is induced with a local temperature greater than 60 °C. Radiofrequency and microwave are the two most frequently used technologies for thermal ablation of the parathyroid gland. The use of laser ablation is relatively limited due to the difficulty in adjusting the optical fiber position.

Preprocedural Evaluation

Parathyroid lesions casing SHPT can be multifocal. Therefore, a careful and thorough evaluation of the size, number, and location of the parathyroid glands is essential before the procedure.

Frequently used imaging modalities include ultrasonography, radionuclide imaging, computed tomography (CT), and magnetic resonance imaging (MRI) [23]. Ultrasonography is considered the primary imaging modality, readily available for evaluating anatomical structures. Also, procedures are performed under ultrasound guidance. Therefore, detecting all lesions beforehand is crucial [17]. However, ultrasonography is operator-dependent. Also, it cannot visualize the lesion when it is located in the retrosternal space. On the other hand, radionuclide imaging is a functional imaging modality for detecting hypersecretory parathyroid glands. While the specificity of radionuclide imaging is very high for assessing hyperparathyroidism, it has low sensitivity. CT and MRI are commonly used for the evaluation of anatomical structures, especially for retrosternal ectopic parathyroid glands. However, they cannot detect a parathyroid gland smaller than 1 cm due to their limited resolution. In general, for preprocedural evaluation, ultrasonography and radionuclide imaging are routinely used. CT and MRI can be considered for cases with suspicious retrosternal ectopic parathyroid glands.

Indications and Contraindications

Indications

Currently, there are no consensus guidelines specific for the parathyroid thermal ablation. For PHPT, the National Institutes of Health's surgical standards in the United States are used. For SHPT, the K/DOQI guidelines and recommendations are used [24].

Indications for PHPT Thermal Ablation

1. Symptomatic PHPT: Including coexisting conditions such as kidney stones, neuromuscular symptoms, neuropsychiatric symptoms, bone diseases, peptic ulcer disease, etc.
2. Asymptomatic PHPT: Parathyroid ablation can be considered for those who meet one of the following conditions:

   (1) Significant hypercalcemia (the blood calcium level is higher than the upper limit of normal blood calcium by 0.25 mmol/L).
   (2) Significantly high urine calcium (24-h urine calcium >400 mg).
   (3) The creatinine clearance rate is reduced by 30% compared with the same age group.

(4) The T score of the dual-energy X-ray absorptiometry of the lumbar spine, hip, or forearms is less than -2.5.
(5) Age <50 years old.
(6) For patients who do not want medical treatment or follow-ups.

Indications for SHPT Thermal Ablation

1. Intact PTH level >800 pgml persistently
2. Resistance to medications such as active vitamin D and its analogs
3. When medication is ineffective with persistent hypercalcemia and/or hyperphosphatemia
4. Progressive extraosseous calcification
5. Imaging indicators:

    (1) Four or more hyperplastic parathyroid glands found on ultrasonography.
    (2) For patients with three or less hyperplastic parathyroid glands on ultrasound, radionuclide imaging, and CT or MRI are required to exclude ectopic parathyroid glands.

Contraindications:

Excluded if any of the following is met:

1. Body temperature >37.5 °C
2. Systemic or local acute infection
3. Severe bleeding tendency or coagulopathy
4. Severe abnormal heart and lung function
5. Presence of hoarseness or abnormal vocal cord activity
6. Parathyroid glands with an excessive size or deep location (for those who cannot tolerate surgery or anesthesia, partial ablation or palliative treatment may be considered)
7. Patients with retrosternal ectopic parathyroid glands that are difficult to be visualized with ultrasonography
8. Patients who either have mental disorders or cannot cooperate during the procedure

Preparation Before Thermal Ablation

Equipment Preparation

1. Ultrasound equipment:
    A Doppler ultrasound supporting contrast-enhanced imaging with a high-frequency probe is generally used. The probe frequency range of 5–12 MHz is recommended.

2. Ablation equipment:

   Radiofrequency and microwave ablation systems suitable for superficial organs are used. Generally, an ablation electrode length between 7 and 10 cm with an outer diameter of 17–19 G and electrode tip length of 5–10 mm are recommended. A radiofrequency ablation system with cold circulation is preferred.

Preparation of Medication and Needles

1. Medication preparation: Ultrasound contrast agents (such as sulfur hexafluoride microbubbles), local anesthetics (such as lidocaine and bupivacaine), and sterile isolation fluid for hydrodissection or liquid isolation (such as 5% glucose solution) are recommended. Intraoperative antihypertensives should be prepared for patients with high blood pressure.
2. Needle preparation: A 5–7 cm, 21–23 G, Chiba needle is mainly used for injecting isolation fluid for hydrodissection or liquid isolation.

Patient Preparation

1. Physical examinations and medical history: patients undergo physical examinations, and pertinent medical history is obtained. Medical history should include cardiac, pulmonary and brain diseases, hypertension, and diabetes. Before the procedure, all patients should actively be engaged in the treatment of their underlying diseases and improving their physical health.
2. Preoperative laboratory tests: including complete blood count, urine culture and urinalysis, blood type and screen, coagulation function, liver function, renal function, electrolytes, parathyroid hormones, tumor markers, and infectious disease examination.
3. Preprocedural examination: including parathyroid ultrasound imaging, parathyroid radionuclide imaging, chest X-ray or chest CT, bone density, electrocardiogram, echocardiogram, etc.
4. All medications for anticoagulation need to be discontinued. Aspirin and warfarin need to be stopped a week and 4–5 days before the procedure, respectively.
5. For hemodialysis patients, the last hemodialysis immediately before the procedure (including the first hemodialysis after the procedure) should be performed without heparin.
6. If the patient has a history of neck surgery, especially a history of recurrent laryngeal nerve damage, laryngoscopy is required to evaluate the vocal cords.
7. Informed consent: the patient and their family members should be informed of the patient's condition before treatment, alternative treatments, the procedure details of thermal ablation and possible complications during and after the procedure, and the additional treatments.

Thermal Ablation Procedure

Patient Position

The patient is positioned in supine, with a soft cushion below the neck, so that the head is slightly tilted back to fully expose the front of the neck. The operator is by the bed on one side of the patient, holding the patient's head with one hand and the ablation needle or puncture needle with the other hand.

Ultrasound Evaluation Before Ablation

Before the procedure, the size, number, location, and internal structure of the bilateral parathyroid glands are evaluated using ultrasound. Contrast-enhanced ultrasonographic imaging is then performed to evaluate the parathyroid gland's microcirculation. At this point, a needle access route is determined.

Local Anesthesia

There are two methods of anesthesia, including local anesthesia and cervical plexus block. Local anesthesia is done via a skin puncture site by injecting lidocaine or bupivacaine under ultrasound guidance. Local anesthetics are injected before the ablation of each parathyroid gland. Additionally, an ultrasound-guided cervical plexus block can be performed. The needle is inserted from the posterior edge of the sternocleidomastoid muscle at the third and fourth cervical spine levels, and lidocaine or bupivacaine is injected into the superficial cervical nerve plexus in the prevertebral fascia located behind the sternocleidomastoid muscle.

Liquid Isolation

The parathyroid glands are located posterior to the thyroid glands, lateral to the trachea and esophagus, and medial to the carotids, internal jugular veins, and vagus nerves. The parathyroid glands are also close to the longus colli muscle and sympathetic nerves. Therefore, it is crucial to protect the surrounding structures from heat damage during the procedure. Hydrodissection or liquid isolation is one of the most critical and widely used techniques. Under ultrasound guidance, a 20–23 G needle is inserted into the space around the parathyroid gland and infuse 10–50 ml of 5% glucose solution to create a liquid "isolation zone" with a distance greater than 5 mm between the parathyroid gland and the carotid artery, trachea, esophagus, and recurrent laryngeal nerve. The parathyroid gland is isolated into either an "island shape" or a "peninsula shape" (Fig. 17.1); thereby, the heat spread is prevented during the procedure.

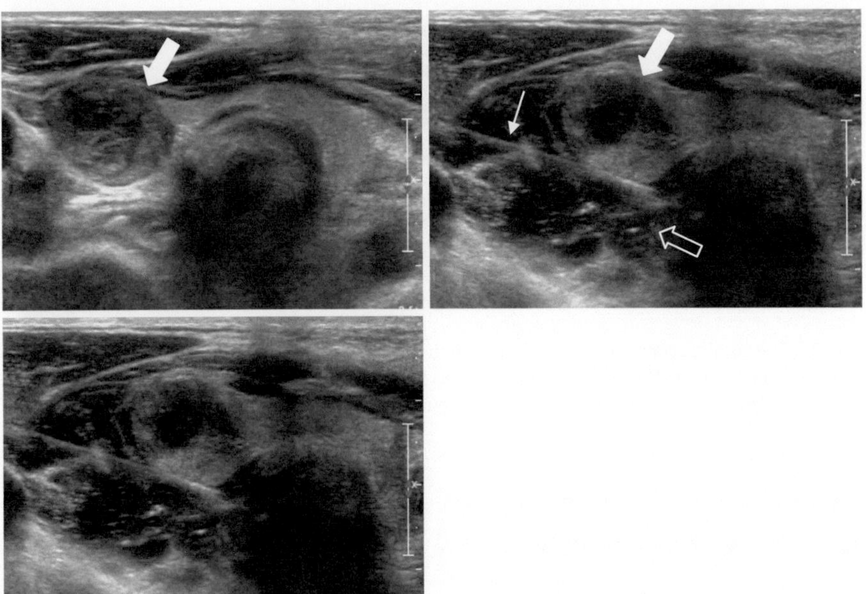

Fig. 17.1 Left image: An ultrasound image shows the parathyroid gland (solid white arrow) located close to the trachea, esophagus, and carotid artery. Right image: 5% glucose solution (hollow arrow) is injected through the needle (thin arrow) into the region between the parathyroid gland (solid white arrow) and surrounding structures, including the trachea, esophagus, and the carotid artery to create a liquid isolation zone. The parathyroid gland is effectively isolated into a "peninsula shape"

Thermal Ablation

Once a liquid isolation zone is successfully created around the parathyroid gland, an electrode is percutaneously inserted into the parathyroid gland under ultrasound guidance. There are two types of ablation techniques: (1) moving-shot and (2) fixed electrode techniques. For patients with SHPT, a 1-mm preservation technique is used to protect a small portion of the gland tissue within 1 mm from the capsule.

1. Moving-shot and fixed electrode techniques: In the moving-shot technique, an electrode is inserted into the gland with the electrode tip positioned at the far end of the gland close to the capsule. Once the position of the tip is confirmed under ultrasound, the ablation is initiated while the electrode is being slowly withdrawn. When the tissue vaporization creates a hyperechoic zone (Fig. 17.2) inside the gland, the electrode is slowly moved backward from the distal to the proximal and from the deep to the shallow locations until the entire gland is successfully ablated. If the target gland is smaller than 1 cm, the fixed electrode technique is used. In this technique, the gland is ablated with the electrode's tip at the distal capsule without withdrawing. Successful ablation is confirmed when the gland is completely covered with hyperechoic vaporization under ultrasound.

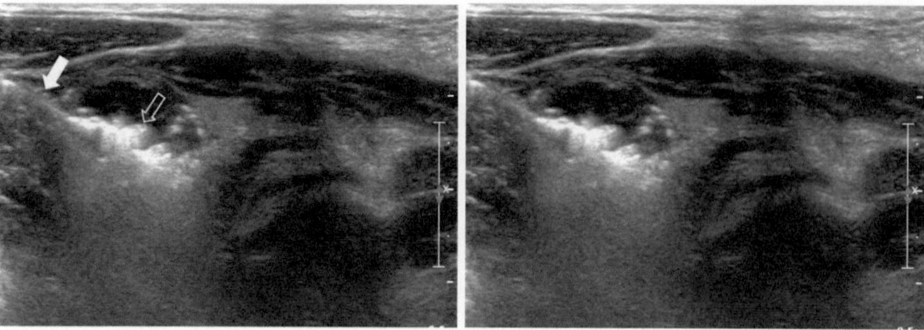

Fig. 17.2 Radiofrequency ablation of the parathyroid gland. Ultrasound image shows the radiofrequency electrode (solid white arrow) and the hyperechoic area of tissue vaporization (hollow arrow) caused by tissue coagulation necrosis from ablation

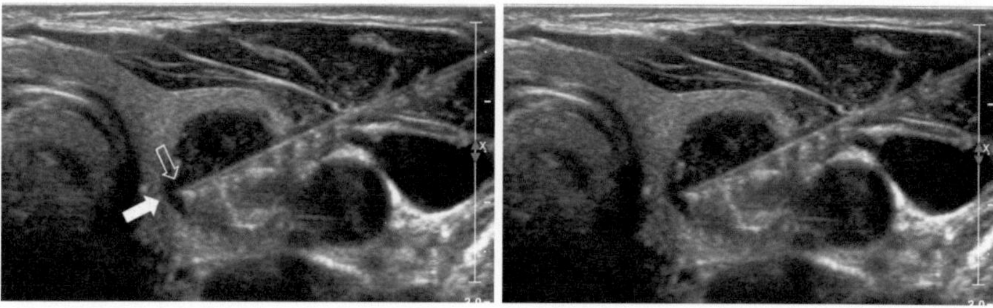

Fig. 17.3 1-mm preservation technique: Ultrasound image shows the electrode's tip (hollow arrow) positioned at the far side of the gland approximately 1 mm from the distal capsule (solid white arrow) of the parathyroid gland

2. "1 mm" preservation technique [17]: This technique is used for patients with SHPT to avoid clinically significant hypoparathyroidism after thermal ablation. Subtotal parathyroidectomy or total parathyroidectomy with arm implantation is frequently used in surgery to maintain a minimum level of PTH. In this 1-mm preservation technique, the electrode's tip is positioned inside the gland approximately 1 mm from the capsule. With this technique, a small portion of the gland tissue near the distal capsule is preserved to maintain the basic PTH level (Fig. 17.3).

Real-Time Evaluation of Ablation Effect

Real-time assessment of the treatment effect is a critical step for achieving the desired outcome. The entire thermal ablation process can be monitored in real time under ultrasound using either basic 2D, color Doppler, or contrast-enhanced method. Rapid PTH assay after the procedure also provides valuable information.

1. Real-Time Ultrasonographic Evaluation

(1) 2D ultrasound evaluation: 2D grayscale ultrasound is the most convenient and commonly used method to evaluate the ablation effect. Microbubbles generated from the tissue coagulation during thermal ablation appear as a hyperechoic area on ultrasound. The hyperechoic area represents the ablation zone (Fig. 17.4). However, diffusion or escape of microbubbles into surrounding structures or vessels can lead to incorrect estimation of the ablation zone. Therefore, 2D ultrasound needs to be limited only to the early screening phase.

(2) Color Doppler ultrasound evaluation: After completion of the ablation resulting in coagulation necrosis of the target tissue, all blood vessels are also damaged and thrombosed. Therefore, no color Doppler signal is observed inside the ablation zone (Fig. 17.5). However, due to the limitations of the color Doppler ultrasound in visualizing small vessels, caution is required for the evaluation of the ablation effect. It is recommended to use color Doppler ultrasound only for preliminary screening.

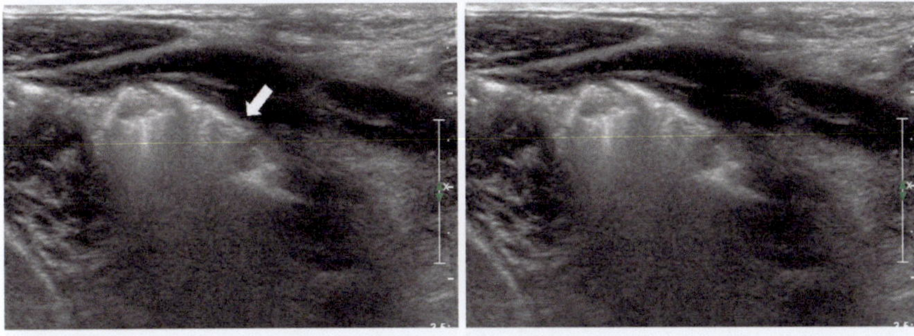

Fig. 17.4 2D grayscale ultrasound image shows the ablation range as a hyperechoic area (solid white arrow) created by microbubbles from tissue vaporization. Covering the entire gland with hyperechoic area confirms successful ablation

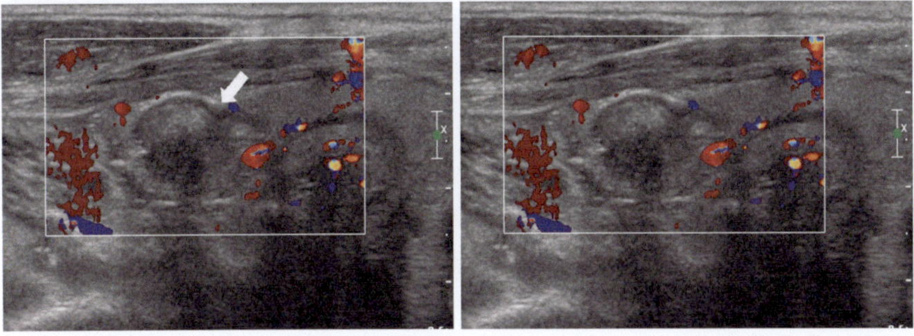

Fig. 17.5 Color Doppler ultrasound image shows no blood flow signal inside the ablation zone (solid white arrow)

(3) Contrast-enhanced ultrasound: Contrast-enhanced ultrasound is considered the most reliable method to evaluate the target lesion's microcirculation, thereby predicting the effect of ablation. Preprocedural ultrasound with contrast enhancement shows rich perfusion in the parathyroid glands (Fig. 17.6). After complete ablation, the treated area no longer shows an enhancement due to occluded or damaged vessels (Fig. 17.7). If a residual enhancement is detected inside the ablation zone, additional ablation is required for complete ablation.

2. Quick Intraoperative Intact PTH Assay

The half-life of the intact PTH (iPTH) is only 2–5 min. Although it can theoretically provide information regarding the ablation effect, its actual use for real-time monitoring is limited due to PTH assay time [25–27]. McLeod et al. proposed a PTH assay in the post-anesthesia care unit for predicting hypocalce-

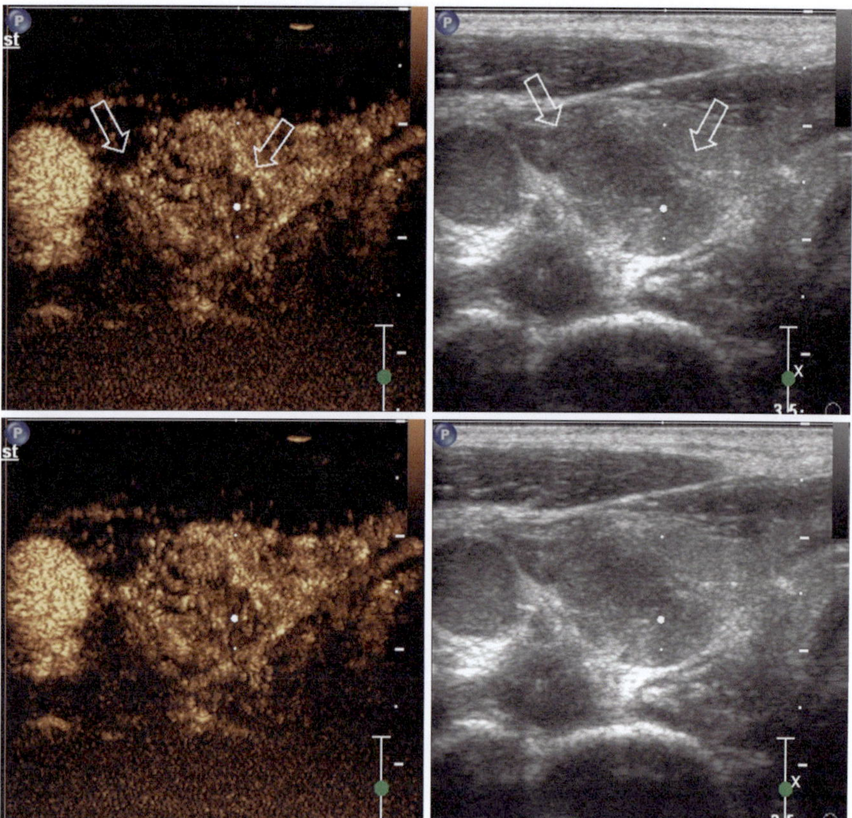

Fig. 17.6 Left: Contrast-enhance ultrasound image before the ablation shows strong enhancement in the hyperplastic parathyroid gland. Right: 2D grayscale ultrasound image shows hyperplastic parathyroid gland (hollow arrows)

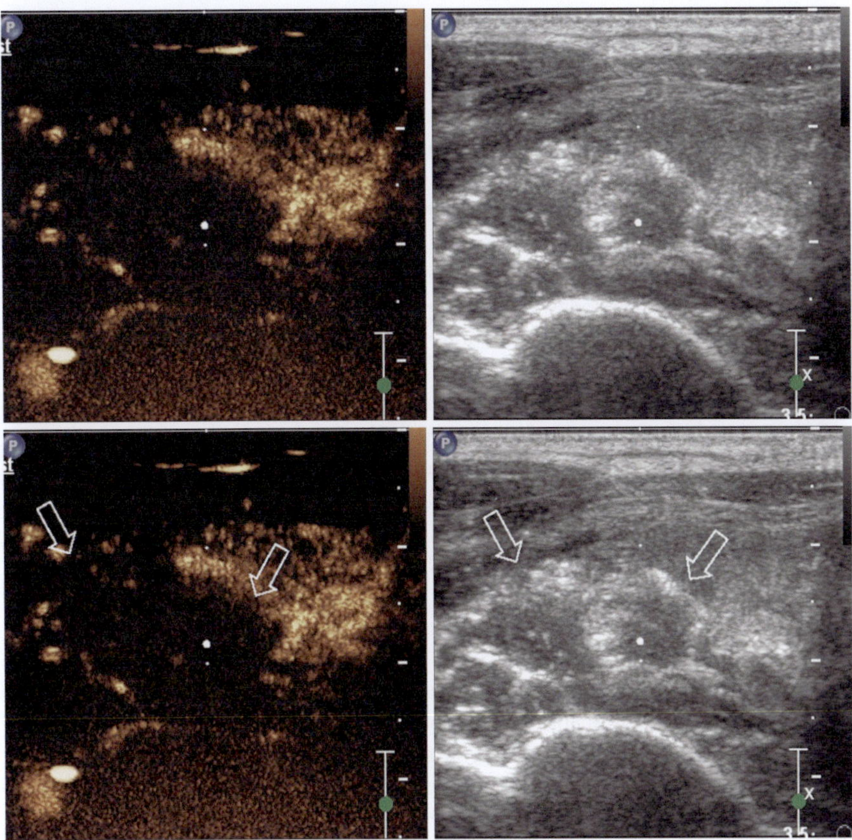

Fig. 17.7 Left: Contrast-enhanced ultrasound image shows complete ablation of the target gland (hollow arrows) without evidence of residual enhancement. Right: 2D grayscale ultrasound image shows the parathyroid gland (hollow arrows) after ablation

mia in patients who underwent thyroidectomy [28]. With a PTH cutoff value of <12 pg/ml and PTH drop >75%, they reported sensitivity and specificity of 100%, 92% and 100%, 88%, respectively.

Complications and Prevention Strategies

Complications are associated with the target glands' size and location, the patient's underlying diseases, the equipment's energy, and the operator's experience and skills.

1. Pain: Most patients experience a certain degree of transient pain during the procedure. It includes local pain and radiating pain or discomfort to the back of the

ear, tooth root, shoulder, and back. The pain is usually not significant and resolves shortly after the procedure. Some patients may experience mild to moderate degree of odynophagia due to thermal injury to the surrounding tissues. The pain is self-limiting and usually resolves within several days.

2. Nausea and vomiting: Mild nausea and vomiting may occur in some patients but usually resolve a few hours after the procedure. These symptoms are believed to be related to local anesthetics or analgesics.

3. Fever: Some patients may experience mild fever after the procedure, due to the glands' coagulation necrosis. In general, the body temperature does not exceed 38 °C. If the fever persists with a temperature higher than 38 °C, further examination is needed to rule out infection.

4. Infection: If a patient shows any infection signs, the procedure should be delayed until the infection is resolved. All procedures should be performed under strict sterile conditions. Infection associated with ablation is rare. If an infection is suspected, immediate antibiotics treatment is required.

5. Bleeding: There are rich blood vessels both inside and around the parathyroid glands, including the inferior thyroid artery and vein. Percutaneous access requires careful ultrasound guidance to avoid vascular injuries. If bleeding occurs, either manual compression or cauterization should be performed immediately. For patients with ongoing hemodialysis, heparin should be avoided before the ablation.

6. Nerve injury: Recurrent laryngeal or superior laryngeal nerve injury is one of the most common complications of the parathyroid ablation with the incidence of 11–18%. Unilateral recurrent laryngeal nerve injury can result in hoarseness and difficulty in swallowing. Bilateral recurrent laryngeal nerve injury can cause aphonia, difficulty in breathing, and even death from suffocation. The superior laryngeal nerve injury causes deep voice and swallowing impairment. To avoid bilateral recurrent laryngeal nerve injury, the patient's voice needs to be monitored in real time during the procedure. If the patient's voice changes, the ablation needs to be paused. The procedure may continue after recovery of the patient's voice. Recurrent laryngeal nerve or superior laryngeal nerve injury usually does not require additional treatment, although neurotrophic medications can be considered in some cases. Most patients recover within 2–3 months.

7. Trachea or esophagus injury: Although the parathyroid glands are close to the trachea and esophagus, the injury can be avoided by using a liquid isolation technique.

8. Hypocalcemia: Hypocalcemia after ablation is common. Severe hypocalcemia may occur a few hours after the procedure and lasts for 1 week or longer. Clinical symptoms include fatigue, abnormal skin sensation, numbness of hands and feet, convulsions, etc. Some patients may have bronchial or gastrointestinal spasms resulting in cough, asthma, and abdominal pain. After ablation, blood calcium levels need to be closely monitored. Some patients may need to take supplemental calcium. Sever hypocalcemia can be avoided by using 1-mm preservation technique.

9. Persistent or recurrent hyperparathyroidism: Persistent hyperparathyroidism is a condition where serum iPTH levels decrease after ablation but are persistently higher than the upper limit of the normal range. Recurrent hyperparathyroidism is a condition that the serum iPTH level is decreased to the normal range after ablation, but rebounds to the upper limit of the normal range. Persistent or recurrent hyperparathyroidism is related to incomplete ablation or undetected ectopic parathyroid glands. In 2017, Peng et al. reported follow-up results in 34 patients with SHPT who underwent thermal ablations [16]. After 1 year, the authors performed repeat ablation in four patients with recurrent or persistent SHPT to achieve the desired treatment outcome.

Percutaneous Parathyroid Injection

Under ultrasound guidance, a needle is inserted percutaneously into the parathyroid gland, and ethanol or calcitriol is injected for treating hyperparathyroidism. Ethanol injection results in coagulation necrosis through dehydration and ischemic change. Calcitriol inhibits PTH secretion by direct binding to the vitamin D receptors. Percutaneous parathyroid injection is used mostly for patients who underwent a thermal ablation but failed or for those who could not undergo a thermal ablation due to the location of the parathyroid gland.

Indications and Contraindications [29]

Indications

1. Persistent hyperparathyroidism with iPTH $\geq$400 pg/ml despite medical treatment. Patients with hyperphosphatemia and/or hypercalcemia resulted from the medical treatment.
2. Enlarged parathyroid glands with suspected nodular hyperplasia on ultrasonography.

Contraindications

1. Enlarged parathyroid gland located where ultrasonographic-guided access is impossible
2. Paralysis of the recurrent laryngeal nerve on the opposite side
3. When neck surgery is scheduled for thyroid carcinoma, etc.

Preparation Before Treatment

1. An ultrasound machine with color Doppler and contrast-enhanced imaging capabilities with the high-frequency probe is recommended. The probe frequency range of 5–12 MHz is preferred.
2. Anhydrous ethanol suitable for injection or intravenous calcitriol.
3. Ultrasound contrast agent: sulfur hexafluoride microbubbles (SonoVue).
4. 20-G, 10-cm Chiba needle.

Patient preparation: Before the procedure, patients should undergo thorough laboratory analysis including complete blood count, coagulation function, liver function, renal function, electrolytes, parathyroid hormones, tumor markers, and infectious disease indicators such as hepatitis, syphilis, and HIV.

Procedure

1. The patient is positioned in supine with a pillow under the neck for full exposure of the neck. Preprocedural ultrasound with a high-frequency probe is performed to evaluate the bilateral parathyroid glands.
2. The neck is prepared and draped using sterile technique. The access site is then injected with local anesthetics including the skin and subcutaneous tissue under ultrasound guidance.
3. Under ultrasound, the needle is inserted close to the distal capsule of the parathyroid gland. Anhydrous ethanol or calcitriol is then slowly injected. If needed, the needle is withdrawn and repositioned to treat the entire gland. The ethanol injection volume is determined based on the volume of the gland. For a gland greater than 1 cm^3, ethanol of 70% of the gland volume is used. For a gland less than 1 cm^3, ethanol of 80% of the gland volume is injected. For calcitriol, 70–90% of the gland volume is used. During ethanol injection, continuous monitoring is essential to prevent a leakage and damage to the surrounding structures. Complications from the leakage of ethanol include local pain and hoarseness.
4. Contrast-enhanced ultrasonography is used for real-time evaluation of the treatment effect.

Treatment Strategy

1. Ethanol injection: Ethanol injection is scheduled between hemodialysis sessions. The first injection is to treat only one or two glands with the greatest volume and richest blood supply. If the iPTH is persistently greater than 200 pg/ml 1 week after the first injection, repeat injection can be considered. For the second

procedure, ethanol is injected either into the untreated portion of the previously injected gland or the new glands that have not been treated. Although repeated procedure can be performed if the iPTH level is persistently high, the total ethanol injections should not exceed five sessions.

2. Calcitriol injection: Calcitriol injection is also scheduled on the days between hemodialysis sessions. The treatment is performed with three injections per week for 2 consecutive weeks.

References

1. Solbiati L, Giangrande A, De Pra L, et al. Percutaneous ethanol injection of parathyroid tumors under US guidance: treatment for secondary hyperparathyroidism. Radiology. 1985;155(3):607–10. https://doi.org/10.1148/radiology.155.3.3889999.
2. Giangrande A, Castiglioni A, Solbiati L, Allari P. Ultrasound-guided percutaneous fine-needle ethanol injection into parathyroid glands in secondary hyperparathyroidism. Nephrol Dial Transplant. 1992;7(5):412–21.
3. Fukagawa M, Kitaoka M, Kurokawa K. Ultrasonographic intervention of parathyroid hyperplasia in chronic dialysis patients: a theoretical approach. Nephrol Dial Transplant. 1996;11(Suppl 3):125–9.
4. Fukagawa M, Kitaoka M, Yi H, et al. Serial evaluation of parathyroid size by ultrasonography is another useful marker for the long-term prognosis of calcitriol pulse therapy in chronic dialysis patients. Nephron. 1994;68(2):221–8. https://doi.org/10.1159/000188261.
5. Chinnaratha MA, Chuang MA, Fraser RJ, Woodman RJ, Wigg AJ. Percutaneous thermal ablation for primary hepatocellular carcinoma: a systematic review and meta-analysis. J Gastroenterol Hepatol. 2016;31(2):294–301.
6. Mazzoccoli G, Tarquini R, Valoriani A, Oben J, Vinciguerra M, Marra F. Management strategies for hepatocellular carcinoma: old certainties and new realities. Clin Exp Med. 2016;16(3):243–56.
7. Dupuy DE, Fernando HC, Hillman S, et al. Radiofrequency ablation of stage IA non-small cell lung cancer in medically inoperable patients: results from the American College of Surgeons Oncology Group Z4033 (Alliance) trial. Cancer. 2015;121(19):3491–8.
8. Kodama H, Yamakado K, Hasegawa T, et al. Radiofrequency ablation using a multiple-electrode switching system for lung tumors with 2.0-5.0-cm maximum diameter: phase II clinical study. Radiology. 2015;277(3):895–902.
9. Baek JH, Kim YS, Lee D, Huh JY, Lee JH. Benign predominantly solid thyroid nodules: prospective study of efficacy of sonographically guided radiofrequency ablation versus control condition. AJR Am J Roentgenol. 2010;194(4):1137–42.
10. Deandrea M, Sung JY, Limone P, et al. Efficacy and safety of radiofrequency ablation versus observation for nonfunctioning benign thyroid nodules: a randomized controlled international collaborative trial. Thyroid. 2015;25(8):890–6.
11. Bennedbaek FN, Karstrup S, Hegedüs L. Ultrasound guided laser ablation of a parathyroid adenoma. Br J Radiol. 2001;74(886):905–7.
12. Jiang T, Chen F, Zhou X, Hu Y, Zhao Q. Percutaneous ultrasound-guided laser ablation with contrast-enhanced ultrasonography for hyperfunctioning parathyroid adenoma: a preliminary case series. Int J Endocrinol. 2015;2015:673604.
13. Adda G, Scillitani A, Epaminonda P, et al. Ultrasound-guided laser thermal ablation for parathyroid adenomas: analysis of three cases with a three-year follow-up. Horm Res. 2006;65(5):231–4.

14. Andrioli M, Riganti F, Pacella CM, Valcavi R. Long-term effectiveness of ultrasound-guided laser ablation of hyperfunctioning parathyroid adenomas: present and future perspectives. AJR Am J Roentgenol. 2012;199(5):1164–8.
15. Kovatcheva RD, Vlahov JD, Stoinov JI, et al. High-intensity focussed ultrasound (HIFU) treatment in uraemic secondary hyperparathyroidism. Nephrol Dial Transplant. 2012;27(1):76–80.
16. 章建全,仇明, 盛建国, 等.　超声引导下经皮穿刺热消融治疗甲状旁腺结节. 第二军医大学学报. 2013;34(4):362–9.
17. Peng C, Zhang Z, Liu J, et al. Efficacy and safety of ultrasound-guided radiofrequency ablation of hyperplastic parathyroid gland for secondary hyperparathyroidism associated with chronic kidney disease. Head Neck. 2017;39(3):564–71.
18. Zhuo L, Peng LL, Zhang YM, et al. US-guided microwave ablation of hyperplastic parathyroid glands: safety and efficacy in patients with end-stage renal disease-a pilot study. Radiology. 2017;282(2):576–84.
19. Zhuo L, Zhang L, Peng LL, et al. Microwave ablation of hyperplastic parathyroid glands is a treatment option for end-stage renal disease patients ineligible for surgical resection. Int J Hyperth. 2019;36(1):29–35.
20. Zeng Z, Peng CZ, Liu JB, et al. Efficacy of ultrasound-guided radiofrequency ablation of parathyroid hyperplasia: single session vs. two-session for effect on hypocalcemia. Sci Rep. 2020;10(1):6206.
21. Jiang B, Wang X, Yao Z, et al. Microwave ablation vs. parathyroidectomy for secondary hyperparathyroidism in maintenance hemodialysis patients. Hemodial Int. 2019;23(2):247–53.
22. Gong L, Tang W, Lu J, et al. Thermal ablation versus parathyroidectomy for secondary hyperparathyroidism: a meta-analysis. Int J Surg. 2019;70:13–8.
23. Itani M, Middleton WD. Parathyroid imaging. Radiol Clin North Am. 2020;58(6):1071–83.
24. Kidney Disease: Improving Global Outcomes (KDIGO) CKD-MBD Work Group. KDIGO clinical practice guideline for the diagnosis, evaluation, prevention, and treatment of Chronic Kidney Disease-Mineral and Bone Disorder (CKD-MBD). Kidney Int Suppl. 2009;(113):S1–130.
25. Lorenz K, Ukkat J, Sekulla C, et al. Total parathyroidectomy without autotransplantation for renal hyperparathyroidism: experience with a qPTH-controlled protocol. World J Surg. 2006;30(5):743–51. https://doi.org/10.1007/s00268-005-0379-0.
26. Irvin GL 3rd, Dembrow VD, Prudhomme DL. Clinical usefulness of an intraoperative "quick parathyroid hormone" assay. Surgery. 1993;114(6):1019–22; discussion 1022–3.
27. Shawky MS. Quick parathyroid hormone assays: a comprehensive review of their utility in clinical practice. Hormones (Athens). 2016;15(3):355–67. https://doi.org/10.14310/horm.2002.1689.
28. McLeod IK, Arciero C, Noordzij JP, et al. The use of rapid parathyroid hormone assay in predicting postoperative hypocalcemia after total or completion thyroidectomy. Thyroid. 2006;16(3):259–65. https://doi.org/10.1089/thy.2006.16.259.
29. Onoda N, Fukagawa M, Tominaga Y, et al. New clinical guidelines for selective direct injection therapy of the parathyroid glands in chronic dialysis patients. NDT Plus. 2008;1(Suppl 3):iii26–8.

Chapter 18
Interventional Treatment of Thyroid Nodules

Auh Whan Park, Tim Huber, and Jung Hwan Baek

Current Practice on Thyroid Nodules

High-resolution ultrasound (US) detects thyroid nodules in 19–68% of healthy, asymptomatic individuals [1, 2]. The clinical importance of thyroid nodules is to exclude thyroid cancer occurring in 5–15% among the detected thyroid nodules [3, 4].

In the 2015 American Thyroid Association (ATA) Management Guidelines for Adult Patients with Thyroid Nodules and Differentiated Thyroid Cancer [5], an algorithm for evaluation and management of patients with thyroid nodules bases on US pattern and fine-needle aspiration (FNA) cytology was suggested. Three main steps exit for workups in the algorithm.

A. W. Park (✉)
Department of Radiology, University of Virginia Health System, Charlottesville, VA, USA

T. Huber
Dotter Department of Interventional Radiology, Oregon Health and Science University, Portland, OR, USA
e-mail: huberti@ohsu.edu

J. H. Baek
Department of Radiology and Research Institute of Radiology, University of Ulsan College of Medicine, Asan Medical Center, Seoul, South Korea

© The Author(s), under exclusive license to Springer Nature Switzerland AG 2022

H. Yu et al. (eds.), *Diagnosis and Management of Endocrine Disorders in Interventional Radiology*, https://doi.org/10.1007/978-3-030-87189-5_18

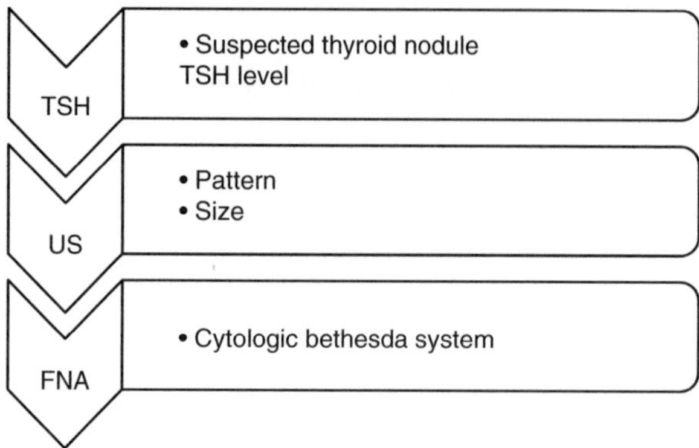

A summary of essential recommendations from the ATA guidelines is as follows.

Workups

Serum Thyroid Stimulation Hormone (TSH)

Serum TSH should be measured during the initial evaluation of a patient with a thyroid nodule (Table 18.1). If the serum TSH is subnormal, a radionuclide (preferably ^{123}I) thyroid scan should be performed. If the serum TSH is normal or elevated, a radionuclide scan should not be performed as the initial imaging evaluation.

Thyroid Sonography

Thyroid sonography with a survey of the cervical lymph nodes should be performed in all patients with known or suspected thyroid nodules. FNA is the procedure of choice in the evaluation of thyroid nodules when clinically indicated. Thyroid nodule diagnostic FNA is recommended (Table 18.2). Thyroid nodules should be assessed for malignancy risk by ATA sonographic risk pattern, not simply by size. Not every thyroid nodule >1 cm needs fine-needle aspiration (FNA), and most nodule <1 cm does not need FNA.

Table 18.1 Evaluation on thyroid stimulation hormone (TSH) with a thyroid nodule

Suspected thyroid nodule	
TSH: normal or elevated	TSH: subnormal
Thyroid/neck sonography	Radionuclide (preferably ^{123}I) thyroid scan

Table 18.2 Sonographic patterns, estimated risk of malignancy, and fine-needle aspiration guidance for thyroid nodules

Thyroid/neck sonography				
High suspicion	Intermediate suspicion	Low suspicion	Very low suspicion	Benign No nodule/size cutoff (1 cm)
FNA ≥ 1 cm		FNA ≥ 1.5 cm	FNA ≥ 2 cm	FNA not required

Table 18.3 American College of Radiology (ACR) Thyroid Imaging, Reporting and Data System (TI-RADS)

Composition (choose 1)		Echogenicity (choose 1)		Margin (choose 1)		Shape (choose 1)		Echogenic foci (choose 1)	
Cystic or almost completely cystic	0	Anechoic	0	Wider than tall	0	Smooth	0	None	0
Spongiform	0	Hyperechoic	1	Taller than wide	3	Ill-defined	0	Large comet tail artifacts	0
Cystic and solid	1	Isoechoic	1			Lobulated	2	Macrocalcifications	1
Solid or almost completely solid	2	Hypoechoic	2			Irregular	2	Peripheral (rim) calcifications	2
		Very hypoechoic	3			Extra-thyroid extension	3	Punctate echogenic foci	3
				↓					

Add points from all categories to determine TI-RADS level

0 points	2 points	3 points	4 points	5 points
TR1	*TR 2*	*TR 3*	*TR 4*	*TR 5*
Benign	Not suspicious	Mildly suspicious	Moderately suspicious	Highly suspicious
No FNA	No FNA	FNA if ≥2.5 cm FNA if ≥1.5 cm	FNA if ≥1.5 cm FNA if ≥1.0 cm	FNA if ≥1.0 cm FNA if ≥0.5 cm

According to a study by Yoon et al. [6], the ATA guidelines were unable to classify 3.4% of 1293 nodules, of which 18.2% were malignant. In 2017, the American College of Radiology (ACR) published a white paper on Thyroid Imaging, Reporting and Data System (TI-RADS), as shown in Table 18.3 [7].

Bethesda System

Thyroid nodule FNA cytologic should be reported using diagnostic groups outlined in the Bethesda system or Reporting Thyroid Cytopathology (Table 18.4) [8].

Table 18.4 Bethesda system revised in 2017 based on post-2010 date

Categories	% Risk of malignancy (*)	Usual management
Nondiagnostic	5–10 (5–10)	Repeat FNA with US
Benign	0–3 (0–3)	Clinical and US follow-up
Atypia of undetermined significance (AUS)/ follicular lesion of undetermined significance (FLUS)	10–30 (6–18)	Repeat FNA, molecular testing, or lobectomy
Follicular neoplasm/suspicious for follicular neoplasm (FN/SFN)	25–40 (10–40)	Molecular testing, lobectomy
Suspicious for malignancy	50–75 (45–60)	Lobectomy or near-total thyroidectomy
Malignant	97–99 (94–96)	Near-total thyroidectomy

*Adjusted risks if noninvasive follicular thyroid neoplasm with papillary-like nuclear features (NIFTP) was not classified as a malignancy. *FNA* fine-needle aspiration, *US* ultrasound

Treatment

Benign Lesion

If the nodule is benign on cytology, further immediate diagnostic studies or treatment is not required.

Malignant Lesion

If a cytologic result is diagnostic for primary thyroid malignancy, surgery is generally recommended.

Thyroid Radiofrequency Ablation

In 1990, percutaneous ethanol ablation (EA) was introduced for treating AFTNs. Although EA is very effective for cystic thyroid nodules and can achieve a volume reduction of more than 85%, it is less effective for solid nodules. It also has several limitations, such as unpredictable diffusion within the tumor, pain, and capsular fibrosis by leaking, making future surgery challenging.

More recently, advances in thermal ablation have allowed effective treatment of solid, benign thyroid nodules. Various energy sources are currently used in thermal ablation, including laser, radiofrequency (RF), microwave, and high-intensity focused ultrasound (HIFU). To date, radiofrequency ablation (RFA) has been the most exhaustively researched and proven therapy in terms of safety and clinical efficacy. Hereafter, RFA will be mainly described in regard to thermal ablation.

The strategy for choosing between EA and thermal ablation depends on the composition of thyroid nodules [9]:

- Cystic nodule: EA
- Predominantly cystic nodule: EA first or combined with thermal ablation
- Predominantly solid or solid nodule: thermal ablation

Indications

Thyroid RFA guidelines are designed to provide scientific information regarding the use of this procedure in clinical practice. Several guidelines have been published [10–17]. A systematic review of clinical practice guidelines for RFA of benign thyroid nodules was published recently [18]. There are subtle differences between these guidelines with indications in common. According to the revised KSThR 2017 guideline [14], the indications and contraindications for treating benign thyroid nodules are as follows.

Indications

- Patients with benign thyroid nodules producing symptoms or patients with cosmetic concerns
- Toxic or pretoxic AFTNs

Thyroid nodules should be confirmed as benign on at least two US-guided FNA or core needle biopsy (CNB) before RFA. A single benign diagnosis on FNA or CNB is sufficient when the nodule has the US features highly specific for benignity and AFTN. In addition, caution should be taken in the use of RFA in pregnant women, patients with serious heart problems, and those with pre-existing contralateral vocal cord palsy.

Contraindications

- Follicular neoplasm or malignancy on FNA or CNB
- A nodule with US criteria suggesting malignancy, despite FNA or CNB results
- Cystic and predominantly cystic thyroid nodules, in which EA has been suggested as a first-line treatment

Anatomy

For a safe and effective procedure, knowledge of neck anatomy, particularly that of the nerves, vessels, and other critical structures, is essential. It is of utmost importance to understand US-based thyroidal and perithyroidal anatomy.

The Thyroid Gland

The *thyroid gland* is a butterfly-shaped midline structure lying anterior and lateral to the trachea in the visceral space of the infrahyoid neck. In adults, each lobe is about 40–60 mm in length, 10–20 mm in width, and 13–18 mm in thickness. The right and left lobes are connected by the isthmus in 2–3 mm in thickness. The limits of normal thyroid volume are 10–15 mL for adult females and 12–18 mL for males [19]. The trachea, esophagus, thyroid gland, and infrahyoid muscles are enclosed by the pretracheal fascia (Fig. 18.1). The pretracheal layer of fascia is situated in the anterior neck, spanning between the hyoid bone superiorly and the thorax inferiorly, where it fuses with the pericardium (Fig. 18.2).

Fig. 18.1 Cross-sectional diagram of the neck with three layers of the deep cervical fascia; T trachea, E esophagus. (With permissions from Park [20])

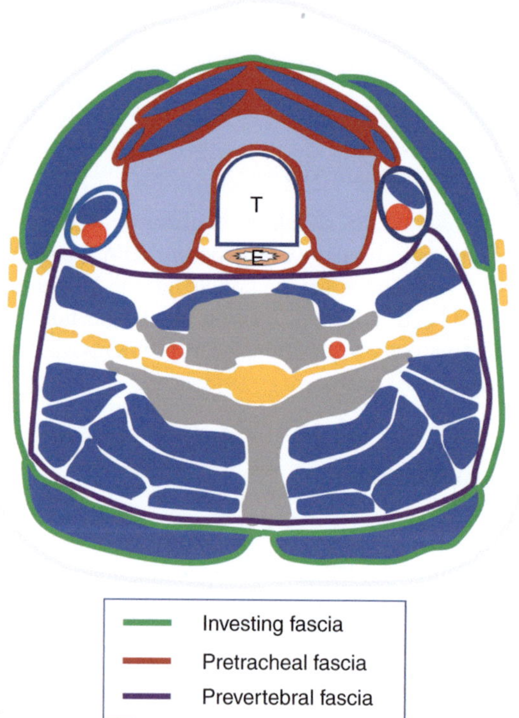

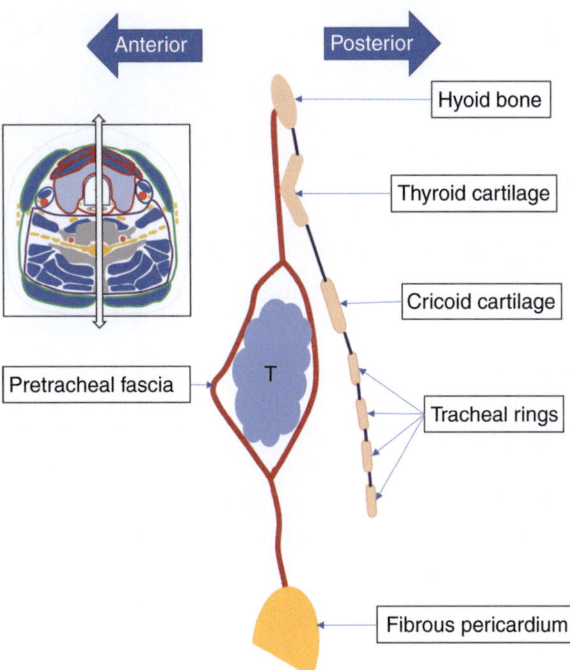

Fig. 18.2 Sagittal view of the pretracheal fascia; T thyroid gland. (With permissions from Park [20])

The false thyroid capsule (also known as the surgical capsule or perithyroidal sheath) has a thin layer of fascia enveloping the thyroid gland, which needs to be dissected away from the thyroid during surgery. Most anatomists and surgeons have described it as a thin capsule deriving from the pretracheal fascia similar to a mesentery in the abdomen. The *true capsule* is formed by condensation of the fibrous stroma of the gland.

The space between the false capsule and the true capsule is a potential space to inject a local anesthetic. For RFA of benign thyroid nodules, perithyroidal lidocaine injection is recommended as a local anesthesia technique [14]. During perithyroidal lidocaine injection, the needle tip should be positioned close to the thyroid gland. Initially, injecting a small amount of lidocaine will create a space between the two capsules. Additional administration of lidocaine injection will dissect the space (Fig. 18.3) and propagate the anesthetic along the posterolateral margin of the thyroid gland.

Vessels

The arteries and veins of the thyroid gland are shown in Table 18.5. The *common carotid artery* (CCA) and *internal jugular vein* (IJV) are located in the posterolateral aspect of the thyroid gland. The *superior thyroidal artery* runs superficially on

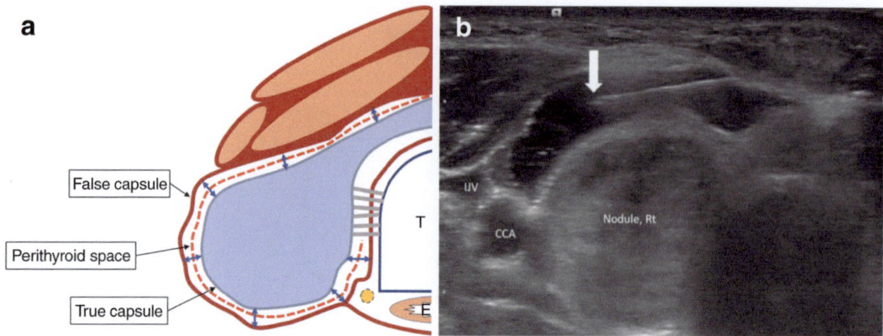

Fig. 18.3 (**a**) Perithyroidal hydrodissection along the pretracheal fascia; T trachea, E esophagus (With permissions from Park [20]). (**b**) Lidocaine injection in the right perithyroidal space; solid white arrow, needle tip; IJV internal jugular vein, CCA common carotid artery

Table 18.5 The vessels of the thyroid gland

Artery	Vein
Superior thyroid	Superior thyroid
	Middle thyroid
Inferior thyroid	Inferior thyroid
Thyroid ima (directly from aortic arch)	Anterior jugular vein

the anterior border of the thyroid gland. This artery runs closely and anterolaterally to the external branch of the superior laryngeal nerve (SLN). The *inferior thyroidal artery* enters the tracheoesophageal groove in a plane posterior to the carotid space, and branches thereof penetrate the posterior aspect of the lateral thyroid lobe (Fig. 18.4).

The *anterior jugular vein* begins near the hyoid bone at the confluence of several superficial veins arising from the submaxillary region (Fig. 18.5). The vein descends along the anterior border of the sternocleidomastoid muscle and passes beneath that muscle to drain into the external jugular vein in the lower part of the neck. This vein is located along the approach route (in front of the isthmus) of the electrode. Although injury to the anterior jugular vein can be easily controlled by simple manual compression, it can disturb the procedure due to persistent oozing.

Muscles

The neck is a cage-like structure encaged by muscles, classified into three groups (Table 18.6). When visualized on US, the neck muscles act as important landmarks for the identification of the nerves (Figs. 18.6 and 18.7).

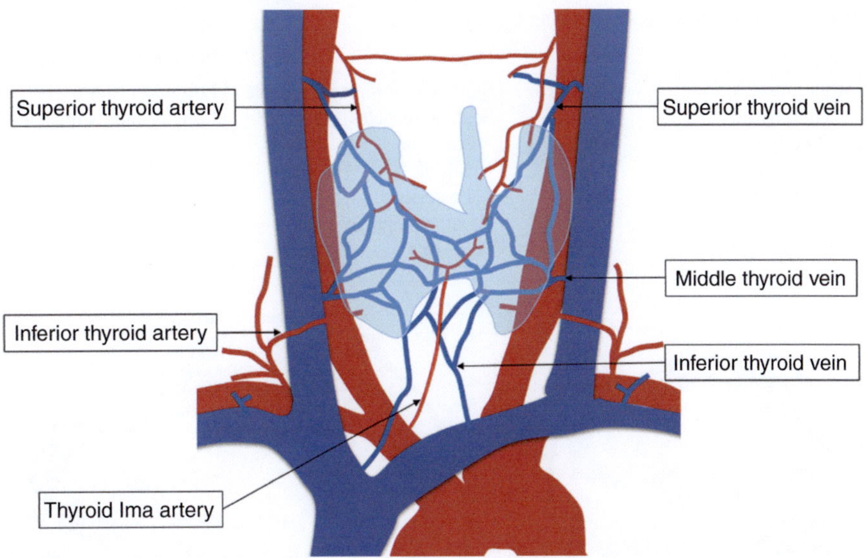

Fig. 18.4 The vessels of the thyroid gland; blue, vein; red, artery. (With permissions from Park [20])

Fig. 18.5 The location of the paired anterior jugular veins. (With permissions from Park [20])

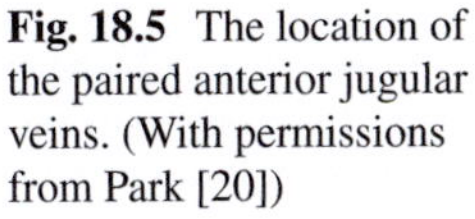

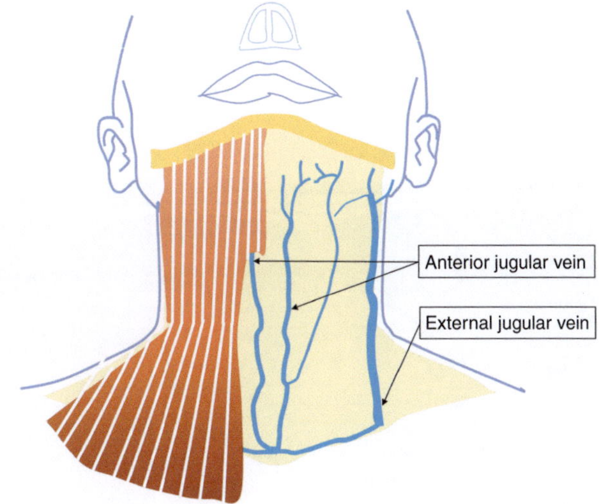

Nerves

Ultrasonographic visibility of the nerve depends on the size of the nerve, the equipment used, and the location in the neck. With high-frequency electrodes (>10–12 MHz), the nerve has a honeycomb-like appearance or displays a reticular

Table 18.6 The muscles surrounding the thyroid gland

Anterior	Lateral	Posterior

Strap muscles: four pairs of muscles:
  Thyrohyoid
  Omohyoid
  Sternohyoid
  Sternothyroid
	Sternocleidomastoid muscle
	Scalene muscles
	  Anterior
	  Middle
	  Posterior
	Levator scapulae muscle
	Trapezius
		Longus colli muscle
		Longus capitis muscle

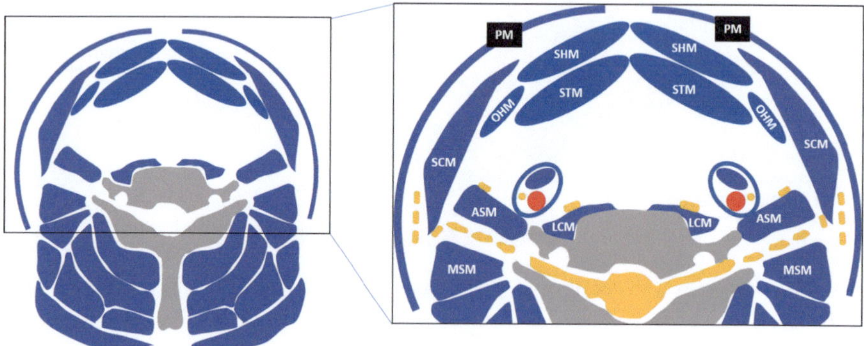

Fig. 18.6 Relationship of the neck muscles to nerves; ASM anterior scalene muscle, LCM longus colli muscle, MSM middle scalene muscle, SCM sternocleidomastoid muscle, SHM sternothyroid muscle, STM sternothyroid muscle, OHM omohyoid muscle, PM platysma muscle. (With permissions from Park [20])

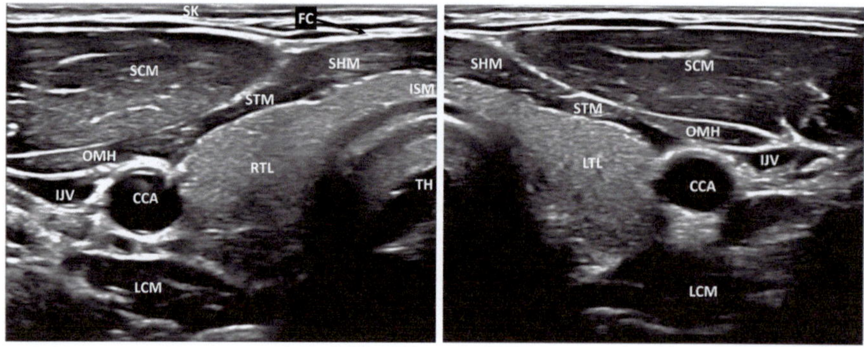

Fig. 18.7 Transverse US scan of the thyroid gland; SK skin, FC fascia cervicalis, SHM sternohyoid muscle, STM sternothyroid muscle, SCM sternocleidomastoid muscle, OHM omohyoid muscle, ISM isthmus, TH trachea, RTL right thyroid lobe, LTL left thyroid lobe, IJV internal jugular vein, CCA common carotid artery, LCM longus colli muscle. (With permissions from Park [20])

pattern created by hypoechoic rounded fascicles. The nerve shows a striated pattern on longitudinal scans, with several parallel echogenic lines from its internal structures. Detection of small nerves may be challenging, but anatomic landmarks such as muscles and vessels are useful in detection and tracking.

Nerve injury is one of the most serious complications during RFA. For ablation of thyroid nodules, the recurrent laryngeal and the vagus nerves are of utmost importance. Other nerves need to be differentiated for ablation of recurrent thyroid cancer or metastatic lymph nodes in the central and lateral compartments [21]. The relationship of neck nerves to adjacent anatomic structures is shown in Fig. 18.8.

Vagus Nerve

The vagus nerve is divided into cranial, cervical, thoracic, and abdominal branches. After leaving the skull through the jugular foramen, the vagus nerve descends in the neck covered by the carotid sheath (Fig. 18.9).

The vagus nerve is usually located posterolateral to the CCA and posteromedial to the IJV. It is easily visualized on US as a 2–3 mm diameter structure. However, variations in its location relative to the carotid sheath have been reported [22]. The vagus nerve can be located anterior, medial, and posterior to the common carotid artery (Fig. 18.10).

In a normal thyroid gland, CCA, the vagus nerve, and IJV are positioned in horizontal alignment. In cases of posterolateral bulging of the thyroid mass, their positions can be changed within the carotid sheath. If the CCA is pushed away inferolaterally and in a vertical alignment, the vagus nerve is positioned anterior or medial to the CCA, with its exposure more prone to thermal injury (Fig. 18.11).

Various symptoms could develop in the case of vagus nerve injury. Because the cervical portion of the vagus nerve is cranial to the origin of the recurrent laryngeal nerve (RLN), vagus nerve injury may cause symptoms resulting from a dysfunction

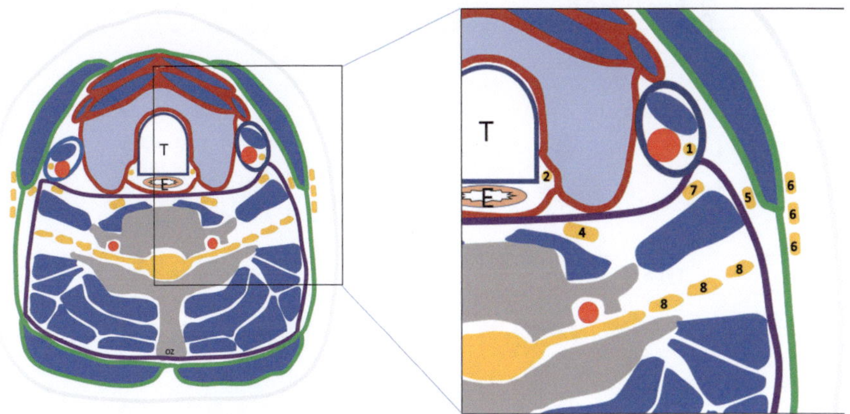

Fig. 18.8 The neck nerves at C6 level; 1, vagus nerve; 2, recurrent laryngeal nerve; 3, superior laryngeal nerve (not in this figure); 4, cervical sympathetic ganglion; 5, spinal accessory nerve; 6, cervical plexus nerve; 7, phrenic nerve; 8, brachial plexus. (With permissions from Park [20])

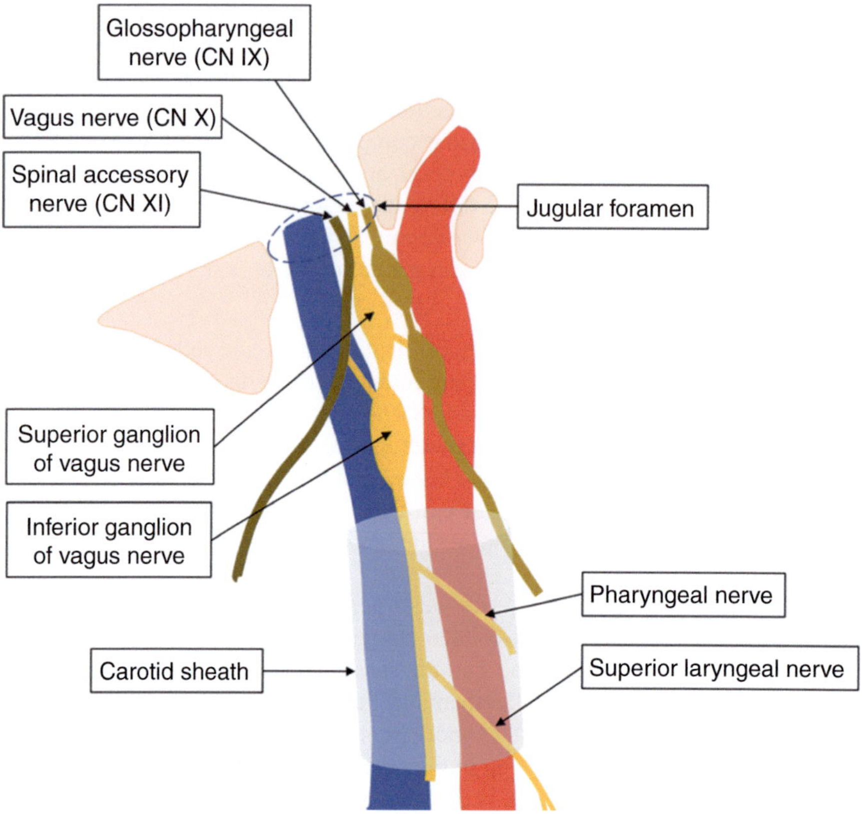

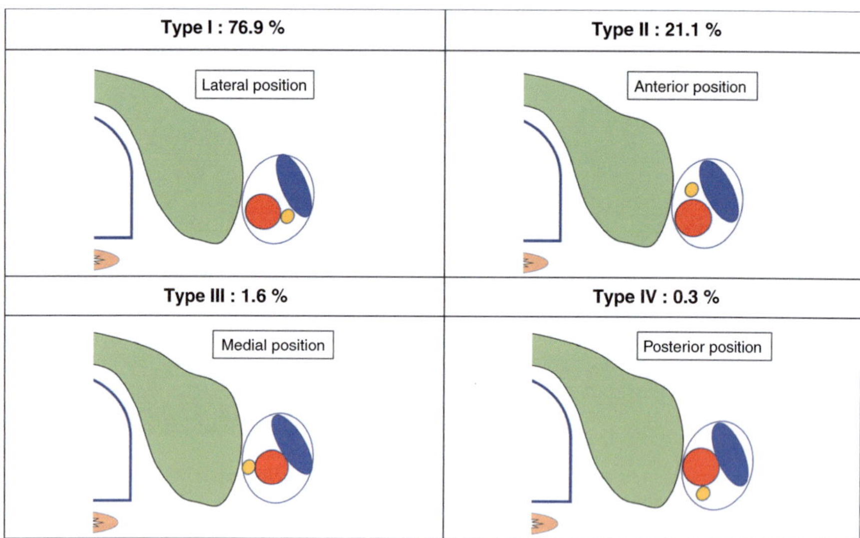

Fig. 18.9 The vagus nerve in the carotid sheath. (With permissions from Park [20])

Fig. 18.10 Variations in the location of the vagus nerve; yellow, the vagus nerve; blue, the internal jugular vein; red, common carotid artery. (With permissions from Park [20])

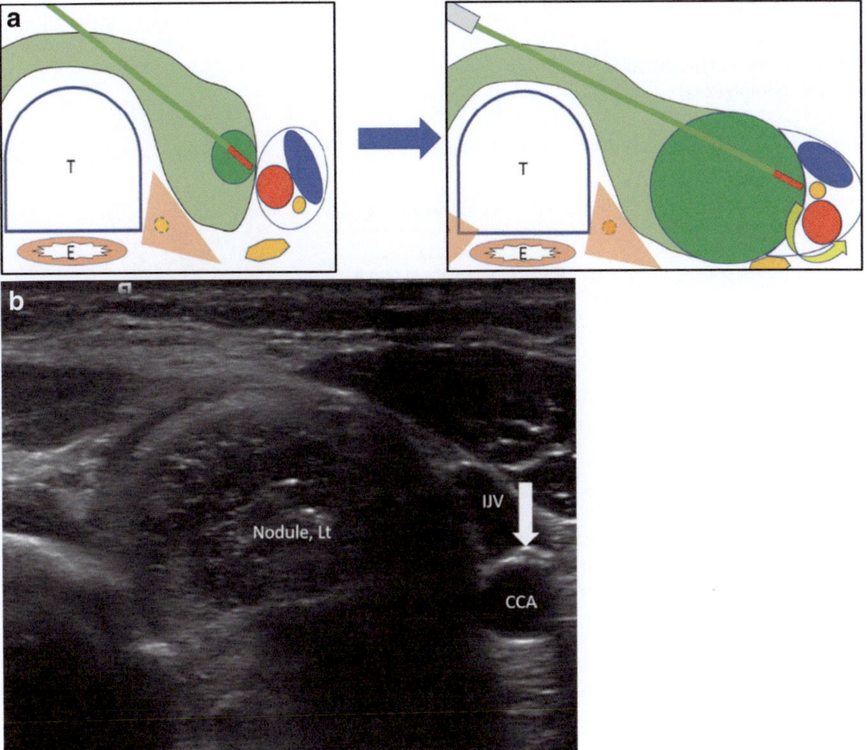

Fig. 18.11 (a) An altered position of the vagus nerve by a bulging thyroid nodule. E esophagus, T trachea; yellow, vagus nerve; blue, internal jugular vein; red, common carotid artery (With permissions from Park [20]). (b) US scan showing an anterior location of the vagus nerve by a bulging nodule in the left lobe of the thyroid gland; solid white arrow, vagus nerve; IJV internal jugular vein, CCA common carotid artery

of the RLN (e.g., cough, voice change) or dysfunction of the vagus nerve itself (e.g., arrhythmia, dysphagia, dyspnea, nausea, hiccups).

The Recurrent Laryngeal Nerve

The Right Recurrent Laryngeal Nerve: The right vagus nerve passes from the posterior aspect of the carotid sheath in the neck base anterior to the first segment of the subclavian artery. At this point, the RLN branches exit from the vagus nerve and first travel inferoposteriorly to loop around this segment of the subclavian artery (the fourth brachial arch remnant). It then progresses superomedially along the neck floor behind the CCA into the right thoracic inlet at the base of the neck and then extends superiorly more obliquely from lateral to medial direction as it ascends the neck. The right RLN finally enters the larynx by penetrating the thyrohyoid membrane at the cricothyroid joint level (Fig. 18.12). The angle between the right RLN and the tracheoesophageal groove is 15–45° in 80% of the patients [23].

Fig. 18.12 The course of the right recurrent laryngeal nerve. (Modified from Randolph [24])

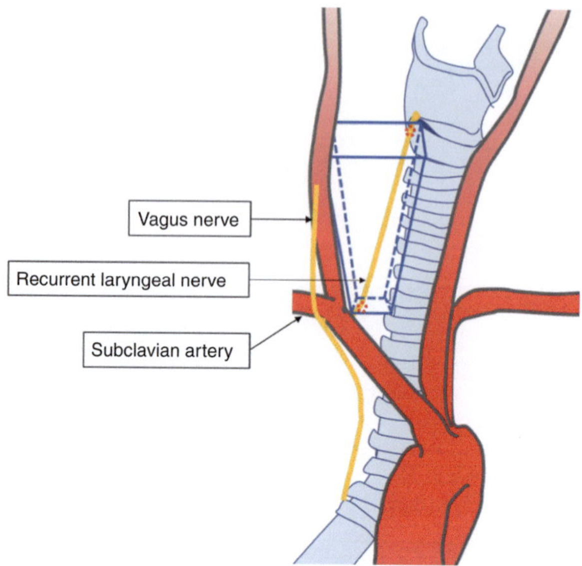

Fig. 18.13 The course of the left recurrent laryngeal nerve. (Modified from Randolph [24])

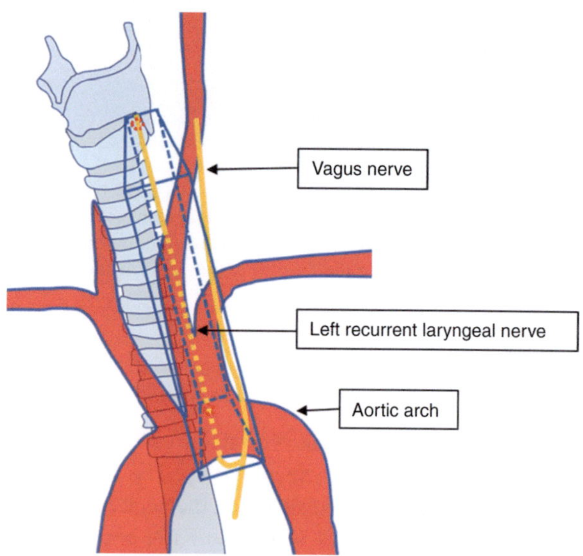

The Left Recurrent Laryngeal Nerve: The left vagus nerve travels from the posterior aspect of the left carotid sheath in the neck base anterior to the aortic arch. Then the left RLN branches underneath the aortic arch just lateral to the obliterated ductus arteriosus and passes posteriorly and superiorly to enter the larynx by penetrating the thyrohyoid membrane at the level of the cricothyroid joint (Fig. 18.13). The left RLN is more medial and ascends into the paratracheal or tracheoesophageal groove [23].

The Dangerous Triangle vs. the Danger Zone

The concept of a "danger triangle" was proposed by Baek et al. to describe an area that encompasses the esophagus, trachea, and medial portion of the thyroid gland around the RLN (Fig. 18.14) [25]. During RFA, the danger triangle should be avoided due to the high risk of thermal injury to these critical structures, especially the RLN. However, this concept has been modified on the right side of the triangle, considering a more oblique course of the right RLN as described above.

The "danger zone" on the right side is an area between the right tracheoesophageal groove and the carotid sheath. This space includes the right RLN and its potential variable locations, the vagus nerve, and the middle cervical sympathetic ganglion (Fig. 18.15). At the mid-to-lower level of the right thyroid gland, the location of the RLN may vary from medial to lateral inside the danger zone.

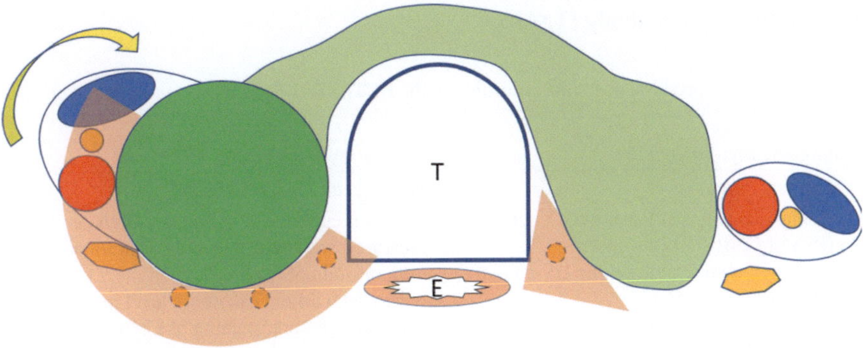

Fig. 18.14 Danger triangle vs. danger zone; E esophagus, T trachea; red circle, common carotid artery; blue oval, internal jugular vein; yellow solid circle, vagus nerve; yellow dotted circle, recurrent laryngeal nerve; yellow heptagon, middle sympathetic ganglion. The dashed yellow circles show the variable locations of the RLN. (With permissions from Park [20])

Fig. 18.15 Volume measurement of an elliptical nodule; $V = abc\pi/6$. a, the longest diameter; b and c, the other two perpendicular diameters

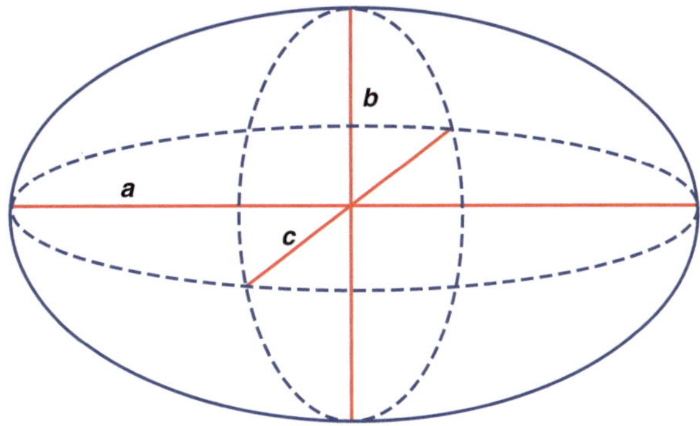

Procedure

Preprocedural Workup

The 2017 KSThR guidelines for the RFA preprocedural checklist are shown in Table 18.7. These are the most detailed guidelines published, to date [14].

Labs
- CBC/coagulation profile
- TSH (thyrotropin)/Free T4/T3
- Calcitonin: increased possibility of medullary carcinoma
- Thyroid autoantibodies: increased possibility of hypothyroidism during follow-up
- Thyroperoxidase antibody (TPOAb)
- Thyroglobulin antibody (TgAb)

Table 18.7 Preprocedural checklist according to the KSThR 2017 guidelines (modified from Kim et al. [14])

Pathologic thyroid nodule	Recurrent thyroid cancer
Pathologic diagnosis	*Pathologic and/or serologic diagnosis*
Benign diagnosis at least two US-guided FNA or CNB Benign diagnosis at least one US-guided FNA or CNB in AFTN Benign diagnosis at least one US-guided FNA or CNB in thyroid nodules with highly specific benign US features	Cancer recurrence at US-guided FNA or CNB Increased washout Tg level in aspirate or Tg immunostain of CNB specimen Increased washout calcitonin level in aspirate or calcitonin immunostaining of CNB specimen in patients with medullary cancer
US	*US*
Features of the nodule and surrounding critical structures Nodule volume	Features of the nodule and surrounding critical structures Tumor volume
Symptom score	
Cosmetic score	
Laboratory tests	*Laboratory tests*

Complete blood count
Blood coagulation battery
Thyroid function test
   Serum TSH
   Serum T3
   Serum fT4
	Complete blood count
	Blood coagulation battery
	Thyroid function test
	   Serum TSH
	   Serum T3
	   Serum fT4

Additional imaging study	*Additional imaging study*
CT or MRI[a] 99mTc pertechnetate or 123I thyroid scan[b]	CT or MRI[a]

AFTN autonomously functioning thyroid nodule, *CNB* core needle biopsy, *CT* computed tomography, *FNA* fine-needle aspiration, *fT4* free thyroxine, *MRI* magnetic resonance imaging, *RFA* radiofrequency ablation, *T3* tri-iodothyronine, *Tg* thyroglobulin, *TSH* thyroid-stimulating hormone (thyrotropin), *US* ultrasound

[a]Selectively indicated

[b]Indicated for AFTN

Pathology

Benign cytopathologic diagnosis (at least two separate times: FNA or CNB) is required. According to the KSThR 2017 guideline, a single benign diagnosis on FNA or CNB is sufficient when the nodule has US features highly specific for benignity.

Imaging

- US features of nodule and neck:

  - Number
  - Location
  - Volume
    Thyroid nodules are round or more elliptical, as shown in Fig. 18.15.
    The formula for calculating the volume of elliptical nodules is as follows:

    $$\text{Ellipsoid volume}\,(V) = \text{height}\,(a) \times \text{width}\,(b) \times \text{length}\,(c) \times \pi\,/\,6$$

  - Composition (Table 18.8)
    The strategy for choosing between EA and thermal ablation depends on the composition of thyroid nodules [9, 14].
  - Vascularity (Table 18.9)
  - Echogenicity
  - Margin
  - Calcifications

- Relationship between the target nodule and adjacent structures (skin, strap muscles, trachea, esophagus, vessels, and nerves).

Table 18.8 Classification of thyroid nodules by composition

Classification	Composition	Selection of ablation
Cystic nodule	>90% cyst	EA
Predominantly cystic nodule	50–90% cyst	EA first or combined with RFA
Predominantly solid nodule	50–90% solid	RFA
Solid nodule	>90 solid	RFA

Table 18.9 Grading of thyroid nodules by vascularity

Grade	Vascularity
0	No intranodular vascularity
1	Intranodular vascularity but peripheral portion only
2	Intranodular vascularity <50%
3	Intranodular vascularity >50%

- Computed tomography (CT) or magnetic resonance imaging (MRI): selectively indicated. CT or MRI examinations may help to evaluate the intrathoracic extent of benign thyroid nodules.
- ^{99m}Tc-pertechnetate or ^{123}I thyroid scan—indicated for AFTN.

Clinical Evaluation

- Symptom score: visual analog scale from 0 to 10 (Fig. 18.16) to rank the severity of discomfort or pain.
- Cosmetic score (Table 18.10).

Informed Consent

The following content should be included in an informed consent statement [14]:

- The change in the size of ablated thyroid nodules may be slow (several months to years).
- The number of expected treatment sessions.
- Possibility of regrowth of the treated nodule and the need for additional treatments.
- Warning for possible pain with various degrees during the ablation.
- Complications of ablation (reported incidence of 3.3%).
- Ask patients about their history of thyroid surgery, the side effects of any drugs they are taking, and whether they are taking drugs such as antiplatelets, anticoagulants, and thyroid hormones. Further observation or admission may be required after ablation, depending on the patients' condition following ablation.

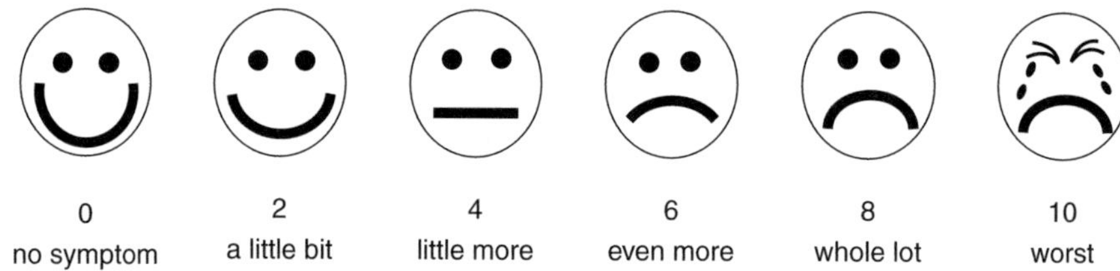

Fig. 18.16 Preprocedural symptom score for RFA

Table 18.10 Cosmetic score features for RFA

Score	Features
1	No palpable mass
2	Palpable mass but no cosmetic problem
3	Cosmetic problem on swallowing only
4	A readily detectable cosmetic problem

The Procedure

Total ablation time usually ranges from 20 to 40 min for a 2–4 cm diameter nodule, but ablation time depends on the operator's experience.

Patient Preparation

The aseptic procedure with sterile technique is recommended.

- Supine position with mild to moderate neck extension: pillow under the shoulder and sponge or thin cushion under the head.
- Skin prep with an antiseptic solution: chlorohexidine or iodopovidone.
- Surgical drape: the opening should be wide enough to allow access to the thyroid and perithyroid structures.
- Grounding pads for a monopolar radiofrequency electrode (MRFE): the electric current runs through the patient's entire body.

Pain Control and Monitoring

Lidocaine (1–3%) is used for local anesthesia at the puncture site and around the thyroid gland and/or thyroid nodule. The skin incision is not needed, thus preventing unnecessary scar formation. If a patient experiences intolerable pain during RFA, the power should be reduced or turned off for several seconds. Pain or discomfort usually disappears rapidly, and the procedure may then be continued. Intravenous (IV) conscious (moderate) sedation could be used for pain control. Voice change should be monitored intermittently during the procedure by having the patient speak a few words when RF power is off [26].

Basic Physics

The term "radiofrequency" refers to a high-frequency alternating electric current oscillating between 200 and 1200 kHz. As shown in Fig. 18.17, a closed electric

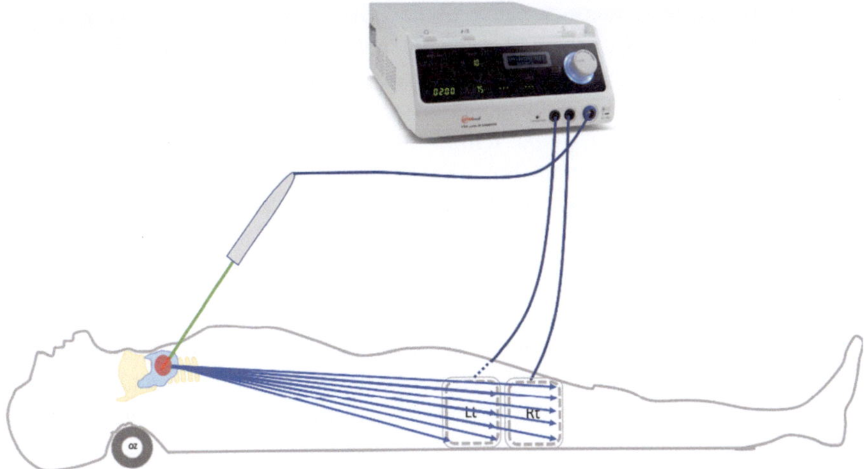

Fig. 18.17 Electric circuit during thyroid RFA. (With permissions from Park [20])

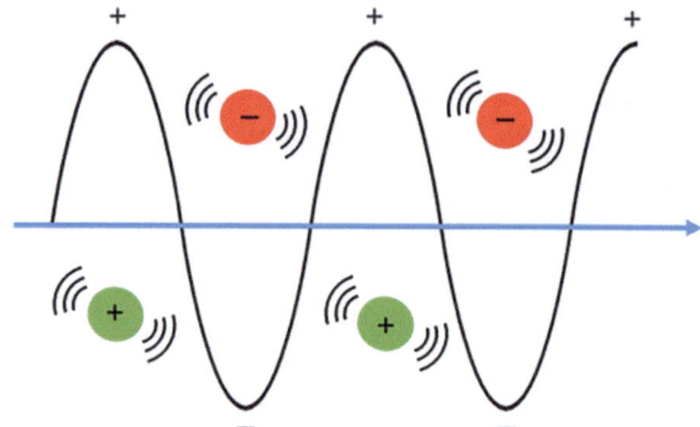

Fig. 18.18 Microscopic phenomena during thyroid RFA

circuit is formed through the body. The RF power agitates tissue ions (i.e., Na+, K+, and Cl) that carry the electric current as they attempt to follow the changes in the direction of the alternating current (Fig. 18.18). For a typical frequency of 500 kHz, the direction of the current (and ion movement) changes a million times per second [25, 27].

There are two heating areas surrounding the RF electrode: the direct heating area and the indirect heating area. The direct heating area is close to the RF electrode and has a high current density. The heat generated in this area is called friction heat. Although this heat causes immediate damage to tumor tissue, the damage is significant only in regions very close to (thus, within a few mm of) the electrode. Simultaneously, tumor tissue that is more remote from the electrode is heated slowly via thermal conduction from the hot region adjacent to the electrode (conduction heat) (Fig. 18.19) [28].

The nature of thermal damage caused by RF is dependent on both the tissue temperature achieved and the duration of heating. Elevation of tissue temperature to 40 °C does not induce tissue damage. Tissue temperatures between 42 and 45 °C, formally termed hyperthermia, cause tissue cells to become more susceptible to damage when exposed to chemotherapeutic agents and/or irradiation. Irreversible cellular damage occurs when temperatures are increased to 46 °C for 60 min or to 50–52 °C for 4–6 min. Near-immediate tissue coagulation is induced at temperatures between 60 and 100 °C, but temperatures greater than 100–110 °C result in vaporization and carbonization (Fig. 18.20) [29, 30]. Microbubbles are produced and represent gases, primarily nitrogen, that are released from the cells (Fig. 18.21), and then the tissue becomes dehydrated [28]. The dehydrated tissue further leads to a noticeable decrease in its electrical conductivity.

Equipment

Generator: An RF generator supplies RF power to the tissue through an electrode. Continuous RF out mode is used for thyroid ablation, which is specially designed for thyroid RFA. In this mode, the RF power is generated continually and controlled by an RF output control.

Electrode: Electrodes have various active tips ranging from several millimeters to a centimeter. Ablation can begin at 5 W (3.8 mm active tip), 10 W (5 mm active

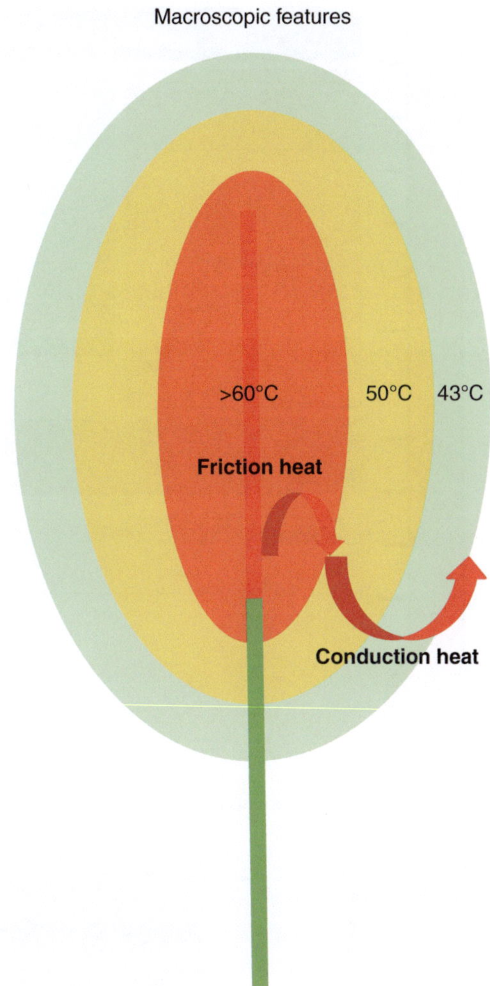

Fig. 18.19 Macroscopic phenomena during thyroid RFA. (With permissions from Park [20])

tip), 20 W (7 mm active tip), or 35 W (10 mm active tip) of RF power under the impedance control mode. If a transient hyperechoic zone at the electrode tip does not appear within 5–10 s, RF power is increased in 5–10 W increments up to 15–80 W [24] (Fig. 18.22). For thyroid RFA, a short shaft length (7 cm) is used, as it allows for more precise control in treating the gland, which is located close to the surface of the neck. An internally cooled electrode is used to prevent or minimize charring (Fig. 18.23).

Pump: Chilled saline (>0 °C) is circulated by a peristaltic pump. The pump continuously reduces the temperature around the electrode tip to prevent or minimize charring (Fig. 18.24). The temperature on the panel of the generator indicates the temperature inside the electrode tip. It is not the actual temperature of the tissue.

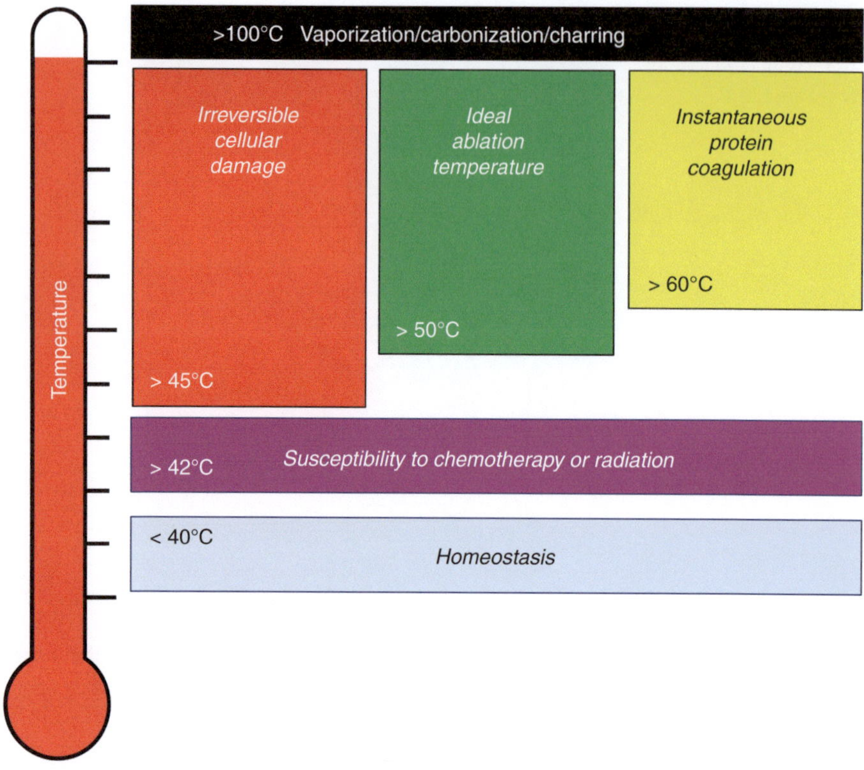

Fig. 18.20 Tissue reaction to heat. (Modified from Hong and Georgiades [28])

Fig. 18.21 Echogenic effects by microbubble

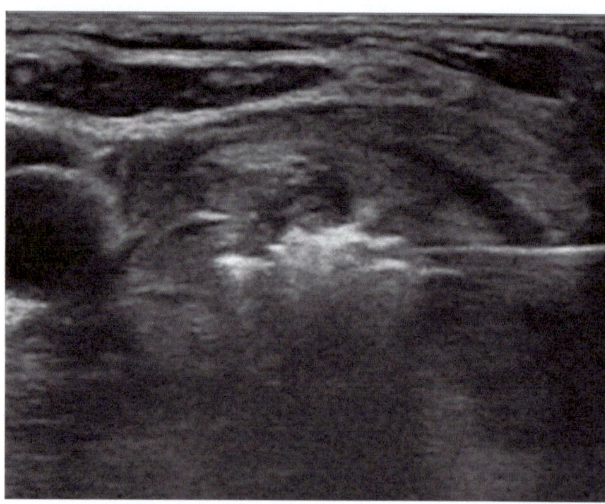

Fig. 18.22 Various sizes for radiofrequency electrode needle tips. (With permissions from STARmed Co., Ltd. Goyang-si, South Korea)

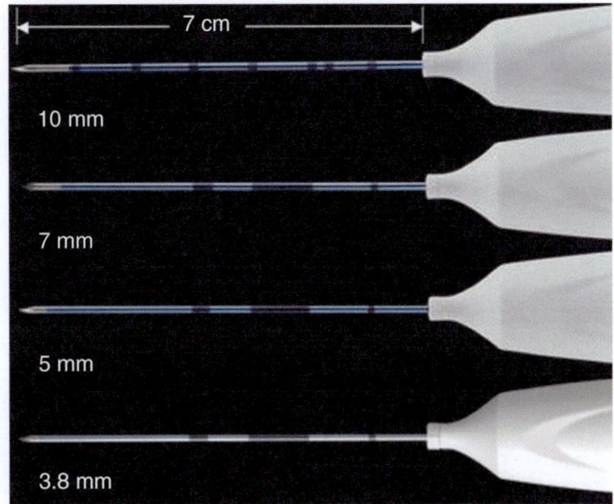

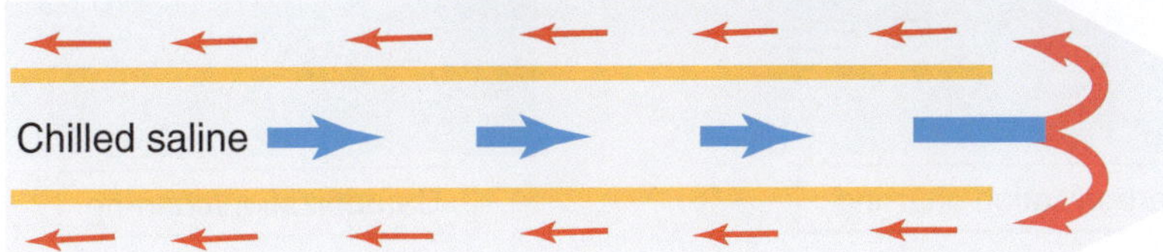

Fig. 18.23 Internal cooling of an electrode tip. (With permissions from Park [20])

Grounding Pads: The grounding pad, which is adhered to the patient's skin away from the ablation site, is intended to safely return the electrical current from the patient back to the generator through a cable (Fig. 18.25). Because the conductive surface area of the grounding pad is much larger than the active electrode, the current is dispersed over a wide area, minimizing the heating of the tissue under the grounding pad. A patient burn risk is increased when contact quality is poor between the grounding pad and the patient because the current is concentrated at the contact points rather than dispersed over the entire grounding pad [29, 31].

Planning the Access Route

Careful observation of the vessels along the approach route is required to prevent an electrode from causing serious hemorrhage. Three approach methods can be used (Fig. 18.26).

The Transisthmic Approach Method Is Recommended: The electrode approach is made from the medial (isthmus) to the lateral (nodule) aspect along the transverse axis of the targeted nodule. The entire length of the electrode and the tip can be easily visualized on the transverse US view. This view allows visualization of the

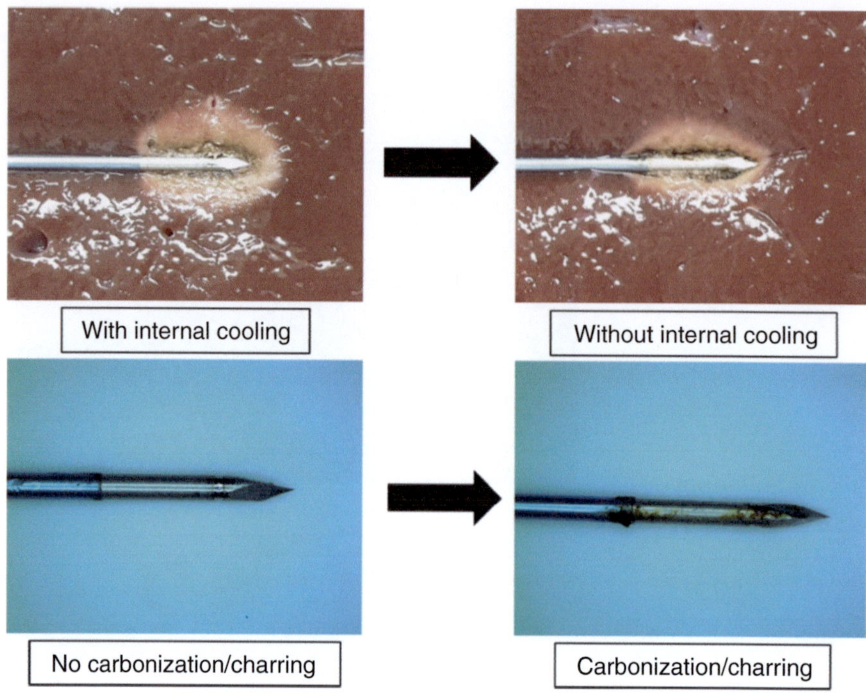

Fig. 18.24 Ex vivo ablation in cow's liver with and without internal cooling; carbonization/charring without internal cooling resulting in a limited ablation

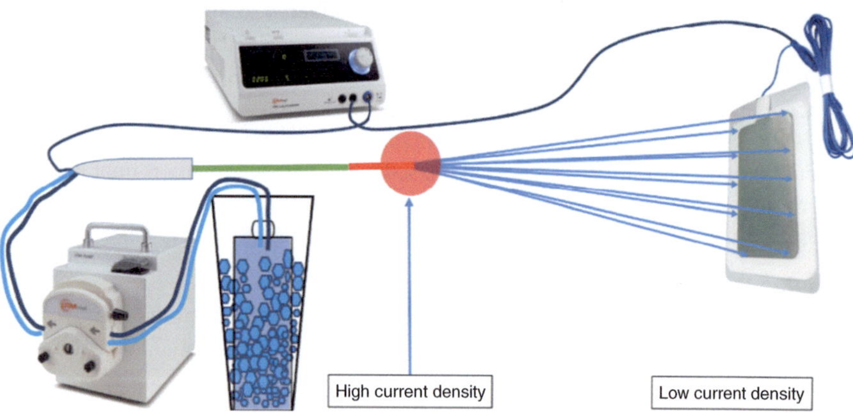

Fig. 18.25 Equipment: generator, pump, monopolar electrode, and grounding pad. (With permissions from STARmed Co., Ltd. Goyang-si, South Korea)

Fig. 18.26 Three approach methods for thyroid RFA; a, transisthmic; b, craniocaudal; c, lateral. (With permissions from Park [20])

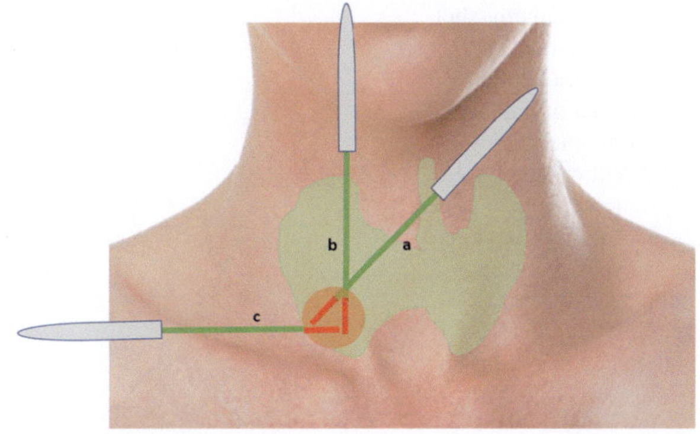

relationship among the electrode tip, the thyroid nodule, the trachea, and the great vessels and may also be used to locate the RLN. Clear visualization of the relationship between the electrode tip and these structures may prevent complications. Passing the electrode through a sufficient amount of thyroid parenchyma (in the isthmus) may prevent the electrode tip's position from moving during swallowing or talking and may also prevent leakage of hot ablated fluid outside the thyroid gland [25, 32].

The Craniocaudal (Longitudinal) Approach Method: The electrode approach is made from the superior to the inferior aspect of a targeted nodule along the long axis of the nodule. It is difficult to determine the relationship between the electrode tip and adjacent structures in the neck. Frequently, movement of the electrode is limited by the mandible or clavicle.

The Lateral Approach Method: If enlarged vessels are present in the isthmus, the lateral approach may prevent serious hemorrhage.

The Moving-Shot Technique

The moving-shot technique for thyroid RFA was designed to avoid thermal injury to surrounding structures [23, 24]. The ablation technique for thyroid nodules should differ from those used to treat tumors in other organs such as the liver or kidneys. For instance, the basic ablation technique for liver tumors requires that the electrode be fixed during ablation. However, the thyroid gland is smaller than other organs, and thyroid nodules are usually ellipsoid rather than round. Therefore, prolonged fixation of the electrode during the ablation of thyroid nodules can cause thermal damage to adjacent structures.

The thyroid nodule is divided into several "conceptual ablating units" of various sizes. These units are smaller at the periphery of the nodule or in areas bordering the adjacent structures around the thyroid gland. The conceptual ablating units are larger in the safer, central portion of the nodule. RFA should be performed unit by unit by moving the electrode, hence the name "moving-shot technique" [25, 32]. Initially, the electrode tip is positioned in the deepest, most remote portion of the nodule, which enables easy monitoring of the electrode tip without disturbances caused by microbubbles. When a transient echogenic area appears in the

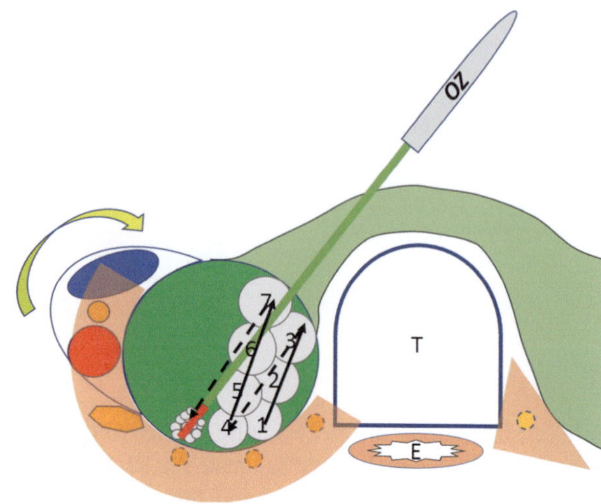

Fig. 18.27 Moving-shot technique; T trachea, E esophagus; red circle, common carotid artery; blue oval, internal jugular vein; yellow solid circle, vagus nerve; yellow dotted circle, recurrent laryngeal nerve; yellow heptagon, middle sympathetic ganglion; numbers 1–7, ablation units. (With permissions from Park [20])

targeted ablating unit, the electrode is continuously moved backward and in the superficial direction to enter untreated ablating units. In predominantly cystic thyroid nodules, the cystic fluid should be aspirated before ablation of the solid portion (Fig. 18.27).

Postprocedural Care and Follow-Up

Immediate Postprocedural Care

Thyroid RFA is an outpatient procedure. The patient will stay in the postprocedural care unit for at least 1 h with monitoring vital signs. After 1–2 h of observation, patients can be discharged. Before the discharge, patients should be evaluated for pain, discomfort, and minor or major complications through physical examination of the thyroid/neck with or without US. The dressing should be changed with a Band-Aid®. Instructions with a follow-up schedule or appointment should be given. Postprocedural medication is not usually required. However, patients who complain of pain or discomfort may benefit from treatment with oral analgesics such as oral acetaminophen or ibuprofen. Admission might be needed when a further observation or clinical care is required in cases of major complications.

For patients experiencing the symptom of difficult breathing by extrinsic compression of the trachea, admission and careful monitoring in an intensive care unit bed might be needed. In severe trachea stenosis, intubation or tracheal stent should also be considered and discussed at a planning stage with ENT surgeons.

During the first day of ablation, neck bulging could be aggravated, and the volume of the ablated nodule may increase. These findings are caused by edema and swelling of the ablated nodule and surrounding soft tissue. Volume reduction usually starts 3–7 days after ablation. The maximal reduction in volume will be observed at the 1-month follow-up, with further gradual reduction anticipated after 3–6 months. Changes in clinical status should be evaluated serially on follow-up visits using symptom and cosmetic scores.

If TSH and thyroid hormones remain abnormal after RFA, they should be re-assayed closely with monthly follow-up interval.

Nonfunctioning Thyroid Nodules
Patients are usually followed up at 1, 3, 6, and 12 months after the procedure and every 6–12 months during the second year after ablation. The physician should check the following items during follow-up visits. For guidelines for monitoring patients after RFA, see [14].

- Any discomfort or complications
- Ablation status of the nodule: volume analysis
- Status of clinical problems: symptom and cosmetic scores, respectively
- Labs: TFT including TSH, freeT4, and T3

US scan is the primary examination tool, with CT or MRI serving ancillary roles. Patients with the intrathoracic extension of the thyroid nodule may require a repeat CT or MRI examination for comparison with CT or MRI data obtained before the procedure.

US findings of successful ablation are as follows:

- Loss of intranodular vascular signal in Doppler US examination
- Decreased nodule volume: >50%
- Decreased echogenicity of the ablated nodule (which looks like a malignancy)

Changes in size, echogenicity, and intranodular vascularity of the nodule should be evaluated on follow-up US examinations. Volume reduction (VR) is calculated using the following equation:

$$VR(\%) = \left[\text{initial volume}(mL) - \text{final volume}(mL) \right] \times 100 \,/\, \text{initial volume}$$

Autonomously Functioning Thyroid Nodules
^{99m}Tc pertechnetate scintigraphy, blood, and US examinations are essential to evaluate the ablation status of AFTN. US examination and laboratory tests for TSH and thyroid hormone should be performed 1, 3, 6, and 12 months after RFA. Measurements of thyroid autoantibodies and ^{99m}Tc pertechnetate scintigraphy should be performed 6–12 months after RFA.

Results

The results of RFA of benign nodules are evaluated by changes in volume (cytoreduction) and clinical problems (pressure symptoms and cosmetic issues). For patients who undergo ablation of AFTNs, the serum concentration of TSH and thyroid hormones in addition to nuclear scan is needed to see the conversion to euthyroidism.

Nonfunctioning Thyroid Nodules

A prospective multicenter study revealed that the mean volume reduction was 80%, 84%, 89%, 92%, and 95% at the 12-, 24-, 36-, 48-, and 60-month follow-ups, respectively [33]. After RFA, symptoms and cosmetic problems improved or disappeared in the majority of patients.

In a retrospective longitudinal observational study, 215 patients were followed up after a single RFA session for >3 years [33]. At 6 months after the procedure, median nodule volume was significantly lower than at baseline, with further progressive volume reduction at 1- and 2-year follow-up. There was no significant change in nodule volume at 3 and 4 years, but at 5 years, there was an additional slight volume reduction. The best response was observed in small nodules with a volume below 10 mL (early reduction of 82%). Large nodules showed a smaller reduction in volume (75% reduction of nodules with a volume of 10 to 20 mL and 65% reduction in those with a volume of ≥20 mL). This shows the difficulty in complete ablation of large nodules with a single-session ablation. Large nodules may require additional treatment of untreated peripheral portions of nodules which can regrow on long-term follow-up.

Autonomously Functioning Thyroid Nodules

In a systemic review and meta-analysis, radiofrequency ablation has proven to be effective in treatment of AFTN. The volume reduction rate was 79% at the 1-year follow-up. TSH normalization or scintigraphically proven efficacy of RFA was about 60% [35]. AFTNs are more likely to respond when their baseline volume is <12 mL and when the volume is reduced by at least 80% after 12 months from the treatment [35, 36]. The result is in line with the concept that the greater the baseline volume, the higher the likelihood to undertreat hyperfunctioning areas, leading to hyperthyroidism or symptom relapse. A tailored patient selection with complete ablation seems the key to successful conversion to euthyroidism in AFTN.

Marginal Regrowth

Even with excellent volume reduction and improved symptomatic and/or cosmetic problems, nodule recurrence has been reported after RFA, which varies from 5% to 35% [37–44]. Regrowth is defined as >50% increase of nodule volume compared to the smallest volume recorded previously during the postprocedural follow-up evaluations [45]. Most cases of regrowth occur as a result of marginal regrowth [46].

Marginal regrowth, also known as regrowth phenomenon, occurs from the under-treated peripheral portion of the tumor. When follow-up US results suggest regrowth of an untreated peripheral portion of the nodule, an additional RFA should be scheduled.

According to Dr. Sim et al., a volume increase of the viable portion was an early indicator of regrowth in treated nodules, which occurred about 1 year earlier than the increase of the total volume [37]. The volume of the viable portion in a treated nodule can be calculated by the following formula (Fig. 18.28).

$$\text{Total volume}\,(Vt) = \text{Viable volume}\,(Vv) + \text{Ablated volume}\,(Va)$$

$$\text{Viable volume}\,(Vv) = \text{Total volume}\,(Vt) - \text{Ablated volume}\,(Va)$$

Ablation of the peripheral portion is the key to achieving a satisfactory volume reduction and preventing regrowth of the nodule, which requires repeat sessions. Because of recurrence induced by marginal regrowth, complete ablation of the nodule margin was emphasized [46].

Several factors were described to influence the nodule regrowth or efficacy [42, 47–51]. It is reported that single-session ablation is effective in most thyroid nodules [33, 52]; however, for nodules larger than 20 mL, additional ablation may be required to achieve sufficient volume reduction [34, 52]. Tumor vascularity was another influencing factor. The tendency to regrow is relatively high for nodules with abundant peripheral vascularity, which can be attributed to incomplete ablation by the heat-sink effect [53]. To prevent this, vascular ablation technique was suggested by Park et al. [26].

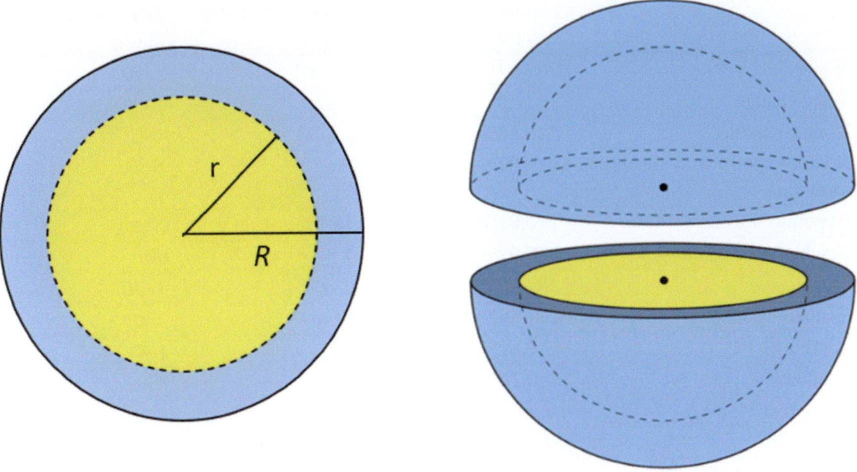

Fig. 18.28 The viable portion (blue outer shell) vs. the ablated portion (yellow inner core) of an ablated tumor. (With permissions from Park [20])

Moreover, possible other influencing factors of the regrowth or efficacy are the tissue characteristics of the thyroid nodule, nodular margin, proximity of the nodule to the critical structures, the total energy deposition during the initial session, and the type of energy source by treatment modalities [23, 47, 52–55].

Complications

Although the complication rate of RFA is low, various complications may still occur. No deaths related to RFA have been reported. The first and largest study of complications in the treatment of benign nodules with US-guided RFA was reported in 2012 by KSThR. From June 2002 to September 2009, 1459 patients underwent RFA of 1543 thyroid nodules with an RF system with internally cooled electrodes at 13 thyroid centers. Twenty (1.4%) major complications were reported, including voice changes in 15 patients, nodule rupture in 3 patients (including 1 patient with abscess formation), hypothyroidism in 1 patient, and brachial plexus injury in Table 18.11 [50].

Pain

Pain is the most common symptom associated with the procedure. Most patients complain of various degrees of pain at the ablated site or pain radiating to the head, ears, shoulders, chest, back, or teeth.

Table 18.11 Complications resulting from thyroid radiofrequency ablation

Complication or side effect	Number of complications	Time of detection (days)	Time to recovery (days)
Major	*20 (1.4%)*	*1–180*	*1–90*
Voice change	15 (1.02%)	1–2	1–90
Nodule rupture	2 (0.14%)	22–30	<30
Nodule rupture with abscess formation	1 (0.07%)	50	None
Hypothyroidism	1 (0.07%)	180	None
Brachial plexus injury	1 (0.07%)	1	60
Minor	*28 (1.92%)*	*1–2*	*1–30*
Hematoma	15 (1.02%)	1	<30
Vomiting	9 (0.62%)	1–2	1–2
Skin burn	4 (0.27%)	1	<7
Side effect	*46 (3.15%)*	*1*	*1–2*
Pain	38 (2.6%)	1	1–2
Vasovagal reaction	5 (0.34%)	1	1
Coughing	3 (0.21%)	1	1

Note: As reported by Baek et al. [50]

Management
- Turn off RF output and stop RFA.

Voice Change

Voice change is one of the most serious complications of RFA ablation and is caused primarily by thermal injury to the RLN, which is different from mechanical injury in the surgical field. Although most patients show complete voice recovery, usually within 60–90 days, some severe injuries can result in permanent RLN palsy [50].

Management
- RF output is turned off immediately.
- Perithyroidal injection of dextrose 5% in water (D5W).
- As a rescue maneuver for voice change during the ablation, chilled D5W can be injected using a 25 G or 27 G needle to cool down the temperature around the nerve. The needle is advanced toward the medial and inferior margin of the carotid artery. Under US guidance, 10–20 cc of the chilled D5W can be quickly injected enough to propagate into the tracheoesophageal groove where the nerve is located (Fig. 18.29). This hydrodissection technique has proven effective not only for a quick recovery of the voice change but also in preventing permanent nerve injury [51, 56].

Hemorrhage

Hemorrhage is usually caused by mechanical injury to the perithyroidal vessels. These vessels can be scanned using color Doppler before insertion of the electrode.

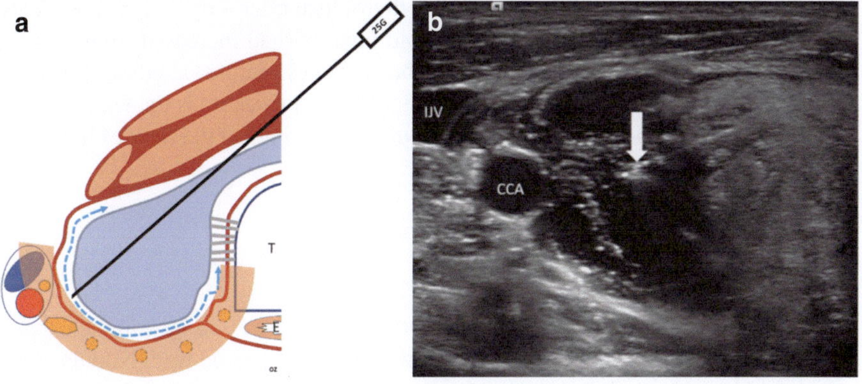

Fig. 18.29 (a) Hydrodissection as a rescue maneuver in voice changes (With permissions from Park [20]). (b) US scan showing D5W injected between the right common carotid artery and posterolateral margin of the thyroid gland; IJV internal jugular vein, CCA common carotid artery

Extraglandular Hemorrhage

Serious perithyroidal hemorrhage can happen when the tip of the electrode perforates the carotid artery or systemic artery. US tracking of the electrode is the key during the moving-shot technique to prevent this. Caution is needed especially when the needle is advanced toward the systemic artery and its branches, such as carotid/subclavian and superior/inferior thyroid arteries. The perithyroidal space can be filled with echogenic blood and can expand when there is an arterial injury. Due to the deep location of the perithyroidal space, manual compression may not be effective in controlling bleeding. The bleeding will usually stop by tamponade in the absence of coagulopathy. But if bleeding is continuous, it could compress or deviate the trachea. It is important to check the patient's vital signs, especially respiration and oxygen level (PaO_2), and maintain the airway. Staff should be well prepared for worst-case scenarios, such as intubation or emergency operation.

Intranodular Hemorrhage

Arterial bleeding is more likely than venous bleeding. Arterial bleeding will appear as an abrupt expansion of the nodule with amorphous new echogenicity on US but can be well controlled by direct ablation of the hemorrhagic focus.

Management

- Use a color Doppler when bleeding is suspected or detected.
- Stop the procedure and apply manual compression

  - If the bleeding continues, stop the ablation and start observing the patient's condition. Cauterize the bleeding focus if feasible.
  - If the bleeding stops, the ablation could be continued.

Hypothyroidism

There have been only a few reports of hypothyroidism after RFA [50, 51]. Patients who developed hypothyroidism after thyroid ablation had increased thyroperoxidase antibody and/or thyroglobulin antibody levels before ablation [56–60]. Although the risks of hypothyroidism are very low and its cause is unclear, patients with elevated antibodies before ablation should be informed of the risks of hypothyroidism after RFA [61].

Rupture

After ablation, rupture of benign thyroid nodules may be caused by volume expansion resulting from delayed hemorrhage or tearing of the nodule wall. Nodular rupture should be suspected in patients who complain of sudden neck bulging and pain during follow-up periods.

Management

- Conservative management:

  - Gentle compression of the bulging site: avoid invasive procedures such as needle aspiration.

- Surgical incision and drainage can be considered if needed.

Tracheal Injury

The initial symptom of tracheal thermal injury is cough. Perforation of the trachea is caused by severe thermal injury.

Management
- Without perforation: observation with conservative management
- With perforation: emergency operation

Esophageal Injury

Esophageal perforation from direct thermal injury may result in neck infection and abscess formation.

Management
- Without perforation: observation with conservative management such as pain control and antibiotics coverage
- With perforation: emergency operation or stent placement

Thermal injury to both the trachea and esophagus may cause neck abscess and tracheoesophageal fistula.

Nausea and Vomiting

Some patients may experience nausea and vomiting after RFA. The cause of these symptoms is unclear. It could be from a disturbance of the autonomic system, especially irritation of the vagus nerve.

Management
- IV antiemetics

Edema and Fever

These are usually transient and self-limited; however, medication may be helpful to alleviate symptoms.

Management
- A single IV bolus of steroid
  - 40–80 mg of methylprednisolone
- A single IV bolus of anti-inflammatory medications
  - IV acetaminophen
- Ice pack

References

1. Tan GH, Gharib H. Thyroid incidentalomas: management approaches to nonpalpable nodules discovered incidentally on thyroid imaging. Ann Intern Med. 1997;126(3):226–31.
2. Guth S, Theune U, Aberle J, Galach A, Bamberger CM. Very high prevalence of thyroid nodules detected by high frequency (13 MHz) ultrasound examination. Eur J Clin Investig. 2009;39(8):699–706.
3. Hegedüs L. Clinical practice. The thyroid nodule. N Engl J Med. 2004;351(17):1764–71.
4. Gharib H, Hegedüs L, Pacella CM, Baek JH, Papini E. Nonsurgical, image-guided, minimally invasive therapy for thyroid nodules. J Clin Endocrinol Metab. 2013;98(10):3949–57.
5. Haugen BR, Alexander EK, Bible KC, Doherty GM, Mandel SJ, Nikiforov YE, et al. 2015 American Thyroid Association Management guidelines for adult patients with thyroid nodules and differentiated thyroid cancer: the American Thyroid Association Guidelines Task Force on thyroid nodules and differentiated thyroid cancer. Thyroid. 2016;26(1):1–133.
6. Yoon JH, Lee HS, Kim E-K, Moon HJ, Kwak JY. Malignancy risk stratification of thyroid nodules: comparison between the thyroid imaging reporting and data system and the 2014 American Thyroid Association management guidelines. Radiology. 2016;278(3):917–24.
7. Tessler FN, Middleton WD, Grant EG, Hoang JK, Berland LL, Teefey SA, et al. ACR thyroid imaging, reporting and data system (TI-RADS): white paper of the ACR TI-RADS committee. J Am Coll Radiol. 2017;14(5):587–95.
8. Cibas ES, Ali SZ. The 2017 Bethesda system for reporting thyroid cytopathology. Thyroid. 2017;27(11):1341–6.
9. Jang SW, Baek JH, Kim JK, Sung JY, Choi H, Lim HK, et al. How to manage the patients with unsatisfactory results after ethanol ablation for thyroid nodules: role of radiofrequency ablation. Eur J Radiol. 2012;81(5):905–10.
10. Na DG, Lee JH, Jung SL, Kim J, Sung JY, Shin JH, et al. Radiofrequency ablation of benign thyroid nodules and recurrent thyroid cancers: consensus statement and recommendations. Korean J Radiol. 2012;13(2):117.
11. Garberoglio R, Aliberti C, Appetecchia M, Attard M, Boccuzzi G, Boraso F, et al. Radiofrequency ablation for thyroid nodules: which indications? The first Italian opinion statement. J Ultrasound. 2015;18(4):423–30.
12. Gharib H, Papini E, Garber JR, Duick DS, Harrell RM, Hegedüs L, et al. American Association of Clinical Endocrinologists, American College of Endocrinology, and Associazione Medici Endocrinologi Medical guidelines for clinical practice for the diagnosis and management of thyroid nodules – 2016 update: appendix. Endocr Pract. 2016;22(Supplement 1):1–60.
13. Interventional-procedure-consultation-document.pdf [Internet]. [cited 2020 June 13]. Available from: https://www.nice.org.uk/guidance/ipg562/documents/interventional-procedure-consultation-document.
14. Kim J, Baek JH, Lim HK, Ahn HS, Baek SM, Choi YJ, et al. 2017 thyroid radiofrequency ablation guideline: Korean Society of Thyroid Radiology. Korean J Radiol. 2018;19(4):632.

15. Dobnig H, Zechmann W, Hermann M, Lehner M, Heute D, Mirzaei S, et al. Radiofrequency ablation of thyroid nodules: "Good Clinical Practice Recommendations" for Austria: an interdisciplinary statement from the following professional associations: Austrian Thyroid Association (ÖSDG), Austrian Society for Nuclear Medicine and Molecular Imaging (OGNMB), Austrian Society for Endocrinology and Metabolism (ÖGES), Surgical Endocrinology Working Group (ACE) of the Austrian Surgical Society (OEGCH). Wien Med Wochenschr 1946. 2020;170(1–2):6–14.
16. Papini E, Pacella CM, Solbiati LA, Achille G, Barbaro D, Bernardi S, et al. Minimally-invasive treatments for benign thyroid nodules: a Delphi-based consensus statement from the Italian minimally-invasive treatments of the thyroid (MITT) group. Int J Hyperth. 2019;36(1):375–81.
17. Papini E, Monpeyssen H, Frasoldati A, Hegedüs L. 2020 European Thyroid Association clinical practice guideline for the use of image-guided ablation in benign thyroid nodules. Eur Thyroid J. 2020;8:1–14.
18. Lee M, Baek JH, Suh CH, Chung SR, Choi YJ, Lee JH, et al. Clinical practice guidelines for radiofrequency ablation of benign thyroid nodules: a systematic review. Ultrasonography. 2021;40(2):256–64. Available from: http://e-ultrasonography.org/journal/view.php?doi=10.14366/usg.20015.
19. Dighe M, Barr R, Bojunga J, Cantisani V, Chammas MC, Cosgrove D, et al. Thyroid ultrasound: state of the art part 1 – thyroid ultrasound reporting and diffuse thyroid diseases. Med Ultrason. 2017;19(1):79–93.
20. Park AW. Thyroid radiofrequency ablation. 1st ed. Charlottesville: Oz & SE; 2020. 114 p.
21. Ha EJ, Baek JH, Lee JH. Ultrasonography-based thyroidal and perithyroidal anatomy and its clinical significance. Korean J Radiol. 2015;16(4):749.
22. Ha EJ, Baek JH, Lee JH, Kim JK, Shong YK. Clinical significance of vagus nerve variation in radiofrequency ablation of thyroid nodules. Eur Radiol. 2011;21(10):2151–7.
23. Fundakowski CE, Hales NW, Agrawal N, Barczyński M, Camacho PM, Hartl DM, et al. Surgical management of the recurrent laryngeal nerve in thyroidectomy: American Head and Neck Society Consensus Statement. Head Neck. 2018;40(4):663–75.
24. Randolph GW. The recurrent and superior laryngeal nerves. 1st ed. Switzerland: Springer; 2016. 313 p.
25. Baek JH, Lee JH, Valcavi R, Pacella CM, Rhim H, Na DG. Thermal ablation for benign thyroid nodules: radiofrequency and laser. Korean J Radiol. 2011;12(5):525.
26. Park HS, Baek JW, Park AW, Chung SR, Choi YJ, Lee JH. Thyroid Radiofrequency Ablation: Updates on Innovative Devices and Techniques. Korean J Radiol. 2017;18(4):615–23.
27. Haemmerich D. Biophysics of radiofrequency ablation. Crit Rev Biomed Eng. 2010;38(1):53–63.
28. Hong K, Georgiades C. Radiofrequency ablation: mechanism of action and devices. J Vasc Interv Radiol. 2010;21(8 Suppl):S179–86.
29. Goldberg SN. Radiofrequency tumor ablation: principles and techniques. [Review] [59 refs]. J Ultrasound. 2001;13(2):129–47.
30. Okhai TA, Smith CJ. Principles and application of RF system for hyperthermia therapy. In: Hyperthermia [Internet]. IntechOpen; 2013 May 15 [cited 2020 June 13]. Available from: https://www.intechopen.com/books/hyperthermia/principles-and-application-of-rf-system-for-hyperthermia-therapy.
31. Goldberg SN, Solbiati L, Halpern EF, Gazelle GS. Variables affecting proper system grounding for radiofrequency ablation in an animal model. J Vasc Interv Radiol. 2000;11(8):1069–75.
32. Shin JH, Baek JH, Ha EJ, Lee JH. Radiofrequency ablation of thyroid nodules: basic principles and clinical application. Int J Endocrinol. 2012;2012:1–7.
33. Jung SL, Baek JH, Lee JH, Shong YK, Sung JY, Kim KS, et al. Efficacy and safety of radiofrequency ablation for benign thyroid nodules: a prospective multicenter study. Korean J Radiol. 2018;19(1):167.
34. Deandrea M, Trimboli P, Garino F, Mormile A, Magliona G, Ramunni MJ, et al. Long-term efficacy of a single session of RFA for benign thyroid nodules: a longitudinal 5-year observational study. J Clin Endocrinol Metab. 2019;104(9):3751–6.

35. Cesareo R, Palermo A, Benvenuto D, Cella E, Pasqualini V, Bernardi S, et al. Efficacy of radiofrequency ablation in autonomous functioning thyroid nodules. A systematic review and meta-analysis. Rev Endocr Metab Disord. 2019;20(1):37–44.
36. Cesareo R, Naciu AM, Iozzino M, Pasqualini V, Simeoni C, Casini A, et al. Nodule size as predictive factor of efficacy of radiofrequency ablation in treating autonomously functioning thyroid nodules. Int J Hyperth. 2018;34(5):617–23.
37. Sim JS, Baek JH, Lee J, Cho W, Jung SI. Radiofrequency ablation of benign thyroid nodules: depicting early sign of regrowth by calculating vital volume. J Hyperth. 2017;33(8):905–10.
38. Lim HK, Lee JH, Ha EJ, Sung JY, Kim JK, Baek JH. Radiofrequency ablation of benign non-functioning thyroid nodules: 4-year follow-up results for 111 patients. Eur Radiol. 2013;23(4):1044–9.
39. Gambelunghe G, Stefanetti E, Colella R, Monacelli M, Avenia N, De Feo P. A single session of laser ablation for toxic thyroid nodules: three-year follow-up results. Int J Hyperth. 2018;34(5):631–5.
40. Valcavi R, Riganti F, Bertani A, Formisano D, Pacella CM. Percutaneous laser ablation of cold benign thyroid nodules: a 3-year follow-up study in 122 patients. Thyroid. 2010;20(11):1253–61.
41. Papini E, Rago T, Gambelunghe G, Valcavi R, Bizzarri G, Vitti P, et al. Long-term efficacy of ultrasound-guided laser ablation for benign solid thyroid nodules. Results of a three-year multicenter prospective randomized trial. J Clin Endocrinol Metab. 2014;99(10):3653–9.
42. Døssing H, Bennedbæk FN, Hegedüs L. Long-term outcome following interstitial laser photocoagulation of benign cold thyroid nodules. Eur J Endocrinol. 2011;165(1):123–8.
43. Spiezia S, Garberoglio R, Milone F, Ramundo V, Caiazzo C, Assanti AP, et al. Thyroid nodules and related symptoms are stably controlled two years after radiofrequency thermal ablation. Thyroid. 2009;19(3):219–25.
44. Sung JY, Baek JH, Jung SL, Kim J, Kim KS, Lee D, et al. Radiofrequency ablation for autonomously functioning thyroid nodules: a multicenter study. Thyroid. 2015;25(1):112–7.
45. Mauri G, Pacella CM, Papini E, Solbiati L, Goldberg SN, Ahmed M, et al. Image-guided thyroid ablation: proposal for standardization of terminology and reporting criteria. Thyroid. 2019;29(5):611–8.
46. Sim JS, Baek JH. Long-term outcomes following thermal ablation of benign thyroid nodules as an alternative to surgery: the importance of controlling regrowth. Endocrinol Metab. 2019;34(2):117.
47. Gambelunghe G, Fede R, Bini V, Monacelli M, Avenia N, D'Ajello M, et al. Ultrasound-guided interstitial laser ablation for thyroid nodules is effective only at high total amounts of energy: results from a three-year pilot study. Surg Innov. 2013;20(4):345–50.
48. Wang B, Han Z-Y, Yu J, Cheng Z, Liu F, Yu X, et al. Factors related to recurrence of the benign non-functioning thyroid nodules after percutaneous microwave ablation. Int J Hyperth. 2017;33(4):459–64.
49. Zhao C-K, Xu H-X, Lu F, Sun L-P, He Y-P, Guo L-H, et al. Factors associated with initial incomplete ablation for benign thyroid nodules after radiofrequency ablation: first results of CEUS evaluation. Clin Hemorheol Microcirc. 2017;65(4):393–405.
50. Baek JH, Lee JH, Sung JY, Bae J-I, Kim KT, Sim J, et al. Complications encountered in the treatment of benign thyroid nodules with US-guided radiofrequency ablation: a multicenter study. Radiology. 2012;262(1):335–42.
51. Kim C, Lee JH, Choi YJ, Kim WB, Sung TY, Baek JH. Complications encountered in ultrasonography-guided radiofrequency ablation of benign thyroid nodules and recurrent thyroid cancers. Eur Radiol. 2017;27(8):3128–37.
52. Cesareo R, Palermo A, Pasqualini V, Simeoni C, Casini A, Pelle G, et al. Efficacy and safety of a single radiofrequency ablation of solid benign non-functioning thyroid nodules. Arch Endocrinol Metab. 2017;61(2):173–9.
53. Rhim H, Goldberg SN, Dodd GD, Solbiati L, Lim HK, Tonolini M, et al. Essential techniques for successful radio-frequency thermal ablation of malignant hepatic tumors. Radiographics. 2001;21(suppl_1):S17–35.

54. Ahn HS, Kim SJ, Park SH, Seo M. Radiofrequency ablation of benign thyroid nodules: evaluation of the treatment efficacy using ultrasonography. Ultrasonography. 2016;35(3):244–52.
55. Gambelunghe G, Bini V, Stefanetti E, Colella R, Monacelli M, Avenia N, et al. Thyroid nodule morphology affects the efficacy of ultrasound-guided interstitial laser ablation: a nested case-control study. Int J Hyperth. 2014;30(7):486–9.
56. Chung SR, Baek JH, Choi YJ, Lee JH. Management strategy for nerve damage during radiofrequency ablation of thyroid nodules. Int J Hyperth. 2019;36(1):203–9.
57. Di Lelio A, Rivolta M, Casati M, Capra M. Treatment of autonomous thyroid nodules: value of percutaneous ethanol injection. AJR Am J Roentgenol. 1995;164(1):207–13.
58. Monzani F, Caraccio N, Goletti O, Lippolis PV, Casolaro A, Del Guerra P, et al. Five-year follow-up of percutaneous ethanol injection for the treatment of hyperfunctioning thyroid nodules: a study of 117 patients. Clin Endocrinol. 1997;46(1):9–15.
59. Baek JH, Moon W-J, Kim YS, Lee JH, Lee D. Radiofrequency ablation for the treatment of autonomously functioning thyroid nodules. World J Surg. 2009;33(9):1971–7.
60. Brkljacic B, Sucic M, Bozikov V, Hauser M, Hebrang A. Treatment of autonomous and toxic thyroid adenomas by percutaneous ultrasound-guided ethanol injection. Acta Radiol. 2001;42(5):477–81.
61. Livraghi T, Paracchi A, Ferrari C, Bergonzi M, Garavaglia G, Raineri P, et al. Treatment of autonomous thyroid nodules with percutaneous ethanol injection: preliminary results. Work in progress. Radiology. 1990;175(3):827–9.

Chapter 19
Arterial Embolization for Thyroid Goiter, Graves' Disease, and Thyroid Malignancy

Alan Alper Sag, Jessica L. Dahle, Jennifer M. Perkins, Hadiza S. Kazaure, Anne Weaver, Sona Sharma, Michael T. Stang, Daniel J. Rocke, Jennifer H. Choe, Tony P. Smith, and Randall P. Scheri

A. A. Sag (✉) · T. P. Smith
Division of Vascular and Interventional Radiology, Department of Radiology, Duke University Medical Center, Durham, NC, USA
e-mail: alan.sag@duke.edu; tony.smith@duke.edu

J. L. Dahle
Endocrine Surgery, Department of Surgery, Ochsner Health, LA, USA
e-mail: jessica.dahle@ochsner.org, jessica.dahle@duke.edu

J. M. Perkins
Division of Endocrinology, University of California San Francisco Medical Center, San Francisco, CA, USA
e-mail: jen.perkins@ucsf.edu

H. S. Kazaure · M. T. Stang · R. P. Scheri
Division of Endocrine Surgery, Department of Surgery, Duke University Medical Center, Durham, NC, USA
e-mail: hadiza.kazaure@duke.edu; michaelt.stang@duke.edu; r.scheri@duke.edu

A. Weaver · S. Sharma
Division of Endocrinology and Metabolism, Department of Medicine, Duke University Medical Center, Durham, NC, USA
e-mail: anne.weaver@duke.edu; sona.sharma@duke.edu

D. J. Rocke
Division of Head and Neck Surgery & Communication Sciences, Department of Surgery, Duke University Medical Center, Durham, NC, USA
e-mail: daniel.rocke@duke.edu

J. H. Choe
Division of Hematology and Medical Oncology, Department of Medicine, Duke University Medical Center, Durham, NC, USA
e-mail: jennifer.choe@duke.edu

© The Author(s), under exclusive license to Springer Nature Switzerland AG 2022

H. Yu et al. (eds.), *Diagnosis and Management of Endocrine Disorders in Interventional Radiology*, https://doi.org/10.1007/978-3-030-87189-5_19

Introduction

Interventional radiology (IR) is built on a legacy of angiography and embolization. Refined over recent decades, these modalities have been successfully applied to acute trauma, elective benign, and elective malignant therapeutics. Applying these methods to the thyroid has the potential to significantly improve patient care by providing minimally invasive options to treat common conditions. For example, in the benign domain, embolization has already been safely demonstrated for a goiter to facilitate surgery or to treat pain, sleep apnea, dyspnea, dysphagia, and/or cosmetic issues. In the malignant domain, angiographic techniques are poised for locoregional therapeutics and synergistic adjuvant therapies.

This chapter aims to create a primer for transarterial locoregional thyroid interventions. Attention is first directed to salient structural relationships succinctly detailed regarding equipment strategies to achieve technical success and avoid complications. An evidence-based framework to guide patient selection and clinical patient care will follow with attention first directed to the benign and then malignant applications. Drug delivery will be reviewed regarding the potential for neoadjuvant radiotherapy and immunotherapy environmental priming. Specific nuances will be discussed, for example, iodine-free transradial angiography in performing radiosensitizing neoadjuvant microenvironment sculpting for I-131 re-treatment.

Practical Anatomic Considerations for Thyroid Embolization

The arterial anatomy of the thyroid is variable because the embryologic thyroid descends simultaneously with aortic arch development [1]. The embryologic thyroid is initially enclosed in a network of arteries, the majority of which disappear [2], giving rise to the conventional four arteries of the thyroid: right superior, right inferior, left superior, and left inferior thyroid arteries, respectively.

The superior thyroid artery (STA) arises from the external carotid artery (ECA) to supply the supero-antero-medial gland and isthmus [3]. The inferior thyroid artery (ITA) arises from the subclavian artery (SCA) to supply the posterolateral gland [4] and, variably, the isthmus [2]. The ITA can arise from the subclavian artery and vertebral artery, or rarely be absent in approximately 5% and 1% and up to 5% of patients, respectively [2]. When absent, a concurrent variant artery, thyroidea ima, arising directly from the aortic arch or brachiocephalic artery (BCA) [3] can replace the ITA to supply its territory [1, 5].

The right lobe is more vascular than the left and is often larger in both health and disease [6], and the ITAs are more prominent than the STAs in mature patients. Blood flow in the thyroid (4–6 mL/minute/gram) is more vigorous than the kidney (3 mL/minute/gram) and especially so in Graves'-associated goiter where it can reach 1 L/minute with a systolic bruit or thrill [6]. This degree of blood flow implies a rich capillary network.

The expected vascular arborization relevant to locoregional drug delivery has incidentally been studied for a different purpose: the creation of surgical neck flaps for wound closure. The neck skin is supplied by a dermal-subdermal plexus derived from myocutaneous perforators of the sternocleidomastoid, strap muscles, and trapezius [7]. The same perforating system supplies the arterial plexus of the thyroid gland and vascular supply to the neck musculature after ligation of the thyroid arteries. The occipital and suprascapular arteries supply the superior and inferior sternocleidomastoid muscle after surgical ligation of the STA [8]. The internal mammary arteries supply the strap muscles after ipsilateral STA and ITA ligation [9]. The thyrocervical trunk, specifically the transverse cervical branch or the superficial cervical branch, supplies the trapezius muscle [9]. Based on the knowledge of this arborization, the thyroid gland can be selectively targeted through each distinct arterial supply.

A comprehensive understanding of this robust arterial supply to the thyroid gland is vital to avoid potential complications. In any embolization procedure, there is a risk of non-target embolization, and anatomic variants impact this risk. In arterial embolization of the thyroid gland, the brain, spinal cord, larynx, face, tongue, parathyroid glands, trachea, esophagus, and hands are at risk for potential non-target embolization.

Anatomic Determinants of Non-target Embolization to the Brain

As noted above, the STA arises from the ipsilateral ECA, and the ITA arises from the ipsilateral thyrocervical trunk. Thus, the radial approach to the thyroid gland is protective in patients with normal anatomic branch patterns as arterial superselection occurs distal to the carotid and vertebral artery origins. In these cases, refluxate-containing particles would embolize the hands, shoulder girdle musculature, face, or tongue, rather than the brain. While this normal anatomic branching pattern occurs in most cases, anomalous arterial branch patterns must be anticipated and ideally identified before the procedure with a CT angiogram or other imaging modality.

Non-ECA origins may benefit from embolic strategies such as flow-controlling catheters or non-particulate embolic agents to allow safe treatment. Specific to the STA, Gupta et al. [9] found an expected or normal origin of the STA in approximately 70% of patients bilaterally, with the remainder variably arising unilaterally from the common carotid artery (CCA) or internal carotid artery (ICA), with less than 10% having aberrant origins bilaterally. However, two cadaveric series by Ozgur [10] and Won [11] provide a less optimistic view demonstrating only 20% have a normal origin of the STA from the ECA, with 40% arising from the CCA and 40% from the carotid bifurcation. Angiographic images at the time of embolization should be carefully reviewed for detecting aberrant extra-thyroidal arterial supply.

Pre-procedure workup and intraprocedural angiography must be utilized to clarify whether cerebral vessels will be at risk at the outset of embolization or during embolization once flow dynamics may have changed. Specific to the ITA, Toni et al. [12] performed a meta-analysis of over 6000 cadaveric analyses concluding that the ITA arises from the thyrocervical trunk in 90%, from the subclavian artery in 9%, and from the vertebral and common carotid arteries (CCA) in the remainder. Toniato reported CCA-origin ITA in 2 out of 8000 thyroidectomies [13], with Nyeki [14] purporting retrovascular goiter position in those cases. When the terminal branch of the ITA is the target in thyroid embolization, rami proximal to this include the ascending cervical artery, which serves the deep neck muscles but more importantly communicates with the vertebral artery [3], placing the posterior cerebral circulation at risk for non-target embolization.

There is extensive communication between the STA and ITA beds [15]. STA-to-STA or STA-to-contralateral ITA communication occurs in 80% of patients [3]. In 20% of patients, all ITA and STA vessels intercommunicate. Therefore, caution should be taken when using very small particles in conjunction with flow cessation devices, such as balloon microcatheters, that may alter hemodynamics and potentially cause left-to-left retrograde embolization subject to the above anatomic variations.

In a small series of thyroid angiograms in patients with thyroid carcinoma, Mojab [16] noted arteriovenous connections likely related to tumor angiogenesis. In the presence of a patent foramen ovale, these connections could result in double-paradoxical embolization reaching the brain via the left-to-right shunt. It is unclear if this is externally generalizable to goiter patients in general; however, the possibility and implications should be noted.

Angiography via femoral access can be beneficial as bilateral thyroid interventions can be accomplished with single cannulation. The thyroidea ima, a variant vessel arising more centrally from the arch vessels serving the isthmus and lobes variably, may also be preferentially accessible via the femoral access. However, specific risks should be considered when utilizing the transfemoral approach. Atherosclerotic plaque may become dislodged along the arterial course to the thyroid target. Again, catheter selection favoring occlusive balloon or umbrella catheters and avoiding embolic agents other than slowly injected particles should be considered to minimize downstream embolization which may reach the brain.

Anatomic Determinants of Non-target Embolization to the Spinal Cord

Spinal cord blood supply is segmental, and branches of the STA and ITA may contribute proximal branches to the spinal cord [17]. To minimize non-target embolization to the spinal cord, the desired treatment target is the terminal thyroid branch. It is important to note that the vertebral arteries also give branches to the spinal cord and the treatment vessel may rarely take off from a vertebral artery. Cone beam CT remains an important technology to delineate spinal cord perfusion once a target vessel has been selected. Direct injection of the target vessel at that level may reveal unnamed collaterals recruited from the spinal cord that may reverse flow during embolization as the downstream territory occludes.

Anatomic Determinants of Non-target Embolization to the Larynx, Face, Tongue, Skin, and Muscles

The STA is usually the first branch from the ECA, originating in a superior trajectory before coursing inferiorly. Cadaveric analysis by Won [11] revealed this expected anatomic origin of the STA from the ECA in approximately 80%, with the remainder arising from either a thyrolingual or linguofacial trunk. After arising from the ECA, the STA can give rise to the infrahyoid artery, supplying infrahyoid strap muscles. The STA can also give rise to the superior laryngeal artery, supplying the laryngeal mucosa and muscles of the larynx [3] before the terminal STA branches reach the thyroid.

The serpentine anatomy of the STA poses specific challenges in thyroid embolization to avoid inadvertent particulate embolization to the larynx, face, tongue, sternocleidomastoid, and strap muscles due to microcatheter kinking and particulate clogging. Embolization targeting the anterosuperior segments of the thyroid risks non-target embolization of the lingual and facial arteries.

Importantly, many of these structures remain unscathed after routine surgical ligation of the vessels implicated. The reason for this difference is that when surgically evident vessels are ligated, this leaves the downstream tissue with reduced arterial blood pressure, but it is also free to seek collateral flow from alternative arteries (as previously detailed), and the tissue does not necrose. In contrast, unintentional particle embolization from the same branches is more harmful because particles are designed to lodge deep in the tissue, and the tissue cannot escape necrosis. Particle size is also relevant as embolic particles <100 micrometers pose the greatest risk for causing skin and mucosal damage [17, 18].

Anatomic Determinants of Non-target Embolization to the Parathyroid Glands

Due to shared arterial blood supply, the parathyroid glands are also at risk for inadvertent ischemia. In normal anatomy, there are four parathyroid glands, with five or more in 10% of patients and three glands in 3% of patients [7]. The position of the superior parathyroid glands is more predictable, and they are symmetric 80% of the time, most frequently at the level of the cricoid [19]. The inferior parathyroid glands are more variable in location.

A well-perfused solitary parathyroid gland is generally considered sufficient to prevent hypocalcemia. If there is clinical concern for hypoparathyroidism, rapid serum PTH testing can reliably confirm the presence of hypoparathyroidism and predict the subsequent risk of hypocalcemia. The rapid PTH testing has an approximately 1-h turnaround time and is available at most major surgery centers.

After embolization, the interventional radiologist should be aware of clinical signs of hypocalcemia, including paresthesia or a positive Chvostek's sign. Severe hypocalcemia can lead to tonic-clonic seizures, laryngeal stridor, and eventual tetany [20]. These factors should be considered especially when performing embolization on the third or fourth quadrant of a patient in whom the other two quadrants have already been embolized.

The superior parathyroid glands are supplied by the STA in only 15% of the time and by the ITA in the remaining 85% of cases [21]. Truncal ligation of the ITA proximal to parathyroid branches does not necessarily result in permanent postoperative hypocalcemia [22] despite the risk of temporary symptomatic hypocalcemia. This is supported by Johansson [23], who noted that ITA occlusion decreased parathyroid blood flow by only 40% on laser Doppler flowmetry. Occlusion of only the STA caused a similar decrease. In contrast, occlusion of the ipsilateral ITA and STA caused profound parathyroid ischemia supporting the idea of a rich paraglandular collateral network [23]. The findings are attributed to STA-ITA intercommunication demonstrated angiographically [24–26], and consistent with this, cases of bilateral ITA embolization resulting in clinical hypoparathyroidism have not been reported thus far. However, in patients who undergo repeated bilateral posterior segment embolizations, there is a risk of causing hypoparathyroidism since each embolization carries a risk of embolizing both the direct and backup collateral arterial supplies to all or many of the parathyroid glands. Therefore, treatment planning should include a consideration of which parathyroid glands are intact and careful consideration of embolization targets.

Anatomic Determinants of Non-target Embolization to the Trachea and Esophagus

Arteries that serve the thyroid can also give rise to branches supplying the trachea and the esophagus. This is a very important anatomic finding to exclude on angiography before particle delivery. Specifically, the ITA gives rise to tracheoesophageal vessels [27] supplying the cervical-level trachea and upper esophagus at the corresponding level. The lower trachea and carina are supplied by the bronchial arteries. The tracheal plexus is formed by the junction of the inferior laryngeal artery and ITA [3] with contribution from the anterior mediastinal branches of the internal mammary arteries and bronchial arteries. The STA does not supply the trachea directly but does contribute to an STA-ITA collateral plexus supplying a small area of the anterior trachea [27]. Thus, inadvertent embolization to the trachea or esophagus may occur during the thyroid-targeted intervention.

Anatomic Determinants of Non-target Embolization to the Hand

In typical arterial configurations, the axillary artery is the first downstream reflux vessel from the thyrocervical trunk. As the ITA arises from the thyrocervical trunk, this anatomic relationship should be noted during thyroid embolization procedures. Accessing the thyroid gland via the radial artery and subsequently the thyrocervical trunk may result in refluxate embolization to the ulnar, or less likely the radial distribution of the hand.

Technical Fundamentals and Equipment Considerations

Intimate knowledge of thyroid anatomy, arterial supply, and available equipment is of paramount importance in successful thyroid embolization. The majority of available clinical studies have reported the use of small sterile microscopic beads made from medical-grade plastics as the embolic agent of choice. These small particle embolics are designed to match the size of the intended target arteriole or capillary bed to result in therapeutic occlusion. The basis for particle-vessel size matching aligns with the goal of embolization in that tissue necrosis is the desired endpoint to reduce the volume of the goiter and allow for physiologic normalization of productive thyroid tissue. As noted above, ideal particle size should be selected based on target and potential non-target tissue as embolic particles <100 micrometers pose the greatest risk for causing skin and mucosal damage [17, 18]. Therapies utilizing particle embolics can be titrated to quantitative endpoints, such as stasis in second-order vessels for five heartbeats on post-embolization angiography. These embolic procedures can also be repeated, which is another favorable aspect of the therapy.

There is extensive collateralization of vessels in the thyroid, which favors particle embolics that deposit in tissue. This extensive collateral vessels can also result in non-target embolization. The option for therapies utilizing drug-eluting particle deposition in the future is enticing. However, the risk of non-target drug delivery through these collaterals should remain a concern and warrant careful utilization.

The choice of contrast should also be carefully considered. Thyroid embolization is ideally performed without the introduction of significant iodine, and gadolinium can be utilized alternatively. Carbon dioxide, on the other hand, carries an unnecessary risk of vapor locking (gas overfilling and occluding blood flow in major vessels) when utilized in the neck and should be avoided. Histoacryl with Lipiodol, while excellently visible, may also not be the optimal agent because its penetration is very distal, and there is a risk of the catheter becoming stuck in the vessel, which is avoidable with the use of particles.

As mentioned above, specific risks should be considered when utilizing the transradial versus transfemoral approaches with respect to potential non-target embolization. The use of a transradial approach for these procedures may significantly reduce the risk of non-target embolization to critical structures in the head and neck.

When utilizing the transfemoral approach, atherosclerotic plaque may become dislodged along the aorta, carotid, or vertebral arteries. Antireflux umbrella- or balloon-style catheters can be used in both approaches. When cannulating the STA specifically, the serpentine course predisposes to kinking the microcatheter and subsequent to particulate clogging. Thus, selecting a RIM-style selection catheter may help avoid this pitfall.

Clinical Considerations for Thyroid Embolization

Goiter Embolization

Despite widespread iodine supplementation, goiter maintains a prevalence of up to 6% [28] of the US population and carries an association with autoimmune disorders such as Graves' or Hashimoto's thyroiditis. Of the 100 million patients from iodine-replete parts of the world with goiter [29], up to 15% will require surgery [30], and if subtotal thyroidectomy is performed, 10% of patients may warrant reoperation [30].

Embolization of goiter can be considered in patients with bulk symptoms (dyspnea, dysphagia, pain, sleep apnea, and cosmetic disfigurement) who are not candidates for a standard surgical option or who would become safer surgical candidates with embolization. For example, embolization can be targeted to shrink a retrosternal goiter component and allow surgical resection without the need for a median sternotomy. For patients who cannot undergo surgery, partial goiter embolization may provide the option to titrate the patient's goiter reduction with staged treatments. Embolization is clinically well tolerated. When applied carefully, it may represent a thyroid-sparing alternative to other treatment options, potentially with a lower risk of vocal paresis, hypoparathyroidism, or thyroid medication dependence.

Support for embolization of goiters has already been demonstrated outside of the United States, but there are less than 200 cases reported in the English-language literature [31]. The first reports are attributed to Galkin in 1994 for primary goiter [32] and recurrent goiter [33]. More definitive studies are needed to delineate patient populations likely to benefit from the embolization, quantify arterial embolization targets to reach the desired clinical effect, and measure the impact of embolization in reducing intraoperative blood loss, operative time, and rate of sternotomy. The existing body of literature supports this direction (Table 19.1).

Embolization as an Alternative to Radioiodide Therapy

Radioiodide therapy is not recommended in several patient populations. Radioiodide treatment is contraindicated in pregnant patients or those who desire pregnancy within 6 months to a year after completing treatment. Patients with local

Table 19.1 Clinical Reports of embolization for goiter with emphasis on novel, large, or recent reports within the last 5 years

Author	Design	Patients	Embolic agent	Outcomes	Major complications
Rohr, 2016 [34]	Case report	1	500–700 micron particles	Resolution of thyroid storm allowing safe thyroidectomy	None
Ducloux, 2016 [31]	Case report	1	300–500 micron particles	TSH low pre-procedure, decreased then reached normal range at 2 months fT4 mildly elevated pre-procedure, normalized at 3 weeks Brief post-embolization mild hyperthyroidism asymptomatic	None
Kaminski, 2014 [35]	Retrospective	22	Histoacryl + Lipiodol mixture or 150–200 micron PVA followed by 200–300 micron PVA	Embolization of bilateral inferior thyroid arteries did not cause significant hypocalcemia Post-embolization syndromes included mild neck pain and elevated temperature Post-embolization rise in fT4 was asymptomatic Graves: Significant decrease in thyrotropin receptor antibody level after treatment	None 5/22 (23%) transient hypocalcemia without supplementation

(continued)

Table 19.1 (continued)

Author	Design	Patients	Embolic agent	Outcomes	Major complications
Brzozowski, 2012 [36]	Retrospective	15	Histoacryl + Lipiodol	Transient asymptomatic elevation of fT3 and fT4 Goiter volume reduction 32% Reduced need for thyreostatic drug usage at 4-year follow-up (2 of 3 patients on Thiamazole no longer needed it after procedure because of euthyreosis)	None 1/15 (7%) transient asymptomatic hypocalcemia
Tartaglia, 2011 [37]	Retrospective	2	100 micron followed by 250 micron particles	Normalization of thyroid hyperfunction at the 6-month follow-up study and reduction of esophagotracheal compressive symptoms durable at 1 year follow-up. No further follow-up available	None One patient needed re-treatment attributed to recanalization of vessels
Zhao, 2009 [38]	Case report	1	Alcohol + Omnipaque (under local anesthesia)	Thyroid bruit resolved immediately post procedure Normalization of thyroid function at 2 months (patient was in thyrotoxic crisis prior to treatment)	None
Zhao, 2008 [39]	Prospective	37	PVA + Papaverine + Omnipaque	At 3-year follow-up: Complete response 26/37 (70%) Partial response 4/37 (11%) Recurrence 7/37 (19%)	None

compressive symptoms or ophthalmopathy may experience progressive and worsening symptoms after radioiodide therapy. Furthermore, some patients may not be appropriate candidates for radioiodide treatment. For example, goiters secondary to Graves' disease may have insufficient iodine uptake to result in effective treatment with radioiodide.

Brito et al. demonstrated in their meta-analysis that multinodular goiter is associated with a lower risk of thyroid cancer than solitary nodules (odds ratio 0.8 with 95% CI 0.67–0.96 including 44,288 patients) [40]. However, Graves' disease and Hashimoto's thyroiditis likely predispose patients to papillary thyroid cancer. Thus, if concern for underlying thyroid malignancy exists, radioiodide treatment may not be the preferred treatment option as the resultant scarring would make the future surgical intervention more challenging and increase the risk of hypoparathyroidism or recurrent laryngeal nerve injury.

Thyroid Embolization in Treatment of Graves' Disease

Embolization may be considered for endovascular management of Graves' disease as it can reduce autoimmune antibody load and is neutral to the calcium-phosphate balance [35]. Graves' disease-related goiter embolization has the potential to create long-term immunonormalization in a fashion similar to subtotal thyroidectomy [39]. This is important as lower antibody levels reduce the risk of ophthalmopathy and placental transfer. Zhao et al. [41] performed embolization with priority for the superior thyroid arteries. On day seven, post-embolization biopsy findings included acute infarction and necrosis of the glandular epithelium and interstitium. At 6 months post-embolization, chronic inflammation and fibroplasia were the dominant findings. At 3 years post-embolization, lymphocytic infiltration was superimposed on the interstitial fibroplasia. Clinically, the level of TSAb (thyroid-stimulating antibody) decreased. This is the primary autoantibody in Graves' stimulating thyroid-stimulating hormone receptor (TSHR) to inhibit apoptosis and promote follicle growth and function [41].

Zhao et al. [42], in a partially overlapping study with that above, followed 37 patients for 3 years, and no patients developed hypothyroidism or hypoparathyroidism after embolization. The parathyroid protection was attributed to the embolization of superior thyroid arteries and only one of two inferior thyroid arteries. Massive thyroid storm did not occur despite aggressive embolization, and this was attributed to generous collateral supply limiting the rate of necrosis in the thyroid. However, the levels of thyroid hormones did begin to increase on day three after embolization owing to the necrotic release of these hormones, which also signaled negative feedback on TSH. The same group found on post-embolization biopsies in Graves' disease patients that embolization decreased expression of VEGF (vascular endothelial growth factor) and bFGF (basic fibroblast growth factor) while decreasing MVD (microvessel density) based on CD34 staining [42] and that thyroid embolization in Graves' disease decreased the activity/titer and positive rate of TSAb, normalized the ratio of CD4+ / CD8+ cells by 6 months, and gradually increased (normalized) the CD3+ / CD8+ ratio at 1 year [39]. They also found that recurrent Graves' disease was diagnosable by regression of the above immunologic improvements, suggesting that further embolization may be needed in those patients [39]. Of note, Tian et al. [43] showed that post-embolization thyroid hormone levels reach their nadir by 3 months. If recurrence occurs, it is most commonly biochemically evident at 1 year.

Based on the current level of evidence, embolization therapy may be most helpful in research trials of hyperthyroid patients who have severe adverse reactions with existing antithyroid medications for Graves', including agranulocytosis or the less severe granulocytopenia, rash, hepatotoxicity, vasculitis, or allergic reactions requiring drug withdrawal. It may also be helpful for those who decline surgery or who are not surgical candidates due to uncontrolled hyperthyroidism or comorbidities. Additionally, embolization may be of interest to female patients desiring future fertility or a preference to defer radioactive therapy although suboptimal medical control as women must wait at least 6 months after radioactive iodine treatment to conceive.

Of note, Graves' disease is not fully understood but felt significant to be a disease of thyroid-specific autoimmunity. To simplify greatly, B cells make antibodies. B cells have a surface marker called CD19; therefore CD19 is synonymous with B cell. In the study by Zhou [39] the CD19 levels did not change after embolization, corroborating with prior reports [44] that the culprit CD19 cells actually reside within the thyroid and do not circulate peripherally. This begs the question of locoregional immunotherapies for Graves' that may not require embolization but could rely on the first-pass extraction of medication injected slowly in a pressure-modified arterial tree using balloon-expandable or umbrella-shaped flow limitation microcatheters. T helper cell to T stimulating cell ratio normalized with clinically successful embolization of Graves' disease (owing to Ts or CD3 + CD8+ cell down-regulation); however, the mechanism is unclear. Finally, natural killer cells (also called CD16 + CD56+ were upregulated in the same study, attributed to a nonspecific inflammatory reaction to "clean up" necrotic embolized thyroid tissue. Large series will be needed to establish the complication rates from this procedure.

Thyroid Embolization and Thyroid Storm

Thyroid storm is frequently mentioned as a feared complication of thyroid embolization. However, Rohr et al. [34] reported the use of embolization to treat a patient with thyroid storm. In that case, recent cardiac catheterization with iodinated contrast prevented radioactive iodine treatment. The condition was refractory to all medical therapies, and surgical therapy was not an option due to concern for thyroid storm. Complete resolution of thyroid storm was evident at 7 days, and the patient underwent surgical resection on day 11.

Antineoplastic Drug Delivery to the Thyroid

Endovascular drug delivery intends either to slowly infuse a medication to rely on the first-pass extraction or to perform a micro-embolic load of drug-eluting particles that can deploy from an ischemic microenvironment. Minimizing ischemia during neoadjuvant radiosensitizing endovascular environment sculpting is an important concept as the mechanism of tumor destruction in radiation therapy is the formation of oxygen free radicals, which require intact blood supply. These concepts will be further explored in the upcoming section of this review.

It is foreseeable that post-surgical patients requiring adjuvant radiosensitizing drug delivery will have altered vascular anatomy after surgical ligation of the major vessels serving the thyroid bed. In these cases, a diagnostic arteriogram may be necessary to reliably identify candidate vessels for drug delivery as the collateralization patterns are not predictable. The nuances described below will become increasingly relevant in that setting.

Dedecjus et al. [45] reported on pre-surgical embolization of 20 patients with thyroid cancer (7 inoperable anaplastic cancer with palliative intent, 13 differentiated thyroid carcinoma with neoadjuvant pre-surgical intent). Both superior thyroid arteries were embolized with 100–750 micron polyvinyl alcohol (PVA) particles and coils, and one inferior thyroid artery was embolized with 100–750 micron PVA. No major complications were observed. It was noted through case-control comparison that embolization significantly reduced blood loss, reduced operating time, and reduced postoperative drainage. Specific to the previously inoperable patients, embolization improved breathing, swallowing, and pain symptoms as well as tumoral bleeding. Thyroid hormones did not significantly increase until 36 h post-embolization, and the authors suggested the operative window to be within this range [45].

Rulli et al. [18] reported a patient in respiratory distress from rapidly enlarging aggressive thyroid lymphoma who was emergently treated with bilateral superior thyroid artery PVA embolization ranging from 150 to 300 microns. The patient was able to tolerate surgery 48 h later with thyroidectomy and was noted to have minimal bleeding and facilitated cleavage planes from thyroid edema. The pathologic diagnosis of lymphoma was possible even though the gland had been embolized 48 h earlier. Beers et al. [46] reported a case of trachea-invasive medullary thyroid carcinoma presenting with hemoptysis for which embolization was therapeutic. Despite initial hemostasis with PVA embolization, tumor revascularization was noted at 2 months post-embolization. Tazbir et al. [47] performed palliative thyroid embolization with 500–710 micron PVA on five patients with anaplastic thyroid carcinoma which temporized hemorrhage and pain from the inoperative condition. Ramos et al. [48] used PVA and Histoacryl to embolize a goiter harboring medullary carcinoma, facilitating surgery for the retrosternally extending gland 7 days later.

Advanced medullary thyroid carcinoma is an especially difficult cancer to treat when inoperable, as surgery is the mainstay of treatment [8]. Two potential techniques of combining angiographic techniques in the salvage or palliative setting have not yet been reported. The first technique for chemoembolization of medullary thyroid cancer is with drug-eluting beads bound to doxorubicin (DEB-DOX) in order to prime the field for radiotherapy. Ideally, this would be minimally embolic as the mechanism of tumor death by radiotherapy is oxygen free radical formation, an important distinction from the embolic endpoint in medullary thyroid carcinoma where liver metastases are embolized with DEB-DOX to stasis to obtain best results [49]. DEB-DOX would carry the benefit of minimizing non-target dose in patients with cardiac comorbidities for the cardiotoxic doxorubicin. The second technique that has not yet been reported is the locoregional delivery of antibody-bound radio-immunotherapeutics such as yttrium-90-anti-CEA [8]. Since medullary thyroid carcinomas can express carcinoembryonic antigen (CEA) on their surface, the yttrium-90-anti-CEA therapy has shown to be effective. However, the systemic infusion of radiolabeled antibodies is known to cause dose-limiting hematologic toxicity, usually requiring pre-treatment harvest of peripheral blood stem cells. Endovascular drug delivery, possibly with a flow-limiting catheter to enhance first-pass extraction in the tumor, may one day substantially limit the number of patients in which "myeloablative" protocols of radiolabeled antibody therapy are needed to obtain adequate tumor response such as in patients with locoregional inoperable disease. Additionally, a common pitfall for radioimmunotherapy and nanoparticle-directed therapy is extraction in the reticuloendothelial system, namely, the spleen [50], whereby the aforementioned injection techniques may allow a smaller dose of the therapeutic to be injected directly to the target, in a repeatable fashion if desired. Gene therapies targeted with viral vectors [51] have been developed for medullary thyroid cancer and can also be delivered in the same fashion, although this has not yet been reported.

Immunotherapeutics for thyroid carcinoma have shown promise but have not yet been studied with local delivery. For example, locally advanced medullary thyroid carcinoma has been treated with systemic Vandetanib [52] and Cabozantinib [53]. In the case of Cabozantinib, for example, systemic administration, increased progression-free survival from 4 months to 11 months [53]. These drugs are often dose-limited due to toxicities, and in locally advanced thyroid cancer, locoregional drug delivery has not yet been reported. Of note, early observations regarding risks for tracheoesophageal fistula after radiation combined with immunotherapeutics [54] or tyrosine kinase inhibitors [55] may be tangentially relevant here, because local delivery of the drug may improve target concentrations and may reduce the dose of radiation needed to consolidate the treatment effect.

Vaccine-type immunotherapy for medullary thyroid carcinoma using dendritic cells pulsed with tumor antigen has also been described in systemic applications. However, all patients in early studies developed strong delayed-type hypersensitivity skin reactions [56]. It is possible that locoregional administration of a lower dose may be just as effective and reduce the incidence of these adverse reactions. Therefore, further studies are warranted.

Targeted therapy can change the tumor microenvironment and prime radioactive iodine-resistant thyroid cancer to become sensitive [57]. Dabrafenib, a BRAF inhibitor, restored radioactive iodine uptake in advanced papillary thyroid cancer patients by causing redifferentiation in six of ten patients, with two of six having a partial response [58]. Dabrafenib has a neutral charge and therefore may not be directly chemically bound to existing drug elution bead platforms; however very recently, an immobilizable analogue i-Dabrafenib has been created [59] for adhesion to sepharose beads. Forthcoming trials may study DEB-DAB microenvironmental priming for radio-sensitization or chemo-sensitization of locally advanced PTC. It would be important to mix these with gadolinium so as not to saturate the target thyroid tissue with iodine from iodinated contrast. This would competitively inhibit the binding of radioactive iodine treatment for weeks to follow, delaying the patient's therapy [60].

Summary

As minimally invasive embolic options are applied throughout the body, the applications to the thyroid are emerging for benign and malignant conditions. Embolization of goiter is at the forefront in this domain, with the potential to provide easier surgical resection with decreased blood loss and postoperative drainage and the potential to shrink a retrosternal component to prevent the need for manubriotomy. Partial goiter embolization may be performed in successive titrated treatments to provide outpatient goiter reduction for the treatment of bulk symptoms while sparing vocal function and potentially leaving the patient euthyroid. Comprehensive knowledge of thyroid anatomy, available equipment, and relevant techniques is vital for successfully targeting the thyroid gland arterial supply while avoiding potential pitfalls and complications. Forthcoming applications of transcatheter embolic technology may include immunonormalization of patients with Graves' disease, acute therapy for thyroid storm, and chemoembolic priming for immunotherapy and radiotherapy to allow reduced-dose radiotherapy. Ongoing and forthcoming studies on these topics will likely shape minimally invasive embolic strategies in the years to follow the current report.

References

1. Mariolis-Sapsakos T, Kalles V, Papapanagiotou I, Bonatsos V, Orfanos N, Kaklamanos IG, et al. Bilateral aberrant origin of the inferior thyroid artery from the common carotid artery. Surg Radiol Anat. 2014;36(3):295–7.
2. Lovasova K, Kachlik D, Santa M, Kluchova D. Unilateral occurrence of five different thyroid arteries—a need of terminological systematization: a case report. Surg Radiol Anat. 2017;39(8):925–9.
3. Stewart JD. Circulation of the human thyroid. Arch Surg. 1932;25(6):1157–65.
4. Hoang JK, Middleton WD, Farjat AE, Langer JE, Reading CC, Teefey SA, et al. Reduction in thyroid nodule biopsies and improved accuracy with American College of Radiology Thyroid Imaging Reporting and Data System. Radiology. 2018;287(1):185–93.
5. Mohebati A, Shaha AR. Anatomy of thyroid and parathyroid glands and neurovascular relations. Clin Anat. 2012;25(1):19–31.

6. Kronenberg H, Larsen PR, Melmed S, Polonsky KS, editors. Williams textbook of endocrinology [electronic resource]. Philadelphia: Elsevier; 2016.
7. McHenry C. Thyroidectomy for nodules or small cancers. In: Clark OH, Duh Q-Y, Kebebew E, editors. Atlas of endocrine surgical techniques [electronic resource]. Philadelphia: Saunders/Elsevier; 2010.
8. Sharkey RM, Hajjar G, Yeldell D, Brenner A, Burton J, Rubin A, et al. A phase I trial combining high-dose 90Y-labeled humanized anti-CEA monoclonal antibody with doxorubicin and peripheral blood stem cell rescue in advanced medullary thyroid cancer. J Nucl Med. 2005;46(4):620–33.
9. Gupta P, Bhalla AS, Thulkar S, Kumar A, Mohanti BK, Thakar A, et al. Variations in superior thyroid artery: a selective angiographic study. Indian J Radiol Imaging. 2014;24(1):66–71.
10. Ozgur Z, Govsa F, Celik S, Ozgur T. Clinically relevant variations of the superior thyroid artery: an anatomic guide for surgical neck dissection. Surg Radiol Anat. 2009;31(3):151–9.
11. Won SY. Anatomical considerations of the superior thyroid artery: its origins, variations, and position relative to the hyoid bone and thyroid cartilage. Anat Cell Biol. 2016;49(2):138–42.
12. Toni R, Casa CD, Castorina S, Roti E, Ceda G, Valenti G. A meta-analysis of inferior thyroid artery variations in different human ethnic groups and their clinical implications. Ann Anat. 2005;187(4):371–85.
13. Toniato A, Bernante P, Tamagnini P, Pelizzo MR. Aberrant inferior thyroid artery: two cases. Surgery. 2003;133(5):599.
14. Ngo Nyeki A-R, Peloni G, Karenovics W, Triponez F, Sadowski SM. Aberrant origin of the inferior thyroid artery from the common carotid artery: a rare anatomical variation. Gland Surg. 2016;5(6):644–6.
15. Xiao H, Zhuang W, Wang S, Yu B, Chen G, Zhou M, et al. Arterial embolization: a novel approach to thyroid ablative therapy for Graves' disease. J Clin Endocrinol Metab. 2002;87(8):3583–9.
16. Mojab K, Ghosh BC. Thyroid angiography. Am J Surg. 1976;132(5):620–2.
17. Larson T. Embolization of Extracranial tumors of the head and neck. In: Duffis EJ, Gandhi CD, Prestigiacomo C, editors. Surgical endovascular surgical neuroradiology [electronic resource] : theory and clinical practice. New York: Thieme; 2015.
18. Rulli F, Villa M, Galatà G, Farinon AM. Rapidly enlarging thyroid neoplasm treated with embolization of thyroid arteries. J Surg Oncol. 2007;96(2):183.
19. Akerstrom G, Malmaeus J, Bergstrom R. Surgical anatomy of human parathyroid glands. Surgery. 1984;95(1):14–21.
20. Andersen DK, Billiar TR, Brunicardi FC, Dunn DL, Hunter JG, editors. Schwartz's principles of surgery [electronic resource]. New York: McGraw-Hill Education; 2014.
21. Richards MD, WM, Sosa MD. Surgical anatomy of the thyroid gland. Carty SE, editor. MA: UpToDate Inc. Accessed 16 Sept 2018.
22. Sanabria A, Kowalski LP, Tartaglia F. Inferior thyroid artery ligation increases hypocalcemia after thyroidectomy: a meta-analysis. Laryngoscope. 2018;128(2):534–41.
23. Johansson K, Ander S, Lennquist S, Smeds S. Human parathyroid blood supply determined by laser-Doppler flowmetry. World J Surg. 1994;18(3):417–20.
24. Mallette LE, Gomez L, Fisher RG. Parathyroid angiography: a review of current knowledge and guidelines for clinical application. Endocr Rev. 1981;2(1):124–35.
25. Nobori M, Saiki S, Tanaka N, Harihara Y, Shindo S, Fujimoto Y. Blood supply of the parathyroid gland from the superior thyroid artery. Surgery. 1994;115(4):417–23.
26. Jianu AM, Motoc A, Mihai AL, Rusu MC. An anatomical study of the thyroid arteries anastomoses. Romanian J Morphol Embryol. 2008;50(1):97–101.
27. Furlow PW, Mathisen DJ. Surgical anatomy of the trachea. Ann Cardiothorac Surg. 2018;7(2):255–60.
28. Peloquin JM, Wondisford F. Nontoxic diffuse and nodular goiter. In: Radovick S, Wondisford FE, editors. Clinical management of thyroid disease [electronic resource]. Philadelphia: Saunders/Elsevier; 2009.

29. Moalem J, Suh I, Duh Q-Y. Treatment and prevention of recurrence of multinodular goiter: an evidence-based review of the literature. World J Surg. 2008;32(7):1301–12.
30. Torre G, Barreca A, Borgonovo G, Minuto M, Ansaldo GL, Varaldo E, et al. Goiter recurrence in patients submitted to thyroid-stimulating hormone suppression: possible role of insulin-like growth factors and insulin-like growth factor–binding proteins. Surgery. 2000;127(1):99–103.
31. Ducloux R, Sapoval M, Russ G. Embolization of thyroid arteries in a patient with compressive intrathoracic goiter ineligible to surgery or radioiodine therapy. Ann Endocrinol. 2016;77(6):670–4.
32. Galkin EV, Grakov BS, Protopopov AV. First clinical experience of radio-endovascular functional thyroidectomy in the treatment of diffuse toxic goiter. Vestn Rentgenol Radiol. 1994;(3):29–35.
33. Galkin EV. Interventional radiology in postoperative recurrent goiter. Vestn Rentgenol Radiol. 1995;(6):9–14.
34. Rohr A, Kovaleski A, Hill J, Johnson P. Thyroid embolization as an adjunctive therapy in a patient with thyroid storm. J Vasc Interv Radiol. 2016;27(3):449–51.
35. Kaminski G, Jaroszuk A, Zybek A, Brzozowski K, Piasecki P, Ziecina P, et al. The calcium-phosphate balance, modulation of thyroid autoimmune processes and other adverse effects connected with thyroid arterial embolization. Endocrine. 2014;46(2):292–9.
36. Brzozowski K, Piasecki P, Ziecina P, Frankowska E, Jaroszuk A, Kaminski G, et al. Partial thyroid arterial embolization for the treatment of hyperthyroidism. Eur J Radiol. 2012;81(6):1192–6.
37. Tartaglia F, Salvatori FM, Russo G, Blasi S, Sgueglia M, Tromba L, et al. Selective embolization of thyroid arteries for preresection or palliative treatment of large cervicomediastinal goiters. Surg Innov. 2011;18(1):70–8.
38. Zhao W, Gao BL, Yi GF, Yang HY, Li H. Thyroid arterial embolization for the treatment of hyperthyroidism in a patient with thyrotoxic crisis. Clin Invest Med. 2009;32(1):E78–83.
39. Zhao W, Gao BL, Jin CZ, Yi GF, Yang HY, Li H, et al. Long-term immunological study in Graves' disease treated with thyroid arterial embolization. J Clin Immunol. 2008;28(5):456–63.
40. Brito JP, Yarur AJ, Prokop LJ, McIver B, Murad MH, Montori VM. Prevalence of thyroid cancer in multinodular goiter versus single nodule: a systematic review and meta-analysis. Thyroid. 2013;23(4):449–55.
41. Zhao W, Gao BL, Tian M, Yi GF, Yang HY, Shen LJ, et al. Graves' disease treated with thyroid arterial embolization. Clin Invest Med. 2009;32(2):E158–E65.
42. Zhao W, Gao BL, Liu ZY, Yi GF, Shen LJ, Yang HY, et al. Angiogenic study in Graves' disease treated with thyroid arterial embolization. Clin Invest Med. 2009;32(5):E335–44.
43. Tian JL, Chen SF, Du YH, Li CL, Wang W, Li YS, et al. Changes of serum thyroid hormone levels in Graves' disease patients after thyroid arterial embolization. Chinese J Interv Imaging Ther. 2012;9(7):523–6.
44. McIver B, Morris JC. The pathogenesis of Graves' disease. Endocrinol Metab Clin N Am. 1998;27(1):73–89.
45. Dedecjus M, Tazbir J, Kaurzel Z, Lewinski A, Strozyk G, Brzezinski J. Selective embolization of thyroid arteries as a preresective and palliative treatment of thyroid cancer. Endocr Relat Cancer. 2007;14(3):847–52.
46. Beers GJ, Svendsen P, Carter AP, Bell R. Embolization of medullary carcinoma of the thyroid invading the trachea: report of a case. Acta Radiol Diagn (Stockh). 1985;26(1):21–3.
47. Tazbir J, Dedecjus M, Kaurzel Z, Lewiński A, Brzeziński J. Selective embolization of thyroid arteries (SETA) as a palliative treatment of inoperable anaplastic thyroid carcinoma (ATC). Neuroendocrinol Lett. 2005;26(4):401–6.
48. Ramos HE, Braga-Basaria M, Haquin C, Mesa CO, De Noronha L, Sandrini R, et al. Preoperative embolization of thyroid arteries in a patient with large multinodular goiter and papillary carcinoma. Thyroid. 2004;14(11):967–70.
49. Hughes P, Healy NA, Grant C, Ryan JM. Treatment of hepatic metastases from medullary thyroid cancer with transarterial embolisation. Eur Radiol Exp. 2017;1(1):9.

50. Le Doussal JM, Martin M, Gautherot E, Delaage M, Barbet J. In vitro and in vivo targeting of radiolabeled monovalent and divalent haptens with dual specificity monoclonal antibody conjugates: enhanced divalent hapten affinity for cell-bound antibody conjugate. J Nucl Med. 1989;30(8):1358–66.
51. Drosten M, Putzer BM. Gene therapeutic approaches for medullary thyroid carcinoma treatment. J Mol Med (Berl). 2003;81(7):411–9.
52. Wells SA Jr, Robinson BG, Gagel RF, Dralle H, Fagin JA, Santoro M, et al. Vandetanib in patients with locally advanced or metastatic medullary thyroid cancer: a randomized, double-blind phase III trial. J Clin Oncol. 2012;30(2):134–41.
53. Viola D, Cappagli V, Elisei R. Cabozantinib (XL184) for the treatment of locally advanced or metastatic progressive medullary thyroid cancer. Future Oncol. 2013;9(8):1083–92.
54. Goodgame B, Veeramachaneni N, Patterson A, Govindan R. Tracheo-esophageal fistula with bevacizumab after mediastinal radiation. J Thorac Oncol. 2008;3(9):1080–1.
55. Blevins DP, Dadu R, Hu M, Baik C, Balachandran D, Ross W, et al. Aerodigestive fistula formation as a rare side effect of antiangiogenic tyrosine kinase inhibitor therapy for thyroid cancer. Thyroid. 2014;24(5):918–22.
56. Schott M, Seissler J, Lettmann M, Fouxon V, Scherbaum WA, Feldkamp J. Immunotherapy for medullary thyroid carcinoma by dendritic cell vaccination. J Clin Endocrinol Metab. 2001;86(10):4965–9.
57. Naoum GE, Morkos M, Kim B, Arafat W. Novel targeted therapies and immunotherapy for advanced thyroid cancers. Mol Cancer. 2018;17(1):51.
58. Rothenberg SM, McFadden DG, Palmer EL, Daniels GH, Wirth LJ. Redifferentiation of iodine-refractory BRAF V600E-mutant metastatic papillary thyroid cancer with dabrafenib. Clin Cancer Res. 2015;21(5):1028–35.
59. Phadke M, Remsing Rix LL, Smalley I, Bryant AT, Luo Y, Lawrence HR, et al. Dabrafenib inhibits the growth of BRAF-WT cancers through CDK16 and NEK9 inhibition. Mol Oncol. 2018;12(1):74–88.
60. Padovani RP, Kasamatsu TS, Nakabashi CCD, Camacho CP, Andreoni DM, Malouf EZ, et al. One month is sufficient for urinary iodine to return to its baseline value after the use of water-soluble iodinated contrast agents in post-thyroidectomy patients requiring radioiodine therapy. Thyroid. 2012;22(9):926–30.

Chapter 20
Interventional Treatment of Hepatic Endocrine Tumors

Kurt Zacharias and Osman Ahmed

Introduction

Hepatic neuroendocrine tumors are almost exclusively metastatic in nature and can arise from primary neuroendocrine tumors of the foregut, midgut, or hindgut. Carcinoids represent the most common origin of hepatic neuroendocrine metastases, although gastrinomas, thymomas, and pancreatic islet cell tumors, among others, have been known to metastasize to the liver [1].

Primary hepatic neuroendocrine tumors represent only approximately 0.3% of all hepatic neuroendocrine tumors. These tumors are often slow-growing (without early symptoms) and are usually only detected in the middle and late stages when they have reached a significant size. Primary hepatic neuroendocrine tumors are almost exclusively diagnosed postoperatively [2].

Neuroendocrine neoplasms demonstrate varying malignancy levels and diverse symptomatology; however, they exhibit relatively consistent imaging patterns when metastatic to the liver [1]. They are notably hypervascular to the background liver and are detectable on multiphase CT with a sensitivity of approximately 70–85% [3] (Fig. 20.1).

On MRI, hepatic neuroendocrine tumors typically demonstrate hypointensity on T1-weighted images, moderate hyperintensity on T2-weighted images, and hyperintensity on hepatic arterial phase and portal venous phases of contrast administration [4] (Fig. 20.2).

K. Zacharias (✉)
Department of Radiology, University of Chicago Medical Center, Chicago, IL, USA
e-mail: kurt.zacharias@uchospitals.edu

O. Ahmed
Department of Interventional Radiology, University of Chicago Medical Center, Chicago, IL, USA
e-mail: oahmed@radiology.bsd.uchicago.edu

© The Author(s), under exclusive license to Springer Nature Switzerland AG 2022

H. Yu et al. (eds.), *Diagnosis and Management of Endocrine Disorders in Interventional Radiology*, https://doi.org/10.1007/978-3-030-87189-5_20

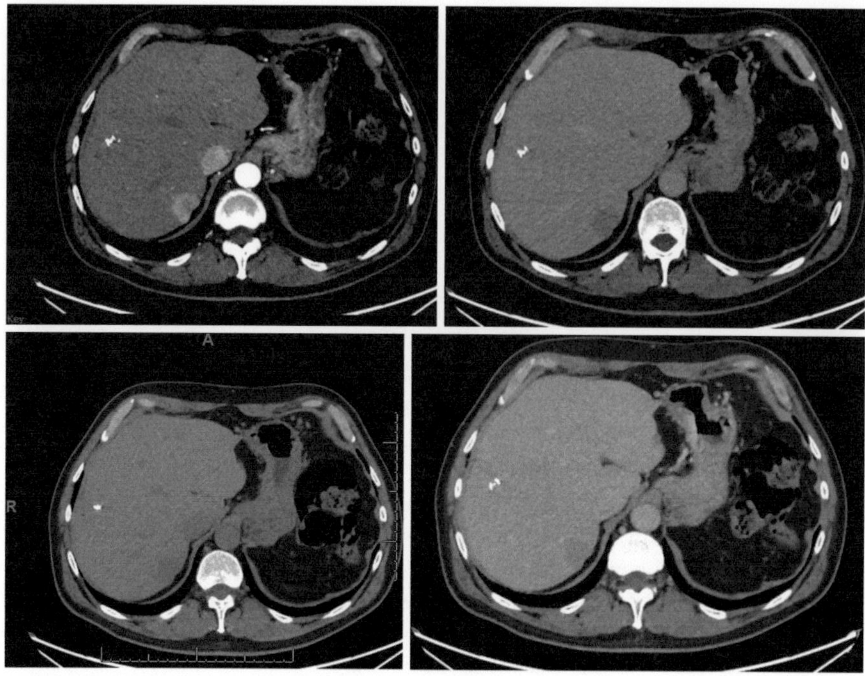

Fig. 20.1 CT of neuroendocrine liver metastases seen in precontrast, arterial, portal venous, and delayed phases. Robust arterial enhancement can be seen, with rapid washout in the portal venous phase and relative hypoattenuation on delayed phase images

Patient Selection for Interventional Treatment

The approach to the treatment of neuroendocrine liver disease is best considered from a multidisciplinary perspective, weighing the input of endocrinologists, surgeons, diagnostic radiologists, radiation oncologists, and interventionalists while taking the patient's own goals of care into account [5]. A relative paucity of data on the management of neuroendocrine liver disease exists, given the rarity of the condition, with most studies being retrospective and utilizing small sample sizes. Certain recommendations can be extrapolated from more robust data that already exists on the treatment of hepatic metastases from other neoplasms, primarily colorectal in origin. While the treatment of neuroendocrine liver disease specifically is a continued topic of research, several recommended criteria for interventional treatment are well-established and include:

- Metastases from non-pancreatic neuroendocrine tumors with resected primary sites
- Absence of or limited burden of extrahepatic metastases (i.e., liver-dominant metastases)
- Preserved underlying synthetic function of the liver with parenchymal burden less than 50%

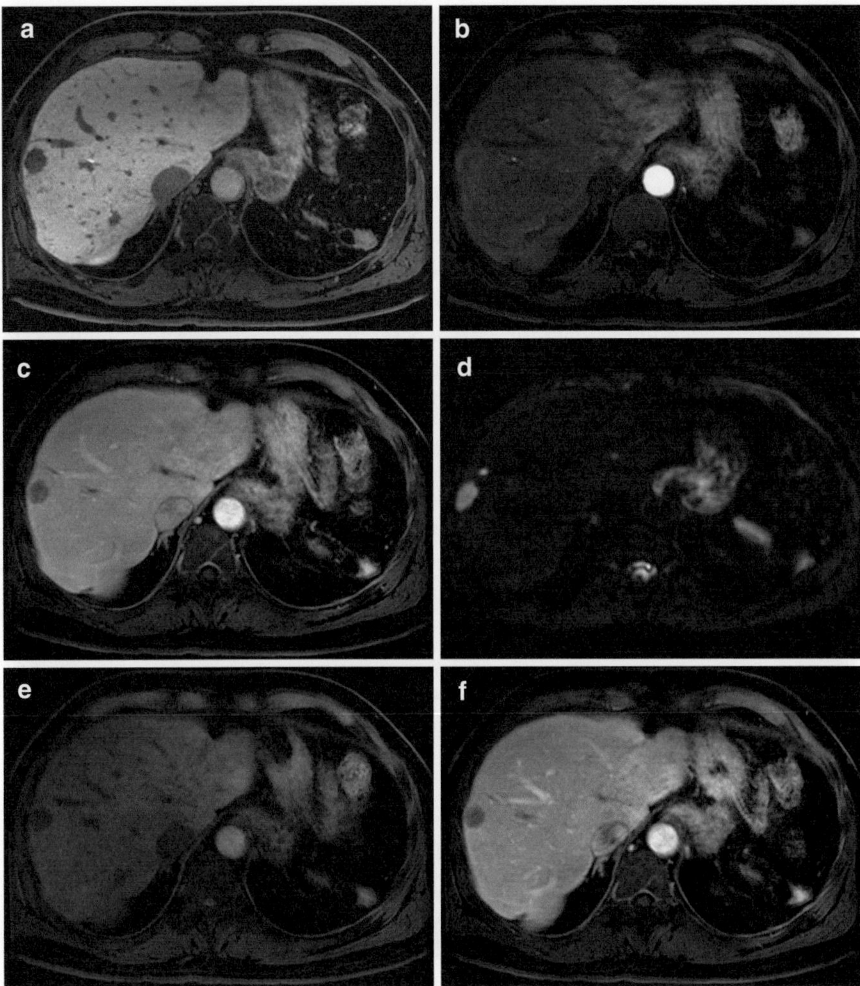

Fig. 20.2 MRI of neuroendocrine liver metastasis. (**a**) T1 pre-contrast phase demonstrates relative hypointensity with arterial enhancement and subsequent washout on (**b**) portal venous and (**c**) delayed phase images. (**d**) Eovist (gadoxetate disodium), the contrast agent used in this sequence, is taken up over time by normal liver parenchyma, but not by the tumor, and (**e**) images at a 20-min delay show marked hypointensity of the tumor as compared to normal liver parenchyma. (**f**) The lesion restricts diffusion on DWI, which is often seen in neuroendocrine metastases

Regardless of the above criteria, it is again worth emphasizing that the decision to treat hepatic neuroendocrine disease should be made on a case-by-case basis, in multidisciplinary fashion, and that a significant number of patients not meeting the above criteria may indeed still benefit from interventional treatment. Goals of interventional treatment include prolongation of life, as liver failure represents the most common cause of mortality in patients with liver-dominant disease, as well as relief of symptoms caused by hormonally active neuroendocrine tumors.

A few relative contraindications to undergoing interventional treatment are as follows:

- History of bilioenteric anastomosis or sphincterotomy
- Decompensated liver disease
- Allergy to iodinated contrast
- Portal venous thrombosis or tumor invasion

If not already obtained, dedicated liver imaging (either CT or MR) is recommended to assess hepatic tumor burden, portal vein involvement, biliary ductal dilatation, and arterial anatomy. More extensive CT, including the chest and pelvis, is also recommended to evaluate for extrahepatic metastases. Laboratory analysis, to include evaluations of liver function, renal function, and coagulation status, is also recommended as a routine part of pre-procedural workup [6].

Interventional techniques which can be used to treat hepatic neuroendocrine tumors range from minimally invasive intra-arterial therapies to percutaneous needle-guided procedures. These include arterial embolization, chemoembolization, selective internal radiation therapy, and percutaneous ablation. Further considerations, indications, and contraindications to specific interventional methods will be discussed in greater detail under their respective headings.

Transarterial Embolization (TAE or "Bland" Embolization)

Basic Principles

Transarterial embolization is a treatment option based on occlusion of small arterioles feeding neuroendocrine tumors. This method, also known as "bland embolization," relies solely on the use of embolic material without an associated infusion of chemotherapeutics, which will be discussed subsequently. Transarterial embolization (TAE) is well established in the treatment of other malignant hypervascular liver tumors and operates off the principle of dual blood supply to the liver. The hepatic arterial and portal venous systems both bring oxygenated blood into the liver. In general, in the case of hypervascular liver neoplasms, the malignancy is supplied to a greater extent by the arterial system, whereas the surrounding liver parenchyma is supplied to a greater extent by the portal venous system [7]. Furthermore, hepatic neuroendocrine tumors demonstrate disorganized angiogenesis with increased vascular permeability as compared to normal parenchyma. These principles allow for the relatively selective destruction of neoplastic tissue and are the foundation upon which transarterial treatment approaches are based.

Technique

Transarterial embolization involves selective angiography to target vasculature supplying tumor and the injection of embolic agents resulting in tissue hypoxia and necrosis [8]. While there is extensive heterogeneity among techniques in use, the basics of procedural technique are as follows:

- Hepatic angiogram to evaluate arterial anatomy and tumor supply
- Anatomic evaluation of arteries in which embolization should be avoided (i.e., right gastric and supraduodenal arteries)
- Advancement of catheter super-selectively into the artery feeding the tumor
- Repeat arteriography (to identify any anomalies which may have been missed on a celiac or SMA arteriogram)
- Injection of embolic material

The endpoint of an embolic procedure is the visualization of the complete blockage of the tumor-feeding branch [9] (Fig. 20.3).

Selection of Embolic Agents

Gelatin Sponge

The first hepatic artery embolization, performed in 1977, utilized absorbable gelatin sponge particles ranging from 1 to 5 mm^3 in size, with reports of persistent occlusion on subsequent angiograms performed 6 weeks after embolization [10]. In these early stages of transarterial treatment techniques, absorbable gelatin powder was also utilized with similar results. However, it has since fallen out of favor given high rates of nontarget embolization [11]. Gelatin sponge (Gelfoam) is no longer utilized as a stand-alone agent for hepatic oncologic interventions as it is regarded as a temporary embolization agent.

Polyvinyl Alcohol Particles (PVA)

Currently available in sizes ranging from approximately 50 to 1000 microns [12], PVA came into subsequent use to treat hepatic tumors and achieved greater degrees of distal embolization and better clinical results than Gelfoam. PVA is compressed and, when rehydrated, can expand up to 15 times. It adheres to blood vessel walls, slowing and eventually stopping blood flow. Additionally, it induces an inflammatory response with subsequent angionecrosis. It is nonbiodegradable and thus considered a permanent embolic agent, and its uses range broadly within interventional radiology. Limitations include inconsistent/inhomogeneous size of the particulate agent with potential for more proximal occlusion.

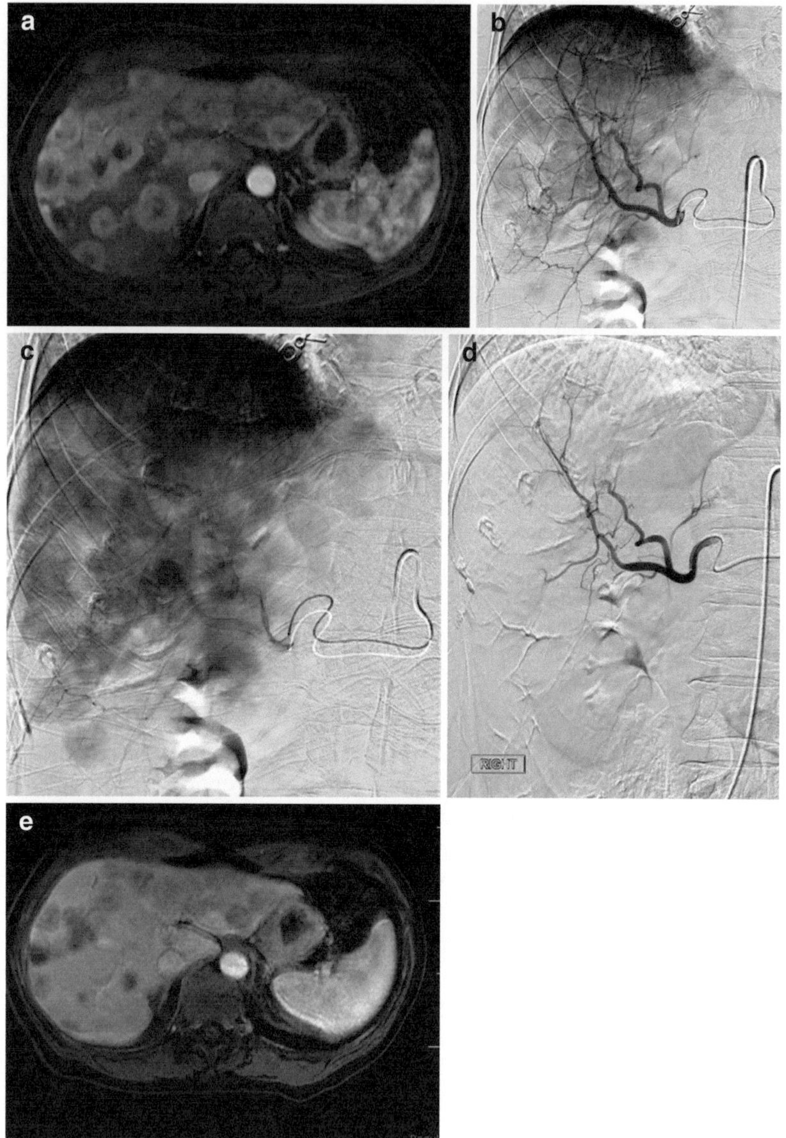

Fig. 20.3 A 48-year-old female with small bowel NET and liver-dominant metastases. The patient underwent bland embolization for carcinoid symptoms, including cutaneous flushing and palpitations. (**a**) Multiphase MRI demonstrates bilobar hypervascular hepatic masses compatible with metastatic disease. (**b**) Arterial phase angiography from the right hepatic artery at the time of bland embolization demonstrates multiple metastatic lesions. (**c**) Parenchymal phase angiography from the right hepatic artery better delineates the numerous hepatic metastases. (**d**) Post bland embolization angiography demonstrates successful vascular occlusion of the tumor-feeding vessels. There is maintained perfusion of the right hepatic artery. (**e**) Follow-up MRI demonstrates a decrease in the number of hepatic lesions with no residual enhancement of the remaining lesions, compatible with necrotic tumor

Microspheres

These newer, spherical agents, which are sometimes made from PVA (although are also manufactured from other polymers, including trisacryl gelatin and polymethylmethacrylate), demonstrate greater uniformity in size and shape, as opposed to the irregularly shaped PVA particles. They show a greater degree of correlation between the size of the particle and the size of the vessel in which embolization occurs, as well as a decreased risk of clumping within the catheter. These are manufactured at industry-standard 200-micron increments, ranging from 300 to 1200 microns, and are the most commonly used TAE agents. The use of microspheres allows for smaller particulate use with more distal occlusion and ischemia-mediated tumor necrosis. Data suggests that smaller (<100 microns) microspheres for neuroendocrine metastases may yield better initial treatment responses [13].

n-Butyl Cyanoacrylate

This tissue glue, mixed with ethiodized oil, is a tissue embolic often used in the treatment of high-flow vascular malformations. However, it has also been examined in at least one trial for the treatment of hepatic neuroendocrine tumors. Experimenters demonstrated complete, distal, permanent embolization, though concerns were raised by two early deaths out of a total population of 29 (7%) [14].

Transarterial Chemoembolization (TACE)

Transarterial chemoembolization (TACE) operates on similar principles as "bland" transarterial embolization, with the added step of selectively administering chemotherapeutic agents to feeding vessels prior to or in conjunction with embolization. When combined with embolization, drug concentration and retention are increased compared to infusion alone, and a decrease in systemic concentrations and systemic side effects can be achieved [15]. TACE is usually performed in one of two ways: the so-called "conventional" method (cTACE) and a second method that utilizes drug-eluting beads (DEB-TACE).

Conventional TACE

Conventional TACE (cTACE) utilizes ethiodized oil, widely available under the trade name Lipiodol (Guerbet). This poppyseed oil, modified for injectability, serves as a radiopaque agent and can be combined with chemotherapeutic agents. While both single chemotherapeutic and combination therapies exist, the most widely used chemotherapeutic agent in TACE is doxorubicin. It is commonly used for hepatocellular carcinoma but also applicable in the cases of neuroendocrine liver tumors [16]. In this latter context, cisplatin, vinblastine, streptozocin, and mitomycin C have also been utilized [17, 18].

Lipiodol demonstrates significant efficacy in tumor-seeking and embolization and appears to be able to cross cancer cell membranes and persist in the tumor for months to years while disappearing from normal parenchyma in as little as 4 weeks. Embolization, performed after administration of the lipiodol-chemotherapy mixture in cTACE, acts to increase drug retention within the tumor and add an element of ischemia to the tumor-killing process. While widely regarded as effective, one of the limitations of cTACE is the significant interinstitutional variability in technique and treatment protocols [16].

Drug-Eluting Beads TACE

TACE performed with drug-eluting beads (DEB-TACE) represents the second major form of TACE. As the name suggests, this method utilizes particles impregnated with chemotherapeutics, thereby achieving embolization and chemotherapy administration in a single step. The most commonly used drug-eluting particles are combined with doxorubicin and release a controlled and steady stream of medication [19]. Beads in the 100–300 micron range appear to work best as there is a more distal embolic effect and increased surface area to elute chemotherapy [20].

Studies report similar overall efficacy as conventional TACE, but DEB-TACE has been associated with an increased risk of biliary injury compared to cTACE [21]. In the specific treatment for hepatic neuroendocrine tumors, at least one retrospective trial has demonstrated decreased treatment response and increased complication rate of DEB-TACE compared to cTACE [22].

Additional Considerations in Embolic Therapy

Tolerance and Complications

Intraprocedural tolerance of embolic therapy, whether TAE or TACE, is generally low, with the majority of patients reporting significant pain as embolization occurs. Most procedures are performed under moderate sedation, although general anesthesia can be considered in some cases. Intra-arterial injection of lidocaine is an additional technique described for reducing patient pain in the immediate post-procedural period [23].

A significant number of patients suffer from a combination of symptoms post-procedurally, which is referred to as post-embolization syndrome (PES). PES is a relatively common, inflammation-mediated response, likely related to tissue necrosis and, if used, systemic side effects of chemotherapeutic agents. It is characterized by fever, anorexia, pain, and nausea/ vomiting. The majority of symptoms occur within 24 h of the procedure. However, there are reports of symptoms up to 2 weeks post-procedurally [24].

While some institutions manage PES expectantly, using antipyretics and anti-emetics as needed, many also administer dexamethasone prophylactically, which appears to limit symptom severity. While generally well-tolerated, dexamethasone administration has important oncological implications, with a reported potential to induce tumor lysis syndrome. Thus, it should be considered carefully in cases where the tumor burden is heavy [25].

Although PES itself is considered benign, some studies suggest that, at least in the case of hepatocellular carcinoma (HCC), increased severity of PES is associated with worse oncologic prognosis [26]. This relationship remains unclear and has not been specifically examined in the case of hepatic neuroendocrine tumors.

Serious adverse effects occur in less than 10% of neuroendocrine embolizations and include [6]:

- *Carcinoid syndrome*: Due to the acute release of vasoactive substances from the necrosing tumor. This may be mitigated by peri-procedure administration of somatostatin.
- *Liver infarction*: Usually segmental. Although rare, there exist reports of total liver ischemia, usually in the case of unrecognized portal venous thrombosis.
- *Nontarget embolization*: Ischemic complications such as cholecystitis may occur from cystic artery embolization.
- *Complications related to angiography*: Dissection, contrast reaction, or other complications common to most interventional procedures.

Outcomes

No large prospective trials have been performed to evaluate the efficacy of embolic therapies in neuroendocrine liver disease. Retrospective analyses indicate between 60% and 90% of patients report improved symptoms with follow-up imaging demonstrating partial response in 50–90% of patients. These changes lasted between 11 and 20 months with one-time therapy and increased duration of effect with repeat embolizations. Studies evaluating overall survival are limited, with studies reporting ranges of 12–84 months post-procedurally.

Some prognostic factors may be predictive of decreased tumor response, including >50% liver involvement, pancreatic primary, male gender, and an ECOG score of 1 or higher. Increased tumor enhancement on arterial phase imaging, indicating a greater degree of tumor vascularity, is likely a favorable prognostic factor and increases the likelihood of response from embolization [6].

TAE vs. TACE

Studies comparing "bland" embolization and chemoembolization for the treatment of neuroendocrine tumors have demonstrated conflicting results, with some showing superiority of one method over the other and others showing equivalent responses. Further confusion may owe itself to the reassessment of neuroendocrine tumor gradation by the World Health Organization in 2010, limiting comparison between studies performed before and after this time.

At the time of this publication, a prospective, multicenter randomized controlled trial comparing cTACE, DEB-TACE, and bland embolization in treating neuroendocrine liver tumors is underway (RETNET), for which results are not yet available [27].

Selective Internal Radiation Therapy (SIRT)

Selective internal radiation therapy (SIRT), also known as transarterial radioembolization, represents a relatively newer treatment modality for hepatic neoplasms, including neuroendocrine tumors, which involves the selective injection of radioactive agents into the tumor.

Technique

As with the embolic techniques, the first stages of SIRT involve angiography and selection of the hepatic artery supplying the hepatic tumor. Then, tumoricidal doses of radiation are injected. Contrary to methods such as cTACE, subsequent embolization is not performed after administration of radiotherapy.

The most commonly used nuclide is the isotope yttrium-90 (^{90}Y). This isotope is either coupled with glass microspheres, sold under the trade name TheraSpheres, or with resin beads, known as SIR-Spheres. Yttrium-90, or Y-90 as it is more commonly known, is a pure beta-radiation emitter that has a mean penetration of approximately 2.5 mm and a maximum penetration of 10 mm, limiting penetration to nontarget patient tissues and allowing for the safety of the operator and any other person the patient might interact with during or after treatment. Holmium-166-labeled microspheres, available under the trade name of QuiremSpheres, represent a third, less commonly used agent for SIRT.

Y90 administration is a two-step process, with an initial procedure for mapping and determining the lung shunt fraction, an integral component of pre-procedural planning. During this phase, technetium-99-labeled macroaggregated albumin (MAA), the same agent used in lung perfusion scans, is injected at the site of anticipated treatment. With a similar size to microspheres, the MAA acts as a marker to predict the expected pattern of microsphere spread. SPECT-CT imaging is performed after MAA administration to assess for extrahepatic spread, including to the lungs, which can occur through shunts created by tumoral neovasculature. The lung shunt fraction is then calculated, representing the percentage of administered MAA that ends up in the lungs. In cases where the shunt fraction is <20%, the value can be used to adjust the dose to minimize lung exposure, ideally below a threshold of 30 Gy. A lung shunt fraction above 20% is a contraindication to the administration of Y90 when using SIR-Spheres [28, 29].

Outcomes

No prospective data exist on SIRT usage in neuroendocrine liver tumors, with retrospective studies showing a wide range in percent response, from 12% to 80%. However, unlike TAE/TACE, which have not demonstrated complete response in any current studies, several studies show a complete response after administration of Y90, although numbers are low at 1–8% of patients [6]. In the case of HCC, for which a larger pool of data is available, Y90 demonstrated longer time-to-progression and decreased toxicity than chemoembolization [30].

Complications and Limitations

In addition to complications associated with angiography, several unique complications can be seen in SIRT as a result of radioactivity:

- *Radiation pneumonitis*: Caused by shunting radioactive material into the lungs, which can often cause irreversible interstitial lung disease. For this reason, dose thresholds of 30 Gy to the lungs, or a lung shunt fraction of >20%, are absolute contraindications to Y90 administration. In patients with lung shunt fractions between 10% and 20%, the dosage can be reduced in an effort to minimize this complication.
- *Radioembolization-induced liver disease (REILD)*: Liver damage that occurs 4–8 weeks after Y90 administration, which is potentially life-threatening. Characterized by jaundice and ascites, this complication is not entirely understood but demonstrates veno-occlusive characteristics on histology and likely represents a form of sino-occlusive disease, exclusively seen in liver treatments that involve radiation. High-radiation doses and extensive tumor burden have been identified as predictive factors for this poorly understood complication [31].
- *Radioembolization-induced chronic hepatotoxicity*: In patients with neuroendocrine tumors and favorable long-term prognosis, those treated by SIRT may be subject to long-term chronic hepatotoxicity due to the delayed radiation-induced effects of the radioactive microspheres [32].
- *Hematologic complications*: Radiation-induced lymphocytopenia and thrombocytosis occur in roughly 3–7% of patients [33].

Percutaneous Ablation

Percutaneous thermal ablation represents another therapeutic modality for hepatic metastases, including neuroendocrine tumors. While cryoablation has been utilized, there have been significant reports of subsequent coagulopathy, some of which have been life-threatening. Thus, radiofrequency ablation (RFA) and microwave ablation (MWA) have become the preferred ablation methods for treating hepatic metastases.

Performed under the guidance of ultrasound or CT, depending on the lesion's location, thermal ablation is performed via placement of ablation probe(s) percutaneously into targeted lesions (Fig. 20.4). RFA and MWA result in heating and destruction of tissue, with a target temperature of 50–100 °C, for 4–5 min. With RFA, temperatures higher than 100 °C can cause carbonization and charring of adjacent tissues [34].

Image-guided RFA has demonstrated a similar response as surgical resection with low mortality and a major complication rate of less than 5%. RFA is limited in its uses, however, as it is most effective in smaller tumors measuring less than 4 cm. The relatively small ablative field achieved with RFA makes complete necrosis of larger lesions difficult. Additionally, the ability to use RFA depends on tumor location, with those located more peripherally representing more ideal targets. Many of these limitations mentioned above may be overcome with MWA, as MWA permits

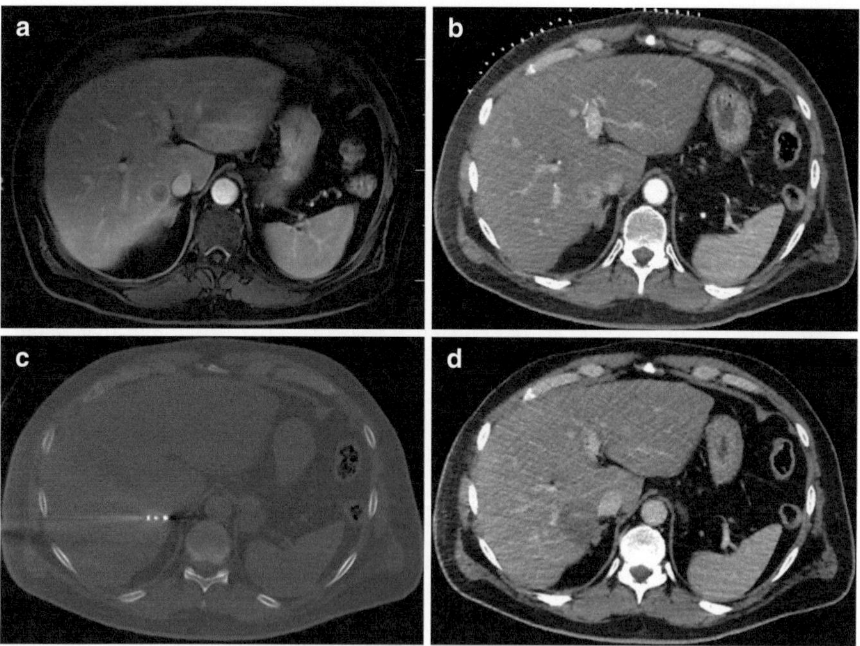

Fig. 20.4 (**a**) Pre-procedure MRI image showing a 2.8 cm metastasis adjacent to the IVC. (**b**) Intra-procedure image demonstrating an enhancing lesion in segment 1. (**c**) Intra-procedure CT image demonstrating the ablation probe in the target lesion. (**d**) Post-ablation contrast CT showing ablation cavity with no evidence of viable tumor

larger ablative zones and is less limited by features such as heat sink and charring [35]. It is worth noting that the severity of symptoms associated with neuroendocrine tumors has been shown to correlate closely with tumor size, and tumor reductions of 90% or greater have shown long-lasting symptomatic benefit, demonstrating that ablation still has utility even in cases where the target lesion cannot be completely destroyed [36, 37].

Summary

Hepatic endocrine tumors may be primary but are more often metastatic, originating from a wide range of primary sites. These tumors demonstrate hypervascularity and derive an increased percentage of their blood supply from the hepatic arterial system compared to normal liver parenchyma, which derives its supply primarily from the portal system. This characteristic allows for transarterial treatment options, which include bland transarterial embolization (TAE), transarterial chemoembolization (TACE), and selective internal radiation therapy (SIRT). Radiofrequency ablation (RFA) represents a second approach, with the percutaneous insertion of probes into a tumor and subsequent heating of tissue, inducing tumor necrosis.

Patients who are not surgical candidates due to heavy hepatic tumor burden or inaccessibility of lesions can be candidates for transarterial and percutaneous therapies. Further study is needed to determine which clinical scenarios would be most appropriate for each treatment option, with the relative advantages and disadvantages of each still not clearly defined.

Regardless, while very few studies of these approaches have yielded complete response, a significant portion of patients experience improvement in symptoms with these interventions, likely due to the fact that endocrine production correlates with tumor size and any significant reduction in tumor burden can improve patient symptoms. Additionally, these treatments often prolong life, as liver failure represents the most significant cause of mortality in patients with liver-dominant neuroendocrine disease. Thus, while rarely curative, the interventions described in this chapter can significantly impact patients' quality of life and will continue to play an important and ever-expanding role in the multidisciplinary treatment of hepatic endocrine tumors.

References

1. Ihse I, Lindell G, Tibblin S. Neuroendocrine tumors metastatic to the liver. In: Holzheimer RG, Mannick JA, editors. Surgical treatment: evidence-based and problem-oriented. Munich: Zuckschwerdt; 2001.
2. Qu C, Qu L, Zhu C, Wang Z, Cao J. Treatment of primary hepatic neuroendocrine tumors with associating liver partition and portal vein ligation for staged hepatectomy. Medicine. 2018;97(37):12408.

3. Paulson EK, McDermott VG, Keogan MT, DeLong DM, Frederick MG, Nelson RC. Carcinoid metastases to the liver: role of triple-phase helical CT. Radiology. 1998;206:143–50.

4. Dromain C, de Baere T, Baudin E, Galline J, et al. MR imaging of hepatic metastases caused by neuroendocrine tumors: comparing four techniques. AJR Am J Roentgenol. 2003;180(1):131–28.

5. Mestier L, Lepage C, Baudin E, Coriat R, Courbon F, et al. Digestive neuroendocrine neoplasms (NEN): French intergroup clinical practice guidelines for diagnosis, treatment, and follow-up. Dig Liver Dis. 2020;52(5):473–92.

6. Barat M, Cottereau A, Kedra A, Dermine S, Palmieri L, et al. The role of interventional radiology for the treatment of hepatic metastases from neuroendocrine tumor: an updated review. J Clin Med. 2020;9(7):2302.

7. Clouse ME, Perry L, Stuart K, Stokes KR. Hepatic arterial chemoembolization for metastatic neuroendocrine tumors. Digestion. 1994;55(Suppl 3):92–7.

8. Tsochatzis EA, Fatourou E, O-Beirne J, Meyer T, Burroughs AK. Transarterial chemoembolization and bland embolization for hepatocellular carcinoma. World J Gastroenterol. 2014;20(12):3069–77.

9. Wang YJ, Baere TD, Idee J, Ballet S. Transcatheter embolization therapy in liver cancer: an update of clinical evidence. Chin J Cancer Res. 2015;27(2):96–121.

10. Allison DJ, Modlin IM, Jenkins WJ. Treatment of carcinoid liver metastases by hepatic-artery embolisation. Lancet. 1977;2(8052–8052):1323–5.

11. Stokes KR, Stuart K, Clouse ME. Hepatic arterial chemoembolization for metastatic endocrine tumors. J Vasc Interv Radiol. 1993;4(3):341–5.

12. ContourTM pva embolization particles [Internet]. www.bostonscientific.com. [cited 2020 Oct 20]. Available from: https://www.bostonscientific.com/en-US/products/embolization/contour-pva-embolization-particles.html.

13. Zener R, Yoon H, Ziv E, Covey A, Brown K, et al. Outcomes after transarterial embolization of neuroendocrine tumor liver metastases using spherical particles of different sizes. Cardiovasc Intervent Radiol. 2019;42(4):569–76.

14. Ang TL, Seewald S, Soehendra N. Endotherapy of gastric fundal varices: intravariceal injection of N-butyl-2-cyanoacrylate. Video J Encycl GI Endosc. 2013;1(1):157–9.

15. Biolato M, Marrone G, Racco S, Di Stasi C, Miele L, et al. Transarterial chemoembolization (TACE) for unresectable HCC: a new life begins? Eur Rev Med Pharmacol Sci. 2010;14(4):356–62.

16. Song JE, Kim DY. Conventional vs drug-eluting beads transarterial chemoembolization for hepatocellular carcinoma. World J Hepatol. 2017;9(18):808–14.

17. Kim YH, Ajani JA, Carrasco CH, Dumas P, Richli W, et al. Selective hepatic arterial chemoembolization for liver metastases in patients with carcinoid tumor or islet cell carcinoma. Cancer Investig. 1999;17(7):474–8.

18. Pelage J, Fohlen A, Mitry E, Lagrange C, Beauchet A, Rougier P. Chemoembolization of neuroendocrine liver metastases using streptozocin and tris-acryl microspheres: embozar (embosphere + zanosar) study. Cardiovasc Intervent Radiol. 2017;40(3):394–400.

19. Poon R, Tso WK, Pang R, Ng K, Woo R, et al. A phase I/II trial of chemoembolization for hepatocellular carcinoma using a novel intra-arterial drug-eluting bead. Clin Gastroenterol Hepatol. 2007;5(9):1100–8.

20. Lewis AL, Taylor RR, Hall B, Gonzalez MV, Willis SL, Stratford PW. Pharmacokinetic and safety study of doxorubicin-eluting beads in a porcine model of hepatic arterial embolization. J Vasc Interv Radiol. 2006;17(8):1335–43.

21. Guiu B, Deschamps F, Aho S, Munck F, Dromain C, et al. Liver/biliary injuries following chemoembolisation of endocrine tumours and hepatocellular carcinoma: lipiodol vs drug-eluting beads. J Hepatol. 2012;56(3):609–17.

22. Kitano M, Davidson GW, Shirley LA, Schmidt CR, Guy GE, et al. Transarterial chemoembolization for metastatic neuroendocrine tumors with massive hepatic tumor burden: is the benefit worth the risk? Ann Surg Oncol. 2016;23(12):4008–15.

23. Cornelis FH, Monard E, Moulin MA, Vignaud E, Laveissiere F, et al. Sedation and analgesia in interventional radiology: where do we stand, where are we heading and why does it matter? Diagn Interv Imaging. 2019;100(12):753–62.
24. Blackburn H, West S. Management of postembolization syndrome following transarterial chemoembolization for primary or metastatic liver cancer. Cancer Nurs. 2016;39(5):E1–18.
25. Ishikawa T. Prevention of post-embolization syndrome after transarterial chemoembolization for hepatocellular carcinoma – is prophylactic dexamethasone useful, or not? Hepatobiliary Surg Nutr. 2018;7(3):214–6.
26. Ubillus WJ, Munoz J, Vekaria M, Wollner IS, Getzen T, et al. Post-embolization syndrome: outcomes regarding the type of embolization. J Clin Oncol. 2011;29(15):e14582.
27. Chen J, Wileyto EP, Soulen MC. Randomized embolization trial for neuroendocrine tumor metastases to the liver (RETNET): study protocol for a randomized controlled trial. Trials. 2018;19:390.
28. Sundram FX, Buscombe JR. Selective internal radiation therapy for liver tumors. Clin Med (Lond). 2017;17(5):449–53.
29. Narsinh KH, Buskirk MV, Kennedy AS, Suhail M, Alsaikhan N, et al. Hepatopulmonary shunting: a prognostic indicator of survival in patients with metastatic colorectal adenocarcinoma treated with 90Y radioembolization. Radiology. 2016;282(1):281–8.
30. Salem R, Lewandowski R, Kulik L, Wang E, Riaz A, et al. Radioembolization results in longer time-to-progression and reduced toxicity compared with chemoembolization patients with hepatocellular carcinoma. Gastroenterology. 2011;140(2):497–507.
31. Sangro B, Gil-Alzugaray B, Rodriguez J, Sola I, Martinez-Cuesta A, et al. Liver disease induced by radioembolization of liver tumors: description and possible risk factors. Cancer. 2008;112(7):1538–46.
32. Currie BM, Hoteit MA, Ben-Josef E, Nadolski GJ, Soulen MC. Radioembolization induced chronic hepatotoxicity: a single-center cohort analysis. J Vasc Interv Radiol. 2019;30(12):1915–23.
33. Braat AJ, Kappadath SC, Ahmadzadehfar H, Stothers CL, Frilling A, et al. Radioembolization with 90y resin microspheres of neuroendocrine liver metastases: international multicenter study on efficacy and toxicity. Cardiovasc Intervent Radiol. 2019;42(3):413–25.
34. Ryan MJ, Willatt J, Majdalany BS, Kielar AZ, Chong S, Ruma JA. Ablation techniques for primary and metastatic liver tumors. World J Hepatol. 2016;8(3):191–9.
35. Lubner MG, Brace CL, Hinshaw JL, Lee FT. Microwave tumor ablation: mechanism of action, clinical results, and devices. J Vasc Interv Radiol. 2010;21(8 Suppl):S192–203.
36. Henn AR, Levine EA, McNulty W, Zagoria RJ. Percutaneous radiofrequency ablation of hepatic metastases for symptomatic relief of neuroendocrine syndromes. Am J Roentgenol. 2003;181(4):1005–10.
37. Mohan H, Nicholson P, Winter DC, O'Shea D, O'Toole D, et al. Radiofrequency ablation for neuroendocrine liver metastases: a systematic review. J Vasc Interv Radiol. 2015;26(7):935–42.

Chapter 21
Special Considerations in Children: Pediatric Renal Vein Sampling

Kent A. Cabatingan

Introduction

Although much less represented than its adult counterpart, pediatric endocrinological disturbances can be further investigated with certain procedures that interventional radiology can provide. Given that primary endocrine pathology has far less prevalence, there has not been a great push to develop tests or protocols in the field of pediatric interventional radiology for this population; however, a mainstay that has not entirely fallen out of favor is renal vein sampling performed for very specific indications. Specifically, pediatric renal vein sampling has been demonstrated to be helpful when troubleshooting cases of pediatric hypertension in cases of renovascular hypertension, of which poorly demarcated fibromuscular dysplasia (FMD) is a common cause among certain age groups. Note, FMD is not a primary endocrine pathology, but it leads to renovascular hypertension by releasing a cascade of measurable hormones causing secondary hypertension.

Pediatric Hypertension

Pediatric hypertension is defined as having greater than 90th percentile in BP according to age, sex, and height as described by the National High Blood Pressure Education Program [1]. Unique to the pediatric age group is that a source for the patient's elevated pressures (secondary hypertension) is identifiable in up to 85% of

K. A. Cabatingan (✉)
Interventional Radiology, Children's Minnesota, Minneapolis, MN, USA
e-mail: Kent.cabatingan@childrensmn.org

© The Author(s), under exclusive license to Springer Nature Switzerland AG 2022

H. Yu et al. (eds.), *Diagnosis and Management of Endocrine Disorders in Interventional Radiology*, https://doi.org/10.1007/978-3-030-87189-5_21

patients [2]. Moreover, renal abnormalities are demonstrated in 75–80% of pediatric patients older than 6 years old with secondary hypertension with FMD considered to account for 10% of cases which can ultimately lead to end-organ renal failure [3, 4].

It can be the interventional radiologist's role to help sample blood to drive further treatment and/or diagnose renovascular hypertension as the cause for the child's hypertension. To better understand the process and rationale for performing the procedure, the operator should have a basic understanding of the disease process.

Pathophysiology

Renovascular hypertension, regardless of its etiology, is a disruption in the renin-angiotensin feedback cascade. Renin is secreted by the juxtaglomerular apparatus, which detects changes within afferent arteriole blood flow to the kidney. When blood flow is decreased, renin is secreted, which converts systemic angiotensinogen to angiotensin I [5]. Following this angiotensin-converting enzyme cleaves angiotensin I to form angiotensin II which goes on to act at different receptors and causes increased water retention, vasoconstriction, and increased sympathetic tone: all of which leads to increased systemic blood pressure to cause an increase in renal artery pressure and, thereby, increasing perfusion to the juxtaglomerular apparatus. The result of this is decreased renin secretion.

Pediatric Fibromuscular Dysplasia

It should be noted that pediatric FMD is poorly understood and beyond the scope of this chapter, but it is suspected to be vastly different from the adult process. Although able to occur anywhere within the body, the most common subset of pediatric FMD is the focal fibroplasia variety which causes a long, narrow, and smooth focal stenosis anywhere within the arterial bed [6]. In the setting of pediatric FMD or any disease process affecting the vasculature, there is decreased perfusion to the juxtaglomerular apparatus via upstream stenosis. The result is that the apparatuses are hypoperfused, and renin secretion is upregulated by the affected kidney. This allows the operator to detect the unilateral differences in the amount of renin when venous sampling. The best candidates for pediatric renal vein sampling are ones that could benefit from treatment should there be a positive result, but also where there is a strong clinical suspicion that there the cause of the child's hypertension is stemming from a renal etiology without imaging findings.

Diagnosis of Fibromuscular Dysplasia

A large number of pediatric FMD cases can be detected by CT angiogram of the renal arteries or MR angiogram. Even if those modalities do not visualize a stenosis which may be leading to hypertension, conventional angiography of the renal arteries could be performed with the added benefit of being able to treat the lesion in the same setting depending on its etiology. It has been the author's practice to sample renal veins when no visualized arterial stenosis can be detected in a pediatric patient that continues to have hypertension in the setting of increasing or maximum dose requirements of three antihypertensive medications. Additionally, any end-organ kidney damage, as evidence by a renal size discrepancy, may also warrant the need for testing. In either setting, there must be no other discernable cause for hypertension prior to intervention.

Pediatric Renal Vein Sampling

Another component of patient selection that is unique to the practice of pediatric interventional radiology is the patient's size. If the patient is below the age of 2 years old and is not on maximum doses of three antihypertensive medications, it has been suggested to defer to procedure until the patient reaches this age as the patient's vasculature is likely to accommodate catheters with less of a chance of injury during sampling or any other subsequent arterial procedure. The procedure can still technically be performed should the patient not fit these criteria on a case-by-case basis.

Preprocedural Preparation

Prior to starting the procedure, a few steps must be taken to ensure optimization of sampling during the procedure as slight variations in medication and patient position could affect the results. Patients are asked to discontinue medication for 2 weeks prior to the procedure to allow for a valid renin baseline to be achieved. This is especially important if the patient is taking angiotensin-converting enzyme (ACE) inhibitors and β-blockers as these would directly affect the values by either causing pre-dilation of the renal artery or directly decreasing adequate renal plasma flow and glomerular filtration rate, respectively. If the patient's condition does not allow for the cessation of all antihypertensive medications, it is crucial that these two classes must be held at a minimum.

On a procedural day, the patient should remain in a supine position for at least 2 h to ensure normalization of the heart rate and profusion to the kidneys

[7]. Given a pediatric patient population, additional support from families or a child life specialist within the hospital may be required to keep the patient as calm as possible. It is discouraged to utilize any medications for this purpose. One hour before the onset of the procedure, enalapril is administered at 40 mcg/kg over 3–5 min and not exceeding 2.5 mg to accentuate any difference in renin levels between the sides. The mechanism of action is akin to a captopril renogram [8].

Procedure Technique

The right common femoral vein is accessed, using ultrasound guidance, with a 21 G needle followed by the placement of a 5-F sheath (Glidesheath Slender®, Terumo). Following this, a 4-F Cobra 2 catheter is used to select the right renal vein first. The right renal vein is selected prior to the left due to the increased anatomical variability, which may manifest as multiple renal veins within 8–30% of the population [9]. With the catheter in the mid-portion of the right renal vein, a total of two separate, 8 ml samples are withdrawn. Following this, the catheter is disengaged, and the left renal vein is selected.

If there is difficulty catheterizing the left renal vein at the L1-2 level, one should consider the possibility of a retroaortic or circumaortic left renal vein which is present in 5–7% of the population. A duplicated IVC can also be present in less than 1% of the population [10]. The tip of the catheter should be placed distal to the left gonadal vein. Of note, the left gonadal vein typically has its origin along the proximal to middle third of the left renal vein. Venous inflow from the gonadal vein could artificially decrease the concentration of renin within the blood pool. A small quantity of contrast should be utilized to confirm the catheter positioning. Once the location is confirmed, a total of two separate 8 mL samples should be collected. If there is a questionable segmental disease, a 2.8-F microcatheter may be used to sample segmental renal veins for a more targeted study in cases of suspected tertiary FMD or Ask-Upmark kidney [7].

Lastly, the catheter is placed within the infrarenal IVC, and two blood samples are collected at this location. This sequence of venous sampling allows the operator to sample renin levels, which may fluctuate rapidly during a procedure in a time-efficient manner. A plasma renin activity ratio of a diseased kidney to unaffected kidney greater than 1.5:1 is considered suggestive of renovascular hypertension with a 63–75% sensitivity and a 60–100% specificity as unilateral pathologic secretion of renin usually results in contralateral suppression of renin production. If segmental measurements are performed, the ratio is usually far greater than 1.5:1 when compared to unaffected ipsilateral segments [11].

Summary

The process of renal vein sampling in the setting of refractory pediatric hypertension can be a powerful diagnostic tool for interventional radiologists to have in their armamentarium and can help drive clinical care for these patients. This technique has been falling out of favor due to the advances of medical imaging to visualize the stenotic arterial segments, but still remains a troubleshooting tool for hinting at questionable tertiary or more distal, segmental arterial stenosis leading to elevated renin levels, in turn leading to renovascular hypertension. The power of the examination is its positive predictive value as a large unilateral discrepancy points to the diagnosis of FMD or other focal renal abnormality within these patients. On the other hand, the ratio of less than 1.5:1 between the two renal veins cannot entirely exclude renovascular hypertension as operator error may be present; however, other causes for hypertension should be considered more likely.

References

1. Patel N, Walker N. Clinical assessment of hypertension in children. Clin Hypertens. 2016;22:15.
2. Viera AJ, Neutze DM. Review diagnosis of secondary hypertension: an age-based approach. Am Fam Physician. 2010;82(12):1241–8.
3. Behrman R, Kliegman R. Nelson textbook of pediatrics. 14th ed. Philadelphia: W.B. Saunders; 1992. p. 251–306.
4. Meyers KE, Sharma N. Fibromuscular dysplasia in children and adolescents. Cath Lab Digest. 2007;15(10):6–11.
5. Sparks MA, Crowley SD, Gurley SB, Mirotsou M, Coffman TM. Classical renin-angiotensin system in kidney physiology. Compr Physiol. 2014;4(3):1201–28.
6. Tullus K. Renovascular hypertension-is it fibromuscular dysplasia or Takayasu arteritis. Pediatr Nephrol. 2013;28(2):191–6.
7. Monroe EJ, Carney BW, Ingraham CR, Johson GE, Valji K. An interventionist's guide to endocrine consultations. Radiographics. 2017;37:1246–67.
8. Thibonnier M, Joseph A, Sassano P, Guyenne TT, Corvol P, Raynaud A, Seurot M, Gaux JC. Improved diagnosis of unilateral renal artery lesions after captopril administration. JAMA. 1984;251(1):56–60.
9. Kaufman JA, Waltman AC, Rivitz SM, Geller SG. Anatomical observations on the renal veins and inferior vena cava at magnetic resonance angiography. Cardiovasc Intervent Radiol. 1995;18(3):153–7.
10. Bass JE, Redwine MD, Kramer LA, Huynh PT, Harris JH Jr. Spectrum of congenital anomalies of the inferior vena cava: cross-sectional imaging findings. Radiographics. 2000;20(3):639–52.
11. Lüscher TF, Greminger P, Kuhlmann U, Siegenthaler W, Largiadèr F, Vetter W. Renal venous renin determinations in renovascular hypertension. Diagnostic and prognostic value in unilateral renal artery stenosis treated by surgery or percutaneous transluminal angioplasty. Nephron. 1986;44(1):17–24.

Correction to: Diagnosis and Management of Endocrine Disorders in Interventional Radiology

Hyeon Yu, Charles T. Burke, and Clayton W. Commander

Correction to:
Hyeon Yu, Charles T. Burke, and Clayton W. Commander (eds.),
Diagnosis and Management of Endocrine Disorders
in Interventional Radiology,
https://doi.org/10.1007/978-3-030-87189-5

This book was inadvertently published with incorrect affiliation of the author Dr. Qian Yang which is corrected as follows:

"Qian Yang, Laboratory for Investigatory Imaging, School of Health and Rehabilitation Sciences, The Ohio State University, Columbus, USA".

The updated version of the book can be found at
https://doi.org/10.1007/978-3-030-87189-5
https://doi.org/10.1007/978-3-030-87189-5_17

© The Author(s), under exclusive license to Springer Nature
Switzerland AG 2022
H. Yu et al. (eds.), *Diagnosis and Management of Endocrine Disorders in
Interventional Radiology*, https://doi.org/10.1007/978-3-030-87189-5_22

Index

© The Author(s), under exclusive license to Springer Nature
Switzerland AG 2022

H. Yu et al. (eds.), *Diagnosis and Management of Endocrine Disorders in
Interventional Radiology*, https://doi.org/10.1007/978-3-030-87189-5

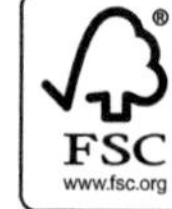

MIX
Papier aus verantwortungsvollen Quellen
Paper from responsible sources
FSC® C105338

If you have any concerns about our products,
you can contact us on
ProductSafety@springernature.com

In case Publisher is established outside the EU,
the EU authorized representative is:
Springer Nature Customer Service Center GmbH
Europaplatz 3, 69115 Heidelberg, Germany

Printed by Libri Plureos GmbH
in Hamburg, Germany